THE COMORBIDITIES OF EPILEPSY

THE COMORBIDITIES OF EPILEPSY

Edited by

MARCO MULA
Consultant in Neurology and Epileptology and Reader in Neurology
St George's University Hospitals NHS Foundation Trust and
St George's University of London
London, United Kingdom

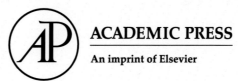

ACADEMIC PRESS
An imprint of Elsevier

Academic Press is an imprint of Elsevier
125 London Wall, London EC2Y 5AS, United Kingdom
525 B Street, Suite 1650, San Diego, CA 92101, United States
50 Hampshire Street, 5th Floor, Cambridge, MA 02139, United States
The Boulevard, Langford Lane, Kidlington, Oxford OX5 1GB, United Kingdom

Notices

Knowledge and best practice in this field are constantly changing. As new research and experience broaden our
understanding, changes in research methods, professional practices, or medical treatment may become necessary.

Practitioners and researchers must always rely on their own experience and knowledge in evaluating and using any
information, methods, compounds, or experiments described herein. In using such information or methods they should be
mindful of their own safety and the safety of others, including parties for whom they have a professional responsibility.

To the fullest extent of the law, neither the Publisher nor the authors, contributors, or editors, assume any liability for any
injury and/or damage to persons or property as a matter of products liability, negligence or otherwise, or from any use or
operation of any methods, products, instructions, or ideas contained in the material herein.

Library of Congress Cataloging-in-Publication Data
A catalog record for this book is available from the Library of Congress

British Library Cataloguing-in-Publication Data
A catalogue record for this book is available from the British Library

ISBN 978-0-12-818620-6

For information on all Academic Press publications
visit our website at https://www.elsevier.com/books-and-journals

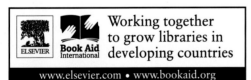

Working together
to grow libraries in
developing countries

www.elsevier.com • www.bookaid.org

Publisher: Nikki Levy
Acquisition Editor: Melanie Tucker
Editorial Project Manager: Carlos Rodriguez
Production Project Manager: Paul Prasad Chandramohan
Cover Designer: Matthew Limbert

Typeset by SPi Global, India

Contents

Contributors

Niruj Agrawal
Department of Neuropsychiatry, St George's Hospital, London, United Kingdom

Stéphane Auvin
Pediatric Neurology Department, Robert-Debré University Hospital, Paris, France

Prisca R. Bauer
Lyon Neuroscience Research Center, Brain Dynamics and Cognition Team, INSERM UMRS 1028, CNRS UMR 5292, Université Claude Bernard Lyon 1, Université de Lyon, Lyon, France

Ettore Beghi
Department of Neuroscience, Istituto di Ricerche Farmacologiche Mario Negri IRCCS, Milano, Italy

Charles E. Begley
Center for Health Services Research, School of Public Health, University of Texas Sciences Center, Houston, TX, United States

Jessica M. Bordenave
Department of Neurology, University of Wisconsin School of Medicine and Public Health, Madison, WI, United States

Christian Brandt
Department of General Epileptology, Bethel Epilepsy Centre, Bielefeld, Germany

Shelly Brett
Department of Neurology, Kingston Hospital NHS Foundation Trust, London, United Kingdom

Paolo Calabresi
Neurology Clinic, University of Perugia—S. Maria della Misericordia Hospital, Perugia; IRCCS "Santa Lucia", Rome, Italy

Stefano Caproni
Azienda Ospedaliera S. Maria, Terni, Italy

Hannah R. Cock
Epilepsy Group, Atkinson Morley Regional Neuroscience Centre, St George's University Hospitals NHS Trust; Institute of Medical & Biomedical Education, St George's University of London, London, United Kingdom

Cinzia Costa
Neurology Clinic, University of Perugia—S. Maria della Misericordia Hospital, Perugia, Italy

Blandine Dozières-Puyravel
Pediatric Neurology Department, Robert-Debré University Hospital, Paris, France

Filippo Sean Giorgi
Department of Clinical and Experimental Medicine, Section of Neurology, University of Pisa and Pisa University Hospital, Pisa, Italy

Fabio Giovannelli
Department of Neuroscience, Psychology, Pharmacology and Child Health (NEUROFARBA), University of Florence, Firenze, Italy

Giuseppe Gobbi
IRCCS—Institute of Neurological Sciences of Bologna, Bologna, Italy

Bruce Hermann
Department of Neurology, University of Wisconsin School of Medicine and Public Health, Madison, WI, United States

Nathalie Jetté
Department of Neurology; Department of Population Health Science and Policy, Icahn School of Medicine at Mount Sinai, New York, NY, United States

Jana Jones
Department of Neurology, University of Wisconsin School of Medicine and Public Health, Madison, WI, United States

Mark Keezer
Research Centre of the University of Montreal Hospital Centre (CRCHUM); Department of Neurosciences, University of Montreal, Montreal, QC, Canada

Rachel Friefeld Kesselmayer
Department of Neurology, University of Wisconsin School of Medicine and Public Health, Madison, WI, United States

Churl-Su Kwon
Department of Neurology; Department of Population Health Science and Policy, Icahn School of Medicine at Mount Sinai, New York, NY, United States

Lady Diana Ladino
Epilepsy Program, Hospital Pablo Tobón Uribe—University of Antioquia, Neuroclínica, Medellín, Colombia

Anna Loussouarn
Pediatric Neurology Department, Robert-Debré University Hospital, Paris, France

Paolo Mainardi
Independent Researcher

Sofia Markoula
Department of Neurology, University Hospital of Ioannina, Ioannina, Greece

Gloria M. Morel
Department of Neurology, University of Wisconsin School of Medicine and Public Health, Madison, WI, United States

Marco Mula
Institute of Medical and Biomedical Education, St George's University of London and Atkinson Morley Regional Neuroscience Centre, St George's University Hospitals NHS Foundation Trust, London, United Kingdom

Daniel Navin Olschewski
Department of Neurology, University Hospital of Cologne, Cologne, Germany

Alberto Preda
Pediatric Neurology and Muscular Diseases Unit, DINOGMI-Department of Neurosciences, Rehabilitation, Ophthalmology, Genetics, Maternal and Child Health University of Genoa, "G. Gaslini" Institute, Genova, Italy

Markus Reuber
Academic Neurology Unit, University of Sheffield, Royal Hallamshire Hospital, Sheffield, United Kingdom

Bastien Rioux
Research Centre of the University of Montreal Hospital Centre (CRCHUM); Department of Neurosciences, University of Montreal, Montreal, QC, Canada

Michele Romoli
Neurology Clinic, University of Perugia—S. Maria della Misericordia Hospital, Perugia, Italy

Josemir W. Sander
NIHR University College London Hospitals Biomedical Research Centre, UCL Queen Square Institute of Neurology, London; Chalfont Centre for Epilepsy, Chalfont St Peter, United Kingdom; Stichting Epilepsie Instellingen Nederland (SEIN), Heemstede, Netherlands

Paola Sarchielli
Neurology Clinic, University of Perugia—S. Maria della Misericordia Hospital, Perugia, Italy

Sharon Shmuely
Stichting Epilepsie Instellingen Nederland—SEIN, Heemstede, The Netherlands; NIHR University College London Hospitals Biomedical Research Centre, UCL Institute of Neurology, London, United Kingdom

Pasquale Striano
Pediatric Neurology and Muscular Diseases Unit, DINOGMI-Department of Neurosciences, Rehabilitation, Ophthalmology, Genetics, Maternal and Child Health University of Genoa, "G. Gaslini" Institute, Genova, Italy

Jose Francisco Téllez-Zenteno
Saskatchewan Epilepsy Program, Department of Medicine, Division of Neurology, University of Saskatchewan, Saskatoon, SK, Canada

Evangelia G. Theochari
Epilepsy Group, Atkinson Morley Regional Neuroscience Centre, St George's University Hospitals NHS Trust, London, United Kingdom

Roland D. Thijs
Stichting Epilepsie Instellingen Nederland—SEIN, Heemstede, The Netherlands; NIHR University College London Hospitals Biomedical Research Centre, UCL Institute of Neurology, London, United Kingdom; Department of Neurology, LUMC Leiden University Medical Centre, Leiden, The Netherlands

Matthew C. Walker
UCL Institute of Neurology, Queen Square, London, United Kingdom

Joanna Whitson
Department of Neuropsychiatry, St George's Hospital, London, United Kingdom

Mahinda Yogarajah
Atkinson Morley Regional Neuroscience Centre, St George's University Hospitals NHS Foundation Trust; Institute of Medical and Biomedical Education, St George's University of London, London, United Kingdom

Gaetano Zaccara
Regional Health Agency of Tuscany, Florence, Italy

Foreword

It is well established that somatic and psychiatric comorbidities are highly prevalent in people with epilepsy. In its new classification of the epilepsies, the International League Against Epilepsy highlights the importance of comorbidities at every stage of the classification process. Furthermore, addressing comorbidities is integral not only to the diagnosis and classification of epilepsy, but also to the management and counselling of people with epilepsy. Yet, epilepsy clinicians working at the coalface may lack awareness of the importance of this broader view of epilepsy care. In some cases, the clinicians' focus may be predominantly on the treatment of the seizures themselves, and comorbidities may be viewed as ancillary events with little consequence on the patient's health. In others, there may be insufficient expertise to manage some of the complex comorbidities. The end result is a high risk of under-diagnosis and suboptimal management of comorbidities and therefore of the patient as a whole. This volume provides a comprehensive view of the comorbidities seen in people with epilepsy.

The study of comorbidities is of crucial importance to our understanding of epilepsy. Not only do they pose questions about association and causality, biology of diseases, and effects of medications (both good and bad), but they also affect our ability to provide comprehensive, rational management of epilepsy itself and also of coexisting clinical conditions. As eloquently stated in the opening chapter of this volume, the relationship between epilepsy and comorbid conditions is complex. We increasingly understand that these associations may point to common predisposing genetic and environmental factors, they may disclose a bidirectional risk, or they may be the direct consequence of the disease or its treatments. This approach highlights important avenues for prevention, diagnosis and treatment.

That different comorbidities affect different groups of people with epilepsy, while some are common to many patients, is illustrated in the sections dealing with different types of illnesses and their management. Common public health problems that are highly relevant in epilepsy care are highlighted, such as obesity, pain, metabolic disorders, bone health and cancer, although infectious disorders are not addressed directly. The central place of mental health, behavioural and cognitive problems is also recognized and addressed.

In this timely publication, Marco Mula has assembled a team of leading experts to address the comorbidities seen in people with epilepsy in a comprehensive manner. The topics range from epidemiological and economic aspects to diagnostic and management guidance for clinicians. Importantly, the essays address methodological issues of the current evidence and point to directions for further scientific enquiry.

The target audience of this volume is broad, ranging from clinicians and researchers to care givers and policy makers. All will gain a better understanding of the scope of comorbidities, their consequences and their management. Our hope is that patients with epilepsy will benefit from this collected wisdom.

Samuel Wiebe, MD
University of Calgary
President International League Against Epilepsy

Preface

Epilepsy is one of the most frequent neurological disorders affecting about 50 million people worldwide. In 1970, Alvin Feinstein defined as "comorbidity" any distinct additional clinical entity that existed during the clinical course of a patient who has the index disease. The practical definition of epilepsy issued by the International League Against Epilepsy in 2014 explicitly recognizes the neurobiological, cognitive, psychological, and social consequences of epilepsy. However, in addition to that, it is becoming evident that patients with epilepsy present with a number of medical problems as a result of the epilepsy itself or because the epilepsy shares some biological links with other medical conditions or as a long-term consequence of the antiepileptic drug treatment.

During the last 15 years, a number of studies have focused on the issue of comorbidities of epilepsy, showing that some disorders are indeed more frequently encountered among patients with epilepsy as compared to the general population. These findings have led to several hypotheses about a shared pathophysiology between epilepsy and these conditions, stimulating research in this area and emphasizing the importance of recognizing this specific group of comorbidities. In fact, although seizure freedom always remains the main goal of the treatment of epilepsy, comorbidities represent an important predictor of quality of life, especially in those patients where seizure freedom is not sustained. But even in those who are in full remission, if comorbidities are not addressed or seizure freedom is achieved at the expense of unacceptable long-term complications, adherence and quality of life remain poor.

For many years, epileptology remained a highly specialized subspecialty focusing on a limited number of technical issues like intracranial monitoring for epilepsy surgery or genetic and advanced neuroimaging techniques. Health professionals are now realizing the importance of comorbidities in patients with epilepsy and the key role of epilepsy centers in addressing these problems in the context of a holistic approach to epilepsy care. This book represents an up-to-date overview of the comorbidities of epilepsy (somatic, neurological, and behavioral), by active international authorities in the field of clinical epileptology, with an emphasis on epidemiology, pathophysiology, diagnosis and management. The book discusses also the problem of comorbidities from a public health point of view and provides the point of view of epilepsy specialist nurses whose role is invaluable in managing complex patients with multiple chronic conditions. This book has a strong clinical perspective and it has been written by clinicians for clinicians with the aim of improving epilepsy care and quality of life of our patients.

Marco Mula
Institute of Medical and Biomedical Education,
St George's University of London and
the Atkinson Morley Regional Neuroscience Centre,
St George's University Hospitals NHS Foundation Trust,
London, United Kingdom

CHAPTER 1

The comorbidities of epilepsy: A conceptual framework

Daniel Navin Olschewski*, Prisca R. Bauer†, Josemir W. Sander‡,§,¶
*Department of Neurology, University Hospital of Cologne, Cologne, Germany
†Lyon Neuroscience Research Center, Brain Dynamics and Cognition Team, INSERM UMRS 1028, CNRS UMR 5292, Université Claude Bernard Lyon 1, Université de Lyon, Lyon, France
‡NIHR University College London Hospitals Biomedical Research Centre, UCL Queen Square Institute of Neurology, London, United Kingdom
§Chalfont Centre for Epilepsy, Chalfont St Peter, United Kingdom
¶Stichting Epilepsie Instellingen Nederland (SEIN), Heemstede, Netherlands

Contents

Abbreviations

AED's	antiepileptic drugs
ICD	International Classification of Diseases
ILAE	International League Against Epilepsy
QOLIE-10	quality of life in epilepsy questionnaire
SCN1A	gene that codes for the alpha subunit of the voltage-gated sodium ion channel
SUDEP	sudden unexpected death in epilepsy

The Comorbidities of Epilepsy
https://doi.org/10.1016/B978-0-12-814877-8.00001-5

Epilepsy, a relatively common neurological condition, is a complex symptom that rarely stands alone. Several large population-based studies have shown that up to 50% of people with epilepsy also have a comorbid condition [1, 2]. In epilepsy, comorbidity implies the coexistence of other medical conditions preceding, co-occurring with, or following the diagnosis of epilepsy, related or unrelated to the underlying potential or putative cause of epilepsy.

The comorbidities of epilepsy encompass somatic and psychiatric conditions, and the prevalence of some of them is up to eight times higher in people with epilepsy than in the general population [3–5]. The comorbidities may impact the diagnosis of epilepsy mainly due to issues of attributions. They can influence treatment decisions as often the choice of antiepileptic medications may positively or negatively affect the comorbid condition, thus complicating a holistic approach to the management of the individual. Comorbidities also affect quality of life and prognosis and result in more frequent visits to health professionals and higher health care-related costs [6].

This chapter provides a theoretical framework for the comorbid associations of epilepsy. It should be seen as a foreword for this topical book on the comorbidities associated with epilepsy, which are responsible for a significant part of the burden epilepsy imposes on the individual and society. It also provides a brief overview of the different potential mechanisms of association between epilepsy and comorbidities and of some recent pathophysiological evidence, which may explain some associations. Most of the comorbid associations of epilepsy mentioned in this chapter will be discussed in more detail in other chapters.

1. Mechanisms of association between epilepsy and comorbid conditions

The comorbidities associated with epilepsy can be subdivided by affected organ system and the International Classification of Diseases [4, 5]. Based on the current understanding of disease mechanisms and temporal associations, epilepsy-associated comorbid conditions can also be divided into five mechanist categories. This type of categorization was initially conceptualized for the classification of migraine and associated comorbid disorders [7]. The categories are: causative mechanisms; resultant mechanisms; shared risk factors; bidirectional effects; and chance and artifactual comorbidities [4, 5]. Table 1 summarizes conditions associated with epilepsy.

1.1 Causative

Some medical conditions can result in epilepsy. This causative relationship is the most straight-forward mechanism of association; for example, stroke, traumatic head injury, and neoplasms are included among the most common causes of symptomatic epilepsy [4]. Some conditions, such as brain tumors [8], alcohol dependence [10],

Table 1 Mechanisms of association between epilepsy and other conditions

Mechanisms of association	Conditions	Pathophysiological link (reference)
Causative	**Direct**	
	Brain tumors (primary, secondary)	Direct cause-and-effect relationship [8]
	Cerebrovascular disease	Direct cause-and-effect relationship [9]
	Alcohol dependence	Changes in brain function/reduction of seizure threshold [10]
	Multiple sclerosis (MS)	High incidence of focal epilepsy as a result of focal MS pathology; extensive cortical inflammation associated with epilepsy in MS [11–13]
	Indirect	
	Risk factors for cerebrovascular and cardiovascular disease	All risk factors for stroke and hypertension may also have independent effects [14, 15]
	Risk factors for brain tumors (metastases)	
Resultant	**Drug-induced**	
	Bone health and density	AEDs affect bone health [16, 17]
	Seizure-induced	
	Fractures	Due to seizure-induced injury [18]
	Headache	Postictal headaches in 50% of people with epilepsy [19]
	Pneumonia	Related to underlying morbidity and seizures, possibly due to aspiration [3]
	Urinary incontinence	Seizure-related or due to underlying conditions [20]
Shared risk factors	**Biological/structural factors**	
	Dementia (Alzheimer's disease, vascular dementia)	Possibly mediated by drugs used for dementia [21]
	Migraine	Excessive cortical hyperexcitability, probably due to function alterations of membrane channels and neurotransmitters [19]
	Systemic lupus erythematosus (SLE)	Mannose-binding lectin (MBL) capacity may mediate pro-inflammatory cytokine production such as IL-6 [22]
	Diabetes mellitus type I	Anti-GAD antibody associated with co-occurrence of temporal lobe epilepsy [23]

Continued

Table 1 Mechanisms of association between epilepsy and other conditions—cont'd

Mechanisms of association	Conditions	Pathophysiological link (reference)
Bidirectional	**Genetic**	
	Dravet syndrome	Development of epilepsy and ataxia due to SCN1A mutation [24]
	Alzheimer's disease	APP, PSEN1, PSEN2 mutations; APP duplications [25, 26]
	Migraine	FHM gene mutations (CACNA1A, ATP1A2, and SCN1A) associated with epilepsy; shared genetic risk factors with BECTS [4, 27, 28]
	Traumatic brain injury	Inheritance of the APOE e4 allele associated with increased risk of late posttraumatic seizures [29]
	Depression	Neurotransmitter, endocrine, and immunologic disturbances likely leading to altered cortical excitability [30, 31]
	Anxiety, suicidality	Possible common underlying pathophysiological mechanisms lowering seizure threshold [30]
	Psychosis/ schizophrenia	Possible neuropathological or genetic association between schizophrenia and epilepsy through LGI1 and CNTNAP2 genes [32]
	Autism spectrum disorder	Genetic, environmental factors, altered neuronal transmission, and structural abnormalities [31, 33, 34]
	Attentional deficit and hyperactivity disorder	Environmental and genetic factors [35]
Chance and artifactual	Arthritis/rheumatism/ back problems	Probably artifactual due to low specificity of radiologic osteoarthritis in people reporting chronic arthritis and rheumatism [36]
	Chronic fatigue	Postictal, depression, AEDs as possible causes [37, 38]
	Asthma	Smoking and/or living conditions [39, 40]
	Peptic ulcers and gastrointestinal bleeding	Possibly induced through co-medication (aspirin, NSAIDs) [3]

multiple sclerosis [11–13], and cerebrovascular disease [9], seem to have a direct cause-and-effect association with epilepsy, whereas risk factors for cardiovascular and cerebrovascular diseases and brain metastases increase the risk of developing epilepsy indirectly [14, 15].

1.2 Resultant

Some conditions can be caused by epilepsy. This category includes the effects of antiepileptic drugs (AEDs) and other medication used in epilepsy [4]. AEDs, particularly enzyme inducers, may play a pivotal role in this mechanism of association and can lead to impaired bone health and density [16, 17]. Consequences of seizures include fractures [18], aspiration pneumonia [3], headache [19] and urinary incontinence [20].

1.3 Shared risk

A shared risk factor is one underlying factor or condition, which results in the development of two or more distinct conditions. The shared risk factor can be of environmental, genetic, neurochemical, physiological, or structural origin [4]. For example, it has been suggested that the co-occurrence of diabetes mellitus type I and some types of temporal lobe epilepsy is mediated through the presence of the anti-glutamic acid decarboxylase (GAD) antibody [23]. Other biological and structural shared risk factors have also been suggested for systematic lupus erythematosus [22] and dementia [21, 25, 26]. Different forms of migraine and epilepsy may be caused by environmental, biological or genetic shared risk factors [4, 19, 27, 28].

1.4 Genetics

Genetic factors can impact the relationship between epilepsy and comorbidities in various ways. They can be either the basis for developing epilepsy or a comorbidity or the source of a shared risk factor for epilepsy and a comorbidity. For instance, mutations in SCN1A, a gene that codes for the alpha subunit of the voltage-gated sodium ion channel, can result in the development of Dravet syndrome (severe myoclonic epilepsy in infancy), as well as a motor disorder [24]. Genetic factors also influence the association between epilepsy and comorbidities [41]. For example, carriers of the APOE e4 allele seem to be at greater risk of developing epilepsy after traumatic brain injury [29]. Genetic predisposition may therefore play an important role in the clustering of comorbid conditions and understanding of these may be of vital importance for a holistic person-centered management approach.

1.5 Bidirectional

A bidirectional, or reciprocal, association arises when one condition can cause another condition and vice versa. These two conditions do not have a strict temporal sequence, meaning that either does not have to precede the other, as could similarly be the case for a shared risk factor. Rather, it involves a complex relationship between two conditions through pathophysiology, genetics, and environment [5]. Bidirectional association with epilepsy has been suggested for depression, anxiety, psychosis, autism spectrum disorder, migraine, and attention deficit and hyperactivity disorder [30–35].

1.6 Chance, artifactual, or spurious association

For some conditions, the frequency of prevalence or incidence in people with epilepsy is the same as in the general population [42]. Information or selection bias can lead to wrongfully attributed links between epilepsy and other conditions [42].

Selection bias is a result of a false representation of the general population in the study population, leading to a misleading relationship between conditions. This includes referral, non-response, and publication bias [42–44]. For example, arthritis [36], chronic fatigue [37, 38], asthma [39, 40], peptic ulcers, and gastrointestinal bleeding [3] may have an artifactual association with epilepsy.

2. The burden of comorbidity

2.1 Diagnosis

Understanding the association between epilepsy and other conditions is necessary to improve care for people with epilepsy [39, 45]. A positive diagnosis of epilepsy should always increase the suspicion that other disorders, either psychiatric or somatic, may be present as it often causes conditions in both domains. Cognitive, psychiatric, and somatic comorbidities are frequently underdiagnosed and undertreated in people with epilepsy [17, 46, 47]. It is important to diagnose and treat comorbidities as early as possible [48]. Regular screening of people with epilepsy for comorbidities, similar to screening for conditions such as depression and osteoporosis in the general population, is therefore important [5, 48].

An important driver for holistic epilepsy care should be the identification and appropriate diagnosis of comorbidities as often assessments in the epilepsy clinic are mostly about seizure control. Screening tools specifically for comorbidities in epilepsy are yet to be developed and implemented.

2.2 Treatment

Comorbidities can strongly influence treatment and outcomes. When treating epilepsy and comorbidities, ideally, a treatment targeting both should be selected. For example, people with migraine and epilepsy might benefit from treatment with topiramate whereas lamotrigine may be the preferred choice for people with epilepsy and a mood disorder [49, 50]. Conversely, some AEDs have a negative effect on certain conditions. The AED perampanel was shown to induce psychiatric adverse reactions in individuals with epilepsy and psychiatric comorbidities [51]. The presence of conditions such as migraine or psychiatric conditions was shown to be associated with a higher risk of pharmacoresistance in people with epilepsy [52].

2.3 Quality of life

The presence of comorbid conditions in people with epilepsy is associated with reduced quality of life [39]. More than half of people with epilepsy and comorbid depression had a reduction in quality of life as measured with the Quality of Life in Epilepsy-10 questionnaire [53]. Depression and attention deficit hyperactivity disorder are important predictors of quality of life, independently from epilepsy and its severity [54]. The primary goal should be seizure freedom, as people who are seizure-free have the same quality of life as the general population, but the prevention and targeted treatment of comorbidities is also necessary to restore quality of life [39, 55].

2.4 Mortality

People with epilepsy have a two- to threefold overall increase in premature mortality rates compared with the general population [56, 57]. Premature mortality risk is highest soon after the first seizures, and it remains elevated even after seizure freedom and off antiepileptic medication [58, 59]. This continuing risk of increased mortality, which seems independent of seizure and drug treatment, is most likely multifactorial, but it is likely that comorbidities play an important role on this. This requires further investigations.

Sudden unexpected death in epilepsy (SUDEP) is the most common cause of epilepsy-related death, it accounts for an estimated 4% of deaths in low-risk groups of people with epilepsy [37, 60]. People who have had a single seizure are attributed to the low-risk group [61]. It is possible that SUDEP shares some commonality with the so-called sudden adult death, and this also requires further investigation.

In people with symptomatic seizures, the majority of deaths within the first year of epilepsy onset are due to the underlying condition rather than the seizures themselves [62]. Most deaths are due to somatic comorbidities, such as cardiovascular or cerebrovascular disease, malignancies, or pneumonia, which are more likely to occur in people with epilepsy than in the general population [58]. Underlying depression and substance abuse in people with epilepsy also lead to increased mortality through suicide [63]. Whether AEDs also have an impact on suicidal behavior in people with epilepsy remains a matter of debate [64].

2.5 Costs

Direct medical costs in people with epilepsy are largely (80%) related to comorbidities rather than to epilepsy [65]. The risk of admission to a hospital is increased, and the medical costs are almost 50% higher than for people with epilepsy without comorbidities [66].

Consequently, early detection and intervention may also result in lower medical costs for those affected.

3. Epilepsy as a systemic condition

The increased prevalence of comorbidities and lifelong elevated risk of premature mortality in people with epilepsy suggest that there might be an underlying systemic dysfunction in some cases [67]. Systemic dysfunction may be a shared risk factor, resulting in the observed associations with other conditions [67].

Through the implementation of validated screening instruments, comorbidities might serve as indicators and prognostic factors for the course of the disease. Developments in this direction are already apparent: comorbidities, such as learning difficulties and psychiatric conditions, were included in the revised classification scheme of epilepsy by the International League Against Epilepsy in 2017 in order to ensure a holistic approach to patient care [68].

In the future, a better understanding of the association between epilepsy and other conditions might make targeted person-centered therapy possible. Therefore, more research in the pathophysiological mechanisms described in this chapter is warranted. Indeed, it could be argued that an important part of all future phenotypic stratification in epilepsy should be the identification of comorbidities as clustering of these could provide insight into common mechanisms, particularly common genetic predispositions.

References

[1] Forsgren L. Prevalence of epilepsy in adults in northern Sweden. Epilepsia 1992;33:450–8.
[2] Novy J, Bell GS, Peacock JL, Sisodiya SM, Sander JW. Epilepsy as a systemic condition: link with somatic comorbidities. Acta Neurol Scand 2017;136:352–9.
[3] Gaitatzis A, Carroll K, Majeed A, Sander JW. The epidemiology of the comorbidity of epilepsy in the general population. Epilepsia 2004;45:1613–22.
[4] Gaitatzis A, Sisodiya SM, Sander JW. The somatic comorbidity of epilepsy: a weighty but often unrecognized burden. Epilepsia 2012;53:1282–93.
[5] Keezer MR, Sisodiya SM, Sander JW. Comorbidities of epilepsy: current concepts and future perspectives. Lancet Neurol 2016;15:106–15.
[6] Starfield B, Lemke KW, Bernhardt T, Foldes SS, Forrest CB, Weiner JP. Comorbidity: implications for the importance of primary care in "case" management. Ann Fam Med 2003;1:8–14.
[7] Lipton RB, Silberstein SD. Why study the comorbidity of migraine? Neurology 1994;44(10 Suppl 7): S4–5.
[8] Japp A, Gielen G, Becker A. Recent aspects of classification and epidemiology of epilepsy-associated tumors. Epilepsia 2013;54:5–11.
[9] Jungehulsing G, Heuschmann P, Holtkamp M, Schwab S, Kolominsky-Rabas P. Incidence and predictors of post-stroke epilepsy. Acta Neurol Scand 2013;127:427–30.
[10] Samokhvalov A, Irving H, Mohapatra S, Rehm J. Alcohol consumption, unprovoked seizures, and epilepsy: a systematic review and meta-analysis. Epilepsia 2010;51:1177–84.
[11] Benjaminsen E, Myhr KM, Alstadhaug KB. The prevalence and characteristics of epilepsy in patients with multiple sclerosis in Nordland county, Norway. Seizure 2017;52:131–5.
[12] Calabrese M, De Stefano N, Atzori M, Bernardi V, Mattisi I, Barachino L, et al. Extensive cortical inflammation is associated with epilepsy in multiple sclerosis. J Neurol 2008;255:581–6.
[13] Burman J, Zelano J. Epilepsy in multiple sclerosis: a nationwide population-based register study. Neurology 2017;89:2462–8.
[14] Ng SK, Hauser WA, Brust JC, Susser M. Hypertension and the risk of new-onset unprovoked seizures. Neurology 1993;43:425–8.
[15] Hesdorffer DC, Hauser WA, Annegers JF, Rocca WA. Severe, uncontrolled hypertension and adult-onset seizures: a case-control study in Rochester, Minnesota. Epilepsia 1996;37:736–41.
[16] Pack A. Bone health in people with epilepsy: is it impaired and what are the risk factors? Seizure 2008;17:181–6.

[17] Lado F, Spiegel R, Masur JH, Boro A, Haut SR. Value of routine screening for bone demineralization in an urban population of patients with epilepsy. Epilepsy Res 2008;78:155–60.

[18] Mahler B, Carlsson S, Andersson T, Tomson T. Risk for injuries and accidents in epilepsy: a prospective population-based cohort study. Neurology 2018;90:e779–89.

[19] Bauer PR, Carpay JA, Terwindt GM, Sander JW, Thijs RJ, Haan J, et al. Headache and epilepsy topical collection on secondary headache. Curr Pain Headache Rep 2013;17(8).

[20] Tellez-Zenteno JF, Matijevic S, Wiebe S. Somatic comorbidity of epilepsy in the general population in Canada. Epilepsia 2005;46:1955–62.

[21] Imfeld P, Bodmer M, Schuerch M, Jick S, Meier C. Seizures in patients with Alzheimer's disease or vascular dementia: a population-based nested case-control analysis. Epilepsia 2013;54:700–7.

[22] Cieslinski J, Skare T, Nisihara R, De Messias-Reason I, Utiyama S. Mannose-binding lectin serum levels in patients with systemic lupus erythematosus: association with thrombocytopaenia and seizure. Lupus 2017;0:1–8.

[23] Malter MP, Frisch C, Zeitler H, Surges R, Urbach H, Helmstaedter C, et al. Treatment of immune-mediated temporal lobe epilepsy with GAD antibodies. Seizure 2015;30:57–63.

[24] Brunklaus A, Ellis R, Reavey E, Forbes GH, Zuberi SM. Prognostic, clinical and demographic features in SCN1A mutation-positive Dravet syndrome. Brain 2012;135(8):2329–36.

[25] Minkeviciene R, Rheims S, Dobszay MB, Zilberter M, Hartikainen J, Fülöp L, et al. Amyloid beta-induced neuronal hyperexcitability triggers progressive epilepsy. J Neurosci 2009;29(11):3453–62. https://doi.org/10.1523/JNEUROSCI.5215-08.2009.

[26] Noebels J. A perfect storm: converging paths of epilepsy and Alzheimer's dementia intersect in the hippocampal formation. Epilepsia 2011;52(Suppl. 1):39–46.

[27] Bianchin MM, Londero RG, Lima JE, Bigal ME. Migraine and epilepsy: a focus on overlapping clinical, pathophysiological, molecular, and therapeutic aspects. Curr Pain Headache Rep 2010;14(4):276–83.

[28] Clarke T, Baskurt Z, Strug LJ, Pal DK. Evidence of shared genetic risk factors for migraine and rolandic epilepsy. Epilepsia 2009;50(11):2428–33.

[29] Diaz-Arrastia R, Gong Y, Fair S, Scott KD, Garcia MC, Carlile MC, et al. Increased risk of late posttraumatic seizures associated with inheritance of APOE e4 allele. Arch Neurol 2003;60 (June):818–22.

[30] Hesdorffer DC, Ishihara L, Mynepalli L, Webb DJ, Weil J, Hauser WA. Epilepsy, suicidality, and psychiatric disorders: a bidirectional association. Ann Neurol 2012;72:184–91.

[31] Kanner AM, Scharfman H, Jette N, Anagnostou E, Bernard C, Camfield C, et al. Epilepsy as a network disorder: what can we learn from other network disorders such as autistic spectrum disorder and mood disorders? Epilepsy Behav 2017;77:106–13.

[32] Chang Y-T, Chen P-C, Tsai I-J, Sung F-C, Chin Z-N, Kuo H-T, et al. Bidirectional relation between schizophrenia and epilepsy: a population-based retrospective cohort study. Epilepsy 2011;52:2036–42.

[33] Su C-C, Chi MH, Lin S-H, Yang YK. Bidirectional association between autism spectrum disorder and epilepsy in child and adolescent patients: a population-based cohort study. Eur Child Adolesc Psychiatry 2016;25:979–87.

[34] Besag FMC. Epilepsy in patients with autism: links, risks and treatment challenges. Neuropsychiatr Dis Treat 2018;14:1–10.

[35] Brikell I, Ghirardi L, D'onofrio BM, Dunn DW, Almqvist C, Dalsgaard S, et al. Archival report familial liability to epilepsy and attention-deficit/hyperactivity disorder: a nationwide cohort study. Biol Psychiatry 2018;83:173–80.

[36] Szoeke CEI, Dennerstein L, Wluka AE, Guthrie JR, Taffe J, Clark MS, et al. Physician diagnosed arthritis, reported arthritis and radiological non-axial osteoarthritis. Osteoarthr Cartil 2008;16 (7):846–50.

[37] Téllez-Zenteno JF, Ronquillo LH, Wiebe S. Sudden unexpected death in epilepsy: evidence-based analysis of incidence and risk factors. Epilepsy Res 2005;65(1–2):101–15.

[38] Şenol V, Soyuer F, Arman F, Öztürk A. Influence of fatigue, depression, and demographic, socioeconomic, and clinical variables on quality of life of patients with epilepsy. Epilepsy Behav 2007;10:96–104.

[39] Elliott JO, Lu B, Shneker B, Charyton C, Moore JL. Comorbidity, health screening, and quality of life among persons with a history of epilepsy. Epilepsy Behav 2008;14:125–9.

[40] Hinnell C, Williams J, Metcalfe A, Patten SB, Parker R, Wiebe S, et al. Health status and health-related behaviors in epilepsy compared to other chronic conditions—a national population-based study. Epilepsia 2010;51:853–61.

[41] Greenland S, Rothman KJ, Lash T. Measures of effect and measures of association. In: Rothman KJ, Greenl S, Lash TL, editors. Modern Epidemiology. Philadelphia, PA: Wolters Kluwer/Lippincott, Williams & Wilkins; 2008. p. 51–70.

[42] Keezer MR, Sander JW. Comorbidity as an epidemiological construct. Lancet Neurol 2016;15:32.

[43] Delgado-Rodriguez M. Bias J Epidemiol Community Health 2004;58:635–41.

[44] Sica GT. Bias in research studies. Radiology 2006;238:780–9.

[45] Gilliam FG, Mendiratta A, Pack AM, Bazil CW. Global care of patients with drug resistant epilepsy epilepsy and common comorbidities: improving the outpatient epilepsy encounter health care considerations in epilepsy. Epileptic Disord 2005;7:27–33.

[46] Barry JJ. The recognition and management of mood disorders as a comorbidity of epilepsy. Epilepsia 2003;44(s4):30–40.

[47] Ott D, Siddarth P, Gurbani S, Koh S, Tournay A, Shields WD, et al. Behavioral disorders in pediatric epilepsy: unmet psychiatric need. Epilepsia 2003;44:591–7.

[48] Institute of Medicine (US) Committee on the Public Health Dimensions of the Epilepsies, England MJ, Liverman CT, Schultz AM, Strawbridge LM, editors. Epilepsy across the spectrum: promoting health and understanding. Washington: National Academies Press; 2012. ISBN-13: 978-0-309-25506-6.

[49] Spritzer SD, Bravo TP, Drazkowski JF. Topiramate for treatment in patients with migraine and epilepsy. Headache 2016;56(6):1081–5.

[50] Šepić-Grahovac D, Grahovac T, Ružić-Baršić A, Ružić K, Dadić-Hero E. Lamotrigine treatment of a patient affected by epilepsy and anxiety disorder. Psychiatr Danub 2011;23(1):111–3.

[51] Kim DW, Oh J. One-year retention study of adjunctive Perampanel treatment in epilepsy patients. Clin Neuropharmacol 2017;0:1–4.

[52] Hitiris N, Mohanraj R, Norrie J, Sills GJ, Brodie MJ. Predictors of pharmacoresistant epilepsy. Epilepsy Res 2007;75:192–6.

[53] Rocamora R, Ley M, Molins A, Toledo M, Sansa G, Bertol V, et al. Effect of lacosamide on depression and anxiety symptoms in patients with focal refractory epilepsy: a prospective multicenter study. Epilepsy Behav 2018;79:87–92.

[54] Boylan L, Flint L, Labovitz D, Jackson S, Starner K, Devinsky O. Depression but not seizure frequency predicts quality of life in treatment- resistant epilepsy. Neurology 2004;62:258–61.

[55] Leidy NK, Elixhauser A, Vickrey B, Means E, Willian MK. Seizure frequency and the health-related quality of life of adults with epilepsy. Neurology 1999;53:162–6.

[56] Cockerell OC, Johnson AL, Sander JWAS, Shorvon SD. Prognosis of epilepsy: a review and further analysis of the first nine years of the British National General Practice Study of epilepsy, a prospective population-based study. Epilepsia 1997;38:31–46.

[57] O'Donoghue MF, Sander JWAS. The mortality associated with epilepsy, with particular reference to sudden unexpected death: a review. Epilepsia 1997;38(s11):S15–9.

[58] Neligan A, Bell GS, Johnson AL, Goodridge DM, Shorvon SD, Sander JW. The long-term risk of premature mortality in people with epilepsy. Brain 2011;134:388–95.

[59] Bell GS, Neligan A, Giavasi C, Keezer MR, Novy J, Peacock JL, et al. Outcome of seizures in the general population after 25 years: a prospective follow-up, observational cohort study. J Neurol Neurosurg Psychiatry 2016;87:843–50.

[60] Surges R, Sander JW. Sudden unexpected death in epilepsy: mechanisms, prevalence, and prevention. Curr Opin Neurol 2012;25(2):201–7.

[61] Kim LG, Johnson TL, Marson AG, Chadwick DW. Prediction of risk of seizure recurrence after a single seizure and early epilepsy: further results from the MESS trial. Lancet Neurol 2006;5:317–22.

[62] Loiseau J, Picot M-C, Loiseau P. Short-term mortality after a first epileptic seizure: a population-based study. Epilepsia 1999;40:1388–92.

[63] Fazel S, Wolf A, Långström N, Newton CR, Lichtenstein P. Premature mortality in epilepsy and the role of psychiatric comorbidity: a total population study. Lancet 2013;382:1646–54.

[64] Mula M, Hesdorffer DC. Suicidal behavior and antiepileptic drugs in epilepsy: analysis of the emerging evidence. Drug Healthc Patient Saf 2011;3:15–20.

[65] Ivanova JI, Birnbaum HG, Kidolezi Y, Qiu Y, Mallett D, Caleo S. Economic burden of epilepsy among the privately insured in the US. PharmacoEconomics 2010;28(8):675–85.

[66] Lee WC, Arcona S, Thomas SK, Wang Q, Hoffmann MS, Pashos CL. Effect of comorbidities on medical care use and cost among refractory patients with partial seizure disorder. Epilepsy Behav 2005;7:123–6.

[67] Yuen AWC, Keezer MR, Sander JW. Epilepsy is a neurological and a systemic disorder. Epilepsy Behav 2018;78:57–61.

[68] Scheffer IE, Berkovic S, Capovilla G, Connolly MB, French J, Guilhoto L, et al. ILAE classification of the epilepsies: position paper of the ILAE Commission for Classification and Terminology. Epilepsia 2017;58:512–21.

CHAPTER 2

Costs of epilepsy: The impact of comorbidities

Churl-Su Kwon*,†, Charles E. Begley‡, Nathalie Jetté*,†
*Department of Neurology, Icahn School of Medicine at Mount Sinai, New York, NY, United States
†Department of Population Health Science and Policy, Icahn School of Medicine at Mount Sinai, New York, NY, United States
‡Center for Health Services Research, School of Public Health, University of Texas Sciences Center, Houston, TX, United States

Contents

Abbreviations

AED	antiepileptic drug
COI	cost of illness
ILAE	International League Against Epilepsy
PPP-US\$	United States Dollar purchasing power parities
QOLIE-10	quality of life in epilepsy inventory-10

1. Introduction

Epilepsy is the second most common neurological disorder estimated to affect 50 million people worldwide [1]. A recent systematic review and meta-analysis of international studies reported a lifetime epilepsy prevalence of 7.60 per 1000 persons (95% CI 6.17–9.38) and an incidence rate of 61.44 per 100,000 person-years (95% CI 50.75–74.38) [2]. Epilepsy has serious health consequences and is associated with increased medical and social service costs

The Comorbidities of Epilepsy
https://doi.org/10.1016/B978-0-12-814877-8.00002-7

and decreased productivity in patients globally [3]. Previous research has recognized the global burden of epilepsy in low- and high-resource countries, enhancing our understanding of the relationship between the economic burden of epilepsy and its epidemiology, somatic/psychiatric comorbidities, stigma, and health policy [3–9].

In the United States total direct and indirect epilepsy cost estimates have ranged from $9.6 billion (2004 dollar) to $12.5 billion (1995 dollar) annually [10]. The estimated cost of epilepsy in Europe in 2004 was €15.5 billion [11]. A recent systematic review of cost of illness (COI) epilepsy studies noted that the direct average annual medical costs related to epilepsy ranged from 40 international United States Dollar purchasing power parities (PPP-US$) in a low-resource country to PPP-US$4748 in a high-resource country [12]. This estimate does not account for all direct expenses in epilepsy nor the indirect costs that can represent up to 85% of the overall cost [12]. The drivers of the direct costs of epilepsy care are multifaceted. Making a diagnosis of epilepsy can involve multiple tests and procedures, medical management, and multiple drugs, and the work-up for and provision of surgery and/or other alternative therapies for more severe epilepsy are cost-intensive [13]. Mean direct medical costs are seen to decrease nearly eightfold within a four-year period from diagnosis, once seizure control is achieved [13]. Health care costs have been shown to decline after successful epilepsy surgery [14].

International cost comparisons are difficult due to disparities in the treatment gap, which has been estimated to result in no treatment or undertreatment of 90% of individuals with epilepsy in some countries [12, 15, 16]. In 2002, as a result of the incongruity between COI studies, the International League Against Epilepsy Commission on the Burden of Epilepsy, Subcommission on the Economic Burden of Epilepsy, published a report providing methodological recommendations for economic analyses in epilepsy [17]. The following were suggested: (1) COI studies should be population-based; (2) studies need to be conducted prospectively; (3) retrospective studies are of value, and need to be population-based rather than focused on subsets of these cohorts; (4) economic analyses studies must be comprehensive, including both direct and indirect costs that can be attributed to epilepsy.

The emphasis on cost control and managed care in health care delivery has increased our awareness of the importance of economic evaluations in epilepsy. COI analysis encompasses various aspects of disease impact on health outcomes for the individual patient, the health care system, and the country as a whole. COI may focus on the longitudinal effects of the disease on morbidity, mortality, and quality of life from onset, or the annual effects of the disease across prevalent cases. Estimating COI is important to help prioritize medical and social service decisions of patients and providers and inform health policymakers in determining appropriate allocation of funds. It has been consistently found that patients with epilepsy have a higher prevalence of somatic and psychiatric comorbidities as compared to those without epilepsy and that they often experience health and social disparities, reduced quality of life, and poorer socioeconomic status [18–21].

Comorbidities associated with epilepsy and their inclusion/exclusion in cost of epilepsy studies explain some of the discrepancies between cost studies due to their influence on the need for services and functioning of people living with epilepsy. Although there have been many studies examining the cost of epilepsy, there are only a few evaluating the impact of comorbidities (medical, neurological, and psychiatric) and the potential impact of prevention strategies from a public health perspective on the cost of epilepsy. In this chapter, we review some basic concepts of COI in epilepsy and the impact of comorbidities on the cost of epilepsy.

2. How is cost measured?

Epilepsy COI studies are challenging as ideally they should consider the direct, indirect, and intangible costs from various perspectives (i.e., the individual, caregivers, third-party payers, and societal perspective) [22]. COI studies that incorporate direct, indirect, and intangible costs are rare. Most research has focused on direct costs and even when indirect and intangible costs are addressed, the components analyzed within studies vary. COI studies are also heterogeneous due to differing geographic regions and health care systems, which subsequently leads to contrasting health care costs between studies. Even studies that are performed in the same country report widely varied epilepsy cost estimates [4, 23, 24]. For example, in the United Kingdom, Swingler et al. [23] looked at patients attending a specialist epilepsy service while Cockerall et al. [4] and Jacoby et al. [24] focused on community-based studies. Thus, comparisons across studies are incredibly difficult, especially when there is a gap in knowledge about overall health resource utilization. Also, most lifetime COI studies are based on statistical modeling since rigorous prospective cohort studies are challenging and costly to perform.

2.1 Direct cost

Direct cost of epilepsy care refers to spending on medical and social services utilized in diagnosing, treating, rehabilitating, and preventing disability. This encompasses outpatient visits, hospitalizations, investigations, medical, surgical, and other alternative therapies, residential care, and so forth. The costs of medical services are typically reported as the average payments made to health care providers and/or facilities. Estimates of direct cost may vary if reported from the patient's (out-of-pocket payments at point of service) or insurance company's (payment for services covered by the plan) point of view. In the United States, patients enrolled in government-funded plans (Medicare for the elderly and disabled, and Medicaid for low-income and disabled) generally incur less out-of-pocket costs than those with private insurance. Most COI studies investigate cost using a payer's point of view because of the availability of data.

There are "bottom-up" and "top-down" approaches to estimating direct health care cost in epilepsy [22]. The "bottom-up" approach uses individual patient records or insurance claims and is recommended especially when accurate cost estimates are needed for different subpopulations. By comparing people with and without epilepsy, it permits estimation of epilepsy-specific costs and cost variation based on sociodemographic characteristics and disease course. However, such studies are arduous and can be expensive as individual medical records and/or claims data must be collected and analyzed for each person identified with epilepsy. Such studies may not be generalizable unless completed on a large population that represents the diversity of epilepsy. [17] The "top-down" approach is useful for highly prevalent conditions that are well represented in national population or provider surveys. These studies utilize diagnostic and procedure coding to classify health resource use and allow comparisons across disease conditions. This methodology is useful in generating estimates that reflect the healthcare costs in the population as a whole. A limitation with these studies is that cost stratification by patient and clinical characteristics are not generally feasible [17].

2.2 Indirect and social service cost

Indirect cost refers to the loss of productivity secondary to morbidity and mortality (unemployment, underemployment), and social service cost refers to cost caregivers (either formal or informal) sustain through their provision of time and in-kind or paid services. Indirect cost studies generally use the "human capital" method, quantifying patients according to their economic capacity. This "human capital" method estimates the present value of the patient's future earnings under the assumption that we use future earnings as a proxy for future productivity, which often is not the case. This approach also assumes that a worker cannot be replaced if unemployment rates are high, which would consequently overestimate value lost [25]. Even with these problems, the "human capital" approach is implemented by most COI researchers since standardized economic models exist for this. In contrast to the "human capital" model, a different economic approach has been the "willingness to pay" strategy that considers indirect and intangible costs by estimating how much the consumer will spend on a unit of good/service, i.e., the amount a patient would be willing to pay to prevent or reduce the likelihood of disease [22]. Intangible costs are those of a non-financial nature. These are reflected in the quality of life of the patient, the side effects of medication, plus the stress and anxiety related to the disease and treatment process. The influence epilepsy has on quality of life in patients is well documented. Loss of independence, co-existing psychiatric comorbidities, stigma, lower welfare, social restrictions, and unemployment, to name a few, are some of the elements that impact persons living with epilepsy. Although theoretically important, estimating intangible costs is difficult due to difficulties acquiring such data.

The day-to-day social care of a person with epilepsy can be a significant burden on the entire family [26, 27]. Epilepsy is disruptive to formal and informal caregivers due to the unpredictable nature of the disease, associations with injuries, comorbidities, stigma, and even sudden death [28]. The importance of social service costs in epilepsy care, although generally acknowledged, is seldom measured due to difficulties estimating their monetary value.

3. Existing cost estimates

The impact of epilepsy on the economy in terms of health resource utilization and loss of productivity has been estimated for the United States and many other, mostly upper income, countries. In one of the earlier studies on this topic, Begley et al. estimated the societal lifetime cost of epilepsy in the United States to be $3 billion (1990 dollar), with drug-resistant epilepsy accounting for 59% of total costs [29]. Lifetime costs were noted to be influenced by epilepsy type, neurological deficits, and response to medication. Total lifetime cost (1990 dollar) ranged from $4272 (patient with remission post-diagnosis) to $138,602 (patient with severe seizures). The total cost of epilepsy in 1995 was estimated at $12.5 billion, of which $1.7 billion represented direct medical costs extrapolated from 608 patient in two metropolitan areas and $10.8 billion in loss of productivity from 1168 surveyed individuals from 18 epilepsy centers [10]. However, in general, the total cost of epilepsy varies greatly between studies. This is in part due to heterogeneity in the methods used in these studies (e.g., different source populations, eligibility criteria, ascertainment methods, etc.).

3.1 Direct costs of epilepsy

Direct costs of epilepsy have been especially studied in the United States and Europe [29–33]. A recent systematic review looked at the direct cost of epilepsy in the United States [31]. Not only did study methods vary widely, cost estimates were noticeably different among studies, with total direct healthcare costs per person ranging from $10,192 to $47,862 (total cost adjusted to 2013 US$) for general epilepsy populations (comprising all clinically defined subgroups). Epilepsy specific costs ranged from $1022 to $19,749 [31]. Other recent population-based studies using claims data have shown similar epilepsy-specific cost estimates ranging from $8412 to $11,354 in the United States [32–35]. Not surprisingly, the above systematic review noted that higher costs were consistently seen in individuals with drug-resistant epilepsy [31]. A narrative review looking at 15 international studies noted the annual direct cost of prevalent epilepsy to be between $55 in India to $3065 in the United Kingdom [36].

Antiepileptic drugs (AEDs) and hospital admissions have been consistently noted to be the greatest factor contributing to direct costs accounting for up to two-thirds of total expenditures in persons with epilepsy [36]. This is especially evident in those with difficult to treat or newly diagnosed epilepsies [12, 37]. The majority of pharmacoeconomic investigations have evaluated direct costs in regards to inpatient, outpatient, emergency care, and medication utilization. Variations in reported costs of epilepsy are great even between high-income countries. In a study of eight European high-income countries, the cost of similar AEDs varied up to 4.4 times [30]. Methodological issues likely give rise to such disparities between estimates [30]. The methods used to evaluate indirect costs are not usually clear. Quantifying intangible costs is complex, and often total societal costs of epilepsy remain undetermined [38].

3.2 Indirect costs of epilepsy

Very few studies provide monetary estimates of indirect costs among persons living with epilepsy. In one study, the investigators used claims data to look at those with epilepsy who were employed and determined their indirect costs of epilepsy from the perspective of an employer, with particular attention to disability and medically related absenteeism [32]. The mean unadjusted annual indirect costs for those employed with epilepsy were higher compared to those without epilepsy (persons with epilepsy [PWE] $3192 vs. control $1242; $P < .0001$) [32]. After adjusting for patient demographics and comorbidities, the mean indirect costs remained significantly higher for those with epilepsy (PWE $2793 vs. control $1578; $P < .001$) [32]. Analogous to this study, employees with focal onset seizures were noted to have significantly greater indirect costs related to absenteeism when compared to those without epilepsy (PWE $3431 vs. control $1511; $P < .001$) [39]. Several European studies have calculated mean annual cost estimates for lost productivity [40, 41]. One Spanish group looked at lost employment to patient and caregiver and provided a mean annual cost estimate of €1528 [40]. A German study estimated the total cost of lost productivity to be €1610 (over a three-month period) based on lost employment to patient [41]. It is well documented that epilepsy affects people's ability to work and that persons with epilepsy face a greater risk of unemployment and underemployment compared to the general population [42]. Although claims data have the ability to elucidate and calculate absenteeism, other nuanced employment outcomes—such as improved work output to cover for lost time, decreased efficiency if recovering from seizures (but decided to continue working), and effect on career trajectory—are not quantifiable. The costs may also be overestimated as claims data cannot always adjust for potential socioeconomic confounders. In order to accurately identify and understand indirect costs, future studies will need to use mixed-methods and collect qualitative data in additional to quantitative data to study the employment related impact of epilepsy. Standardization and development of economic analyses are needed in order to overcome the heterogeneity of indirect cost reporting.

3.3 Intangible costs of epilepsy

Intangible costs, such as the costs associated with stigma, are thought to comprise a substantial fraction of the cost of epilepsy [43]. In persons with epilepsy, social isolation and lack of independence may negatively affect development and self-esteem. They become less likely to wholly integrate into the community, which can lead to serious economic consequences [44–46]. Other intangible burdens include personal injury consequent to a seizure. There are increased rates of injuries in persons with epilepsy compared to those without epilepsy [47]. Injuries are a financial burden not only to patients but also to caregivers who have to learn to cope with the unpredictable nature of the disease and its associations with injuries and comorbidities. Unfortunately, putting a monetary value to such cost cannot be accurately assessed and is theoretical at most. Some studies have attempted to assess burden of illness on patients' wellbeing using a validated Quality of Life in Epilepsy-10 inventory scale [40, 48]. However, there are no studies that truly capture intangible costs in epilepsy.

4. How do comorbidities influence the cost of epilepsy?

Comorbidities increase health care costs significantly, with annual adjusted costs rising exponentially with additional coexisting conditions [49]. It is estimated that up to half of adults with epilepsy have a coexisting comorbid condition [50]. The frequency of psychiatric and medical comorbidities in people with epilepsy has been described in population-based cross-sectional cohorts [18, 19]. In one study, psychiatric and neurological comorbidities affected 30%–50% of persons with epilepsy [18]. Another study reported a lifetime prevalence of 36% of any mental disorder in persons with epilepsy, including suicidal ideation (25%), mood disorder (24%), anxiety disorder (23%), and major depression (17%) [19, 20]. In a Centers for Disease Control and Prevention study, the most commonly comorbid neurological conditions in people with epilepsy were severe headache or migraine affecting 34.7% versus 16.2% in the general population, and stroke affecting 14.3% in persons with epilepsy versus 2.4% in the general population [51]. Persons with epilepsy also have higher prevalence of medical comorbidities including asthma, osteoporosis, obesity, and heart disease as compared to the general population [21, 52, 53].

In a US study where claims data for the privately insured were analyzed, direct epilepsy-related costs accounted on average for 20% of total costs versus 80% that was spent on treating somatic and psychiatric comorbidities [32]. In an adult cohort of persons with drug-resistant focal epilepsy, hospitalizations were 3.7 times greater in those with a Charlson Comorbidity Index ≥1, with treatment costs 136% greater for all medical care compared to those without comorbidities [54]. Depression was seen to have the greatest marginal effect on likelihood of hospitalization and cost; however, somatic comorbidities such as hypertension, anemia, headache, and brain tumors were also noted to have higher associated health care use and cost [54]. This is supported by other studies where epilepsy comorbidities were associated with higher hospital treatment cost [34, 35, 55].

A study that looked at direct health care cost in Medicare fee-for-service beneficiaries in the general US population showed that 65% of participants had two or more chronic conditions, which accounted for 95% of Medicare expenditures [56]. Other studies, not surprisingly, also observed that the number of comorbid conditions increased with an aging population in persons with epilepsy [33]. Comorbidities affect diagnosis and consequent treatment, as well as increase hospitalization length of stay and thus overall costs [33]. Wilner et al. studied health plan costs by comorbidities and noted, as expected, that increasing number of comorbidities significantly increased overall health care costs in persons with epilepsy [33]. Unplanned hospital readmissions are highest in patients older than 65 years of age, secondary to coexisting comorbid conditions which further drive up costs [55]. As part of the Treatment in Geriatric Epilepsy Research study in American veterans, patients with new-onset epilepsy were found to have five times the odds of a medical admission as compared to those without epilepsy [57]. The most significant medical conditions resulting in these hospitalizations included comorbid gall bladder disorders, myocardial infarcts, angina, and anemia. Significant psychiatric disorders associated with medical admissions in the former study included alcohol dependence and schizophrenia [57].

Children with new-onset epilepsy and concomitant comorbid illnesses are at risk of reduced quality of life [27]. Depression and attention deficit hyperactivity disorder are perceived to lead to poor social integration and academic standards, independent of seizure type and severity [58]. Similarly, adults with depression and other psychological comorbidities endure stigma, low self-esteem, and self-efficacy, which are implicated as factors associated with predicting unemployment and underemployment that lead to increasing indirect costs of epilepsy.

Comorbidities will undoubtedly alter treatment plans in those with epilepsy. Patients who have comorbid hepatic or renal disease or an underlying psychiatric disorder are a few examples where different AED therapeutic decisions will have to be considered as compared to those without such comorbidities. Psychiatric comorbidities are linked with a lack of response to AEDs and development of drug resistance [59]. Uncontrolled epilepsy is associated with cognitive decline, psychosocial effects, and increased morbidity, leading to increased health care expenditure [60]. Those patients who are at risk of cognitive decline with surgery may not be able to be offered surgery, which has been noted to decline after successful epilepsy surgery [14].

The relationship between epilepsy and autoimmune mechanisms has been increasingly identified. One study looking at population-level claims data observed that the risk of epilepsy was significantly amplified in patients with autoimmune diseases (type 1 diabetes mellitus, psoriasis, rheumatoid arthritis, Graves disease, Hashimoto thyroiditis, Crohn's disease, ulcerative colitis, systemic lupus erythematosus, antiphospholipid syndrome, Sjörgren syndrome, myasthenia gravis, celiac disease) [61]. Epilepsy and autoimmune diseases frequently coexist, and surveillance of either condition is often necessary. Successful treatment in persons with autoimmune therapy propel treatment costs in persons with epilepsy [62].

Adverse drug events often increase health care costs [63]. The impact of AED adverse events on adherence and dropout are barriers that need to be overcome in order to achieve good seizure control [64]. Adverse effects in persons with epilepsy are associated with 25% discontinuation in early treatment and also contribute to a lack of adherence to treatment [65]. Adverse effects from AEDs are repeatedly seen as one of the strongest predictors of poor quality of life, independent of seizure outcome [66]. This may be especially prominent in older persons with epilepsy. The elderly are at an increased risk of experiencing adverse effects due not only to age-related pharmacokinetics and pharmacodynamics but also to interactions with medications related to their comorbid conditions. For example, AED-provoked cognitive complications can exacerbate preexisting psychiatric conditions as well as impair coordination and induce injuries and falls [67].

Intellectual disability is present in 20% of adults with epilepsy [68]. In children with intellectual disability, the most prevalent chronic condition is epilepsy, with prevalence ranging from 5.5% to 35% depending on the study type and population [69]. Many of these individuals living with epilepsy are drug resistant. Persons with epilepsy with intellectual disability also have features influencing AED adverse effects, such as potential underlying brain injury and inherited metabolic disorders, and have a predisposition to overtreatment and polypharmacy [70]. These comorbid intellectual deficits and behavioral abnormalities may impede the medical assessment/treatment in these populations who are among the most drug exposed groups in society [71].

5. Gaps in care and knowledge

The diagnosis and treatment of comorbid conditions in epilepsy is an important priority identified by the Institute of Medicine 2012 report on epilepsy [72]. The importance of comorbidities, monitoring, and timely treatment in patients with epilepsy cannot be understated [72]. Comorbidities complicate the overall management of epilepsy and can further exacerbate seizures as well as cause further harm to the patient. Early detection of comorbidities will lead to prompt intervention and noticeable health care benefits. Somatic comorbidities, such as osteoporosis, migraine, and psychiatric comorbidities, often go unnoticed and undertreated [73–76]. The Institute of Medicine report in 2012 stated that in order to improve surveillance and prevention of epilepsy, one of the key areas to be addressed includes the establishment and dissemination of standard comorbidity screening tools [72]. Certainly, validated screening tools and guidelines are present for disorders such as osteoporosis and depression in the general population. However, this has not been the case in the epilepsy population [72]. Cost savings are likely to come from better control of seizures, reducing the need for hospitalizations and emergency room visits for seizures and early detection and treatment of comorbid conditions, as well as their prevention. Effective management also depends on early recognition of those most at risk of comorbidities and the targeting of appropriate disease management interventions. These interventions will need to be evaluated through robust clinical trials.

The attribution of costs to epilepsy is challenging to separate from the cost of the primary epileptogenic condition. Well-designed prospective studies for each epilepsy etiology need to be undertaken [17]. An important challenge is differentiating true epilepsy comorbidities from diseases that cause epilepsy and vice versa. A difficulty of attribution of cost occurs, seeing whether the costs faced in persons with epilepsy should be attributed completely/partially to epilepsy or to another underlying comorbid disease. A better understanding of the economic aspects of epilepsy will lead to improved allocation of care for persons with epilepsy [77]. From the most recent systematic review by Begley and Durgin on the direct costs of epilepsy in the United States, it was found that very few studies have looked at subpopulations (i.e., adults, pediatric, well-controlled seizures, drug-resistant epilepsy, presence of comorbidities) within epilepsy cohorts and those that did were too heterogeneous and challenging to perform any comparative analysis [31]. Further research is necessary to delineate the broader economic burden of epilepsy and how it varies across subpopulations.

Additional research is also necessary to better define drivers of health resource utilization and costs in epilepsy and their associations with epilepsy comorbidities. Knowledge gaps in this area exist especially where prospective long-term studies are non-existent, and studies that use appropriate utility weights and incorporating all aspects of COI (e.g., direct, indirect, and intangible costs) are rare. A more collaborative approach between epileptologists, economists and health services researchers is essential to overcome the methodologic issues that arise through cost evaluation within the management of epilepsy.

References

[1] Dua T, Saxena S. Atlas: country resources for neurological disorders. 2017. Geneva, Switzerland: World Health Organization; 2017.
[2] Fiest KM, Sauro KM, Wiebe S, Patten SB, Kwon CS, Dykeman J, et al. Prevalence and incidence of epilepsy: a systematic review and meta-analysis of international studies. Neurology 2017;88(3): 296–303.
[3] de Boer HM, Mula M, Sander JW. The global burden and stigma of epilepsy. Epilepsy Behav 2008;12 (4):540–6.
[4] Cockerell OC, Hart YM, Sander JW, Shorvon SD. The cost of epilepsy in the United Kingdom: an estimation based on the results of two population-based studies. Epilepsy Res 1994;18(3):249–60.
[5] Hamer HM, Spottke A, Aletsee C, Knake S, Reis J, Strzelczyk A, et al. Direct and indirect costs of refractory epilepsy in a tertiary epilepsy center in Germany. Epilepsia 2006;47(12):2165–72.
[6] Thomas SV, Sarma PS, Alexander M, Pandit L, Shekhar L, Trivedi C, et al. Economic burden of epilepsy in India. Epilepsia 2001;42(8):1052–60.
[7] Hong Z, Qu B, Wu XT, Yang TH, Zhang Q, Zhou D. Economic burden of epilepsy in a developing country: a retrospective cost analysis in China. Epilepsia 2009;50(10):2192–8.
[8] Forsgren I, Beghi E, Ekman M. Cost of epilepsy in Europe. Eur J Neurol 2005;12(Suppl 1):54–8.

[9] Leonardi M, Ustun TB. The global burden of epilepsy. Epilepsia 2002;43(Suppl 6):21–5.

[10] Begley CE, Famulari M, Annegers JF, Lairson DR, Reynolds TF, Coan S, et al. The cost of epilepsy in the United States: an estimate from population-based clinical and survey data. Epilepsia 2000;41(3): 342–51.

[11] Pugliatti M, Beghi E, Forsgren L, Ekman M, Sobocki P. Estimating the cost of epilepsy in Europe: a review with economic modeling. Epilepsia 2007;48(12):2224–33.

[12] Strzelczyk A, Reese JP, Dodel R, Hamer HM. Cost of epilepsy: a systematic review. PharmacoEconomics 2008;26(6):463–76.

[13] Begley CE, Lairson DR, Reynolds TF, Coan S. Early treatment cost in epilepsy and how it varies with seizure type and frequency. Epilepsy Res 2001;47(3):205–15.

[14] Langfitt JT, Holloway RG, McDermott MP, Messing S, Sarosky K, Berg AT, et al. Health care costs decline after successful epilepsy surgery. Neurology 2007;68(16):1290–8.

[15] Mbuba CK, Ngugi AK, Newton CR, Carter JA. The epilepsy treatment gap in developing countries: a systematic review of the magnitude, causes, and intervention strategies. Epilepsia 2008;49(9):1491–503.

[16] Meyer AC, Dua T, Ma J, Saxena S, Birbeck G. Global disparities in the epilepsy treatment gap: a systematic review. Bull World Health Organ 2010;88(4):260–6.

[17] Begley CE, Beghi E, Beran RG, Heaney D, Langfitt JT, Pachlatko C, et al. ILAE Commission on the Burden of Epilepsy, Subcommission on the Economic Burden of Epilepsy: final report 1998-2001. Epilepsia 2002;43(6):668–73.

[18] Gaitatzis A, Carroll K, Majeed A, Sander JW. The epidemiology of the comorbidity of epilepsy in the general population. Epilepsia 2004;45(12):1613–22.

[19] Tellez-Zenteno JF, Matijevic S, Wiebe S. Somatic comorbidity of epilepsy in the general population in Canada. Epilepsia 2005;46(12):1955–62.

[20] Tellez-Zenteno JF, Patten SB, Jette N, Williams J, Wiebe S. Psychiatric comorbidity in epilepsy: a population-based analysis. Epilepsia 2007;48(12):2336–44.

[21] Strine TW, Kobau R, Chapman DP, Thurman DJ, Price P, Balluz LS. Psychological distress, comorbidities, and health behaviors among U.S. adults with seizures: results from the 2002 National Health Interview Survey. Epilepsia 2005;46(7):1133–9.

[22] Hodgson TA, Meiners MR. Cost-of-illness methodology: a guide to current practices and procedures. Milbank Mem Fund Q Health Soc 1982;60(3):429–62.

[23] Swingler RJ, Davidson DL, Roberts RC, Moulding F. The cost of epilepsy in patients attending a specialist epilepsy service. Seizure 1994;3(2):115–20.

[24] Jacoby A, Buck D, Baker G, McNamee P, Graham-Jones S, Chadwick D. Uptake and costs of care for epilepsy: findings from a U.K. regional study. Epilepsia 1998;39(7):776–86.

[25] Mincer J. Investment in human-capital and personal income-distribution. J Polit Econ 1958;66(4): 281–302.

[26] Lv R, Wu L, Jin L, Lu Q, Wang M, Qu Y, et al. Depression, anxiety and quality of life in parents of children with epilepsy. Acta Neurol Scand 2009;120(5):335–41.

[27] Taylor J, Jacoby A, Baker GA, Marson AG. Self-reported and parent-reported quality of life of children and adolescents with new-onset epilepsy. Epilepsia 2011;52(8):1489–98.

[28] Ellis N, Upton D, Thompson P. Epilepsy and the family: a review of current literature. Seizure 2000;9 (1):22–30.

[29] Begley CE, Annegers JF, Lairson DR, Reynolds TF, Hauser WA. Cost of epilepsy in the United States: a model based on incidence and prognosis. Epilepsia 1994;35(6):1230–43.

[30] Heaney DC, Sander JW, Shorvon SD. Comparing the cost of epilepsy across eight European countries. Epilepsy Res 2001;43(2):89–95.

[31] Begley CE, Durgin TL. The direct cost of epilepsy in the United States: a systematic review of estimates. Epilepsia 2015;56(9):1376–87.

[32] Ivanova JI, Birnbaum HG, Kidolezi Y, Qiu Y, Mallett D, Caleo S. Economic burden of epilepsy among the privately insured in the US. PharmacoEconomics 2010;28(8):675–85.

[33] Wilner AN, Sharma BK, Thompson A, Soucy A, Krueger A. Diagnoses, procedures, drug utilization, comorbidities, and cost of health care for people with epilepsy in 2012. Epilepsy Behav 2014;41:83–90.

[34] Cramer JA, Wang ZJ, Chang E, Powers A, Copher R, Cherepanov D, et al. Healthcare utilization and costs in children with stable and uncontrolled epilepsy. Epilepsy Behav 2014;32:135–41.

[35] Cramer JA, Wang ZJ, Chang E, Powers A, Copher R, Cherepanov D, et al. Healthcare utilization and costs in adults with stable and uncontrolled epilepsy. Epilepsy Behav 2014;31:356–62.

[36] Pillas D, Selai C. Economic aspects of epilepsy and antiepileptic treatment: a review of the literature. Expert Rev Pharmacoecon Outcomes Res 2005;5(3):327–38.

[37] Begley CE, Beghi E. The economic cost of epilepsy: a review of the literature. Epilepsia 2002;43(Suppl 4):3–9.

[38] Kotsopoulos IA, Evers SM, Ament AJ, de Krom MC. Estimating the costs of epilepsy: an international comparison of epilepsy cost studies. Epilepsia 2001;42(5):634–40.

[39] Ivanova JI, Birnbaum HG, Kidolezi Y, Qiu Y, Mallett D, Caleo S. Direct and indirect costs associated with epileptic partial onset seizures among the privately insured in the United States. Epilepsia 2010;51 (5):838–44.

[40] Pato AP, Perez EC, Hernando IC, Gonzalez JRL, Constenla IR, Sampedro FG. Analysis of direct, indirect, and intangible costs of epilepsy. Neurologia 2011;26(1):32–8.

[41] Strzelczyk A, Haag A, Reese JP, Nickolay T, Oertel WH, Dodel R, et al. Trends in resource utilization and prescription of anticonvulsants for patients with active epilepsy in Germany. Epilepsy Behav 2013;27(3):433–8.

[42] Heaney D. Epilepsy at work: evaluating the cost of epilepsy in the workplace. Epilepsia 1999;40(Suppl 8):44–7.

[43] Beran RG. The burden of epilepsy for the patient: the intangible costs. Epilepsia 1999;40(Suppl 8):40–3.

[44] Hayden M, Penna C, Buchanan N. Epilepsy: patient perceptions of their condition. Seizure 1992;1 (3):191–7.

[45] Carlton-Ford S, Miller R, Brown M, Nealeigh N, Jennings P. Epilepsy and children's social and psychological adjustment. J Health Soc Behav 1995;36(3):285–301.

[46] Jacoby A, Baker GA, Steen N, Potts P, Chadwick DW. The clinical course of epilepsy and its psychosocial correlates: findings from a U.K. Community study. Epilepsia 1996;37(2):148–61.

[47] Kwon CS, Liu M, Quan H, Wiebe S, McChesney J, Wirrell E, et al. The incidence of injuries in persons with and without epilepsy—a population-based study. Epilepsia 2010;51(11):2247–53.

[48] Viteri C, Codina M, Cobaleda S, Lahuerta J, Barriga J, Barrera S, et al. Validation of the Spanish version of the QOLIE-10 quality of life in epilepsy questionnaire. Neurologia 2008;23(3):157–67.

[49] Charlson M, Charlson RE, Briggs W, Hollenberg J. Can disease management target patients most likely to generate high costs? The impact of comorbidity. J Gen Intern Med 2007;22(4):464–9.

[50] Forsgren L. Prevalence of epilepsy in adults in northern Sweden. Epilepsia 1992;33(3):450–8.

[51] Centers for Disease Control and Prevention. Comorbidity in adults with epilepsy—United States, 2010. MMWR Morb Mortal Wkly Rep 2013;62(43):849–53.

[52] Hinnell C, Williams J, Metcalfe A, Patten SB, Parker R, Wiebe S, et al. Health status and health-related behaviors in epilepsy compared to other chronic conditions—a national population-based study. Epilepsia 2010;51(5):853–61.

[53] Shiek Ahmad B, Hill KD, O'Brien TJ, Gorelik A, Habib N, Wark JD. Falls and fractures in patients chronically treated with antiepileptic drugs. Neurology 2012;79(2):145–51.

[54] Lee WC, Arcona S, Thomas SK, Wang Q, Hoffmann MS, Pashos CL. Effect of comorbidities on medical care use and cost among refractory patients with partial seizure disorder. Epilepsy Behav 2005;7 (1):123–6.

[55] Mitchell RJ, Herkes G, Nikpour A, Bleasel A, Shih P, Vagholkar S, et al. Examining health service utilization, hospital treatment cost, and mortality of individuals with epilepsy and status epilepticus in New South Wales, Australia 2012-2016. Epilepsy Behav 2018;79:9–16.

[56] Wolff JL, Starfield B, Anderson G. Prevalence, expenditures, and complications of multiple chronic conditions in the elderly. Arch Intern Med 2002;162(20):2269–76.

[57] Copeland LA, Ettinger AB, Zeber JE, Gonzalez JM, Pugh MJ. Psychiatric and medical admissions observed among elderly patients with new-onset epilepsy. BMC Health Serv Res 2011;11:84.

[58] Dunn DW, Johnson CS, Perkins SM, Fastenau PS, Byars AW, de Grauw TJ, et al. Academic problems in children with seizures: relationships with neuropsychological functioning and family variables during the 3 years after onset. Epilepsy Behav 2010;19(3):455–61.

[59] Hitiris N, Mohanraj R, Norrie J, Sills GJ, Brodie MJ. Predictors of pharmacoresistant epilepsy. Epilepsy Res 2007;75(2–3):192–6.

[60] Devinsky O. Patients with refractory seizures. N Engl J Med 1999;340(20):1565–70.

[61] Ong MS, Kohane IS, Cai T, Gorman MP, Mandl KD. Population-level evidence for an autoimmune etiology of epilepsy. JAMA Neurol 2014;71(5):569–74.

[62] Vincent A, Bien CG, Irani SR, Waters P. Autoantibodies associated with diseases of the CNS: new developments and future challenges. Lancet Neurol 2011;10(8):759–72.

[63] Suh DC, Woodall BS, Shin SK, Hermes-De Santis ER. Clinical and economic impact of adverse drug reactions in hospitalized patients. Ann Pharmacother 2000;34(12):1373–9.

[64] Perucca P, Carter J, Vahle V, Gilliam FG. Adverse antiepileptic drug effects: toward a clinically and neurobiologically relevant taxonomy. Neurology 2009;72(14):1223–9.

[65] Kwan P, Brodie MJ. Early identification of refractory epilepsy. N Engl J Med 2000;342(5):314–9.

[66] Gilliam F. Optimizing health outcomes in active epilepsy. Neurology 2002;58(8 Suppl 5):S9–20.

[67] Loring DW, Marino S, Meador KJ. Neuropsychological and behavioral effects of antiepilepsy drugs. Neuropsychol Rev 2007;17(4):413–25.

[68] McCarron M, O'Dwyer M, Burke E, McGlinchey E, McCallion P. Epidemiology of epilepsy in older adults with an intellectual disability in Ireland: associations and service implications. Am J Intellect Dev Disabil 2014;119(3):253–60.

[69] Oeseburg B, Dijkstra G, Groothoff J, Reijneveld S, Jansen D. Prevalence of chronic health conditions in children with intellectual disability: a systematic literature review. Intellect Dev Disabil 2011;49:59–85.

[70] Perucca E, Kwan P. Overtreatment in epilepsy: how it occurs and how it can be avoided. CNS Drugs 2005;19(11):897–908.

[71] Kerr M, Guidelines Working Group, Scheepers M, Arvio M, Beavis J, Brandt C, et al. Consensus guidelines into the management of epilepsy in adults with an intellectual disability. J Intellect Disabil Res 2009;53(8):687–94.

[72] England MJ, Liverman CT, Schultz AM, Strawbridge LM. Epilepsy across the spectrum: promoting health and understanding. A summary of the Institute of Medicine report. Epilepsy Behav 2012;25(2):266–76.

[73] Lado F, Spiegel R, Masur JH, Boro A, Haut SR. Value of routine screening for bone demineralization in an urban population of patients with epilepsy. Epilepsy Res 2008;78(2–3):155–60.

[74] Kwan P, Man CB, Leung H, Yu E, Wong KS. Headache in patients with epilepsy: a prospective incidence study. Epilepsia 2008;49(6):1099–102.

[75] Barry JJ. The recognition and management of mood disorders as a comorbidity of epilepsy. Epilepsia 2003;44(Suppl 4):30–40.

[76] Ott D, Siddarth P, Gurbani S, Koh S, Tournay A, Shields WD, et al. Behavioral disorders in pediatric epilepsy: unmet psychiatric need. Epilepsia 2003;44(4):591–7.

[77] Pachlatko C. The relevance of health economics to epilepsy care. Epilepsia 1999;40(Suppl 8):3–7.

CHAPTER 3

Bone health in epilepsy

Evangelia G. Theochari*, Hannah R. Cock*,†
*Epilepsy Group, Atkinson Morley Regional Neuroscience Centre, St George's University Hospitals NHS Trust, London, United Kingdom
†Institute of Medical & Biomedical Education, St George's University of London, London, United Kingdom

Contents

1. Introduction

The first concerns about epilepsy and bone health, and the potential effect of antiepileptic drugs (AEDs) in particular, date back to the late 1960s [1]. While initial reports and studies were frequently confounded by other factors, such as immobility or institutionalization, a robust association between AED use and fracture risk is now well established, both in children and adults. Of people with epilepsy on long-term AEDs, 50% or more are reported to have demonstrable bone disorders, either clinical or subclinical [2]. The primary clinical manifestation of bone disorders, most notably osteoporosis, is an increased risk of fracture. Fracture can be a major life event, associated with a significant burden in terms of disability and death [3], and can also carry substantial socioeconomic implications via effects on health care utilization, employment, daily function, and care needs.

The Comorbidities of Epilepsy
https://doi.org/10.1016/B978-0-12-814877-8.00003-9

In 2010 there were an estimated 600,000 incident hip fractures in the European Union, costing €20 billion and accounting for 54% of the total costs of osteoporosis [4]. The risk of osteoporosis increases with age, such that prevention and management is primarily targeted at postmenopausal women and men over 50. More than one in three adult women and one in five men will sustain a fragility fracture (sustained from a fall of standing height or less) in their lifetime. With the aging population, absolute numbers are steadily rising, and associated costs are expected to increase on average by 25% by 2025 [5], so this is a major public health issue. Together with suggestions from recent studies that some of the additional risks of epilepsy and AEDs associated bone disease are potentially avoidable, there is a need for increased awareness and evidence-based guidance on managing epilepsy-associated bone disease. In this chapter, we will review the available literature on the effects of epilepsy and the AEDs on bone health, the potential mechanisms involved, and how best to identify, monitor, and treat those most at risk of metabolic bone disease.

2. Bone functions in health and disease

Bone is a dynamic tissue with multiple roles (Table 1). Cortical bone, accounting for around 80% in adults, is dense and compact and provides the structural stability of the skeleton. Trabecular (also known as cancellous) bone, on the other hand, is more metabolically active through its large surface. Bone undergoes a continuous process of remodeling, also known as bone turnover, as a result of a cycle of activation, bone resorption and then formation as illustrated in Fig. 1.

In an adult, 25% of trabecular bone is resorbed and replaced annually, whereas only 3% of the cortical bone undergoes the same resorption/replacement process. Bone remodeling is crucial for skeleton integrity and tight regulation of calcium homeostasis, and it is regulated by steroid and thyroid hormones, polypeptides, and locally circulating cytokines and growth factors. It is also dependent on available calcium, phosphorous, and vitamin D. Any imbalance of bone formation/resorption can lead to bone disease. In children and young adults, when the skeleton is still developing, an imbalance of bone resorption/formation has a negative effect on bone accumulation, whereas in older adults it leads to bone loss. The primary symptom of metabolic bone disease is an increased risk of fracture, including with minimal or no trauma.

Table 1 Bone functions

Function	Example
Structural support	Essential support for control of posture and movement
Protection of vital organs	Brain inside the skull, heart, and lungs in the ribcage
Biochemical	Storage of lipids and minerals, especially calcium
Hematological	Contains marrow with stem cells producing blood cells and platelets

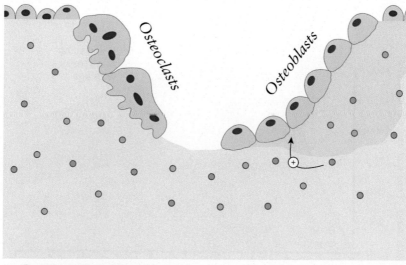

○ TGF-β, transforming growth factor beta
○ IGF, insulin-like growth factor

Fig. 1 Bone remodeling. The cycle starts by activation of precursor osteoclasts to become mature multinucleated osteoclasts, which are responsible for bone resorption, acting on old or damaged bone. In parallel, osteoblasts are activated to produce collagenous and non-collagenous proteins (osteoid, or bone matrix), which are then mineralized. Once embedded in this matrix, the osteoblasts become osteocytes and are responsible for exchange of nutrients, though they eventually die off, stimulating osteoclasts to start the cycle again. *(Figure by Shandristhe azylean; original file: bonemetabolism.png created by JE.at.UWOU|T. Uploaded 05:04, November 17, 2006 (UTC)., CC BY-SA 3.0, https://en.wikipedia.org/w/index.php?curid=28248772.)*

Reduced bone mineral density (BMD), or bone mass, and vitamin D deficiency are established independent risk factors for fracture, the most important clinical manifestation of metabolic bone disease.

2.1 Bone mineral density

During childhood and adolescence, the skeleton grows both in size and density, reaching a peak in early adult life and declining thereafter (Fig. 2).

There is considerable individual variability of which around 75% is due to hereditary factors, including sex and ethnicity: Caucasian women have the highest incidence of reduced bone mass, with African Americans relatively protected (Africans in Africa have been little studied). Bone mass is assessed in practice as BMD, measured noninvasively with dual-energy X-ray absorptiometry (DEXA), which has an accuracy of 1%–2% at any given site and is the agreed gold standard [6, 7]. Values can be obtained for whole bones or joints, or bone cortex or trabecular bone alone. Values taken from sites of potential fracture, ideally the total hip score, are considered the most valid. Results are

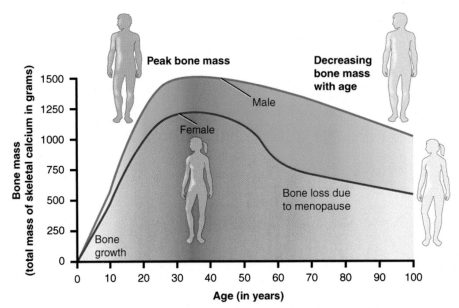

Fig. 2 Bone mass with age and gender in the healthy population. Measured in clinical practice using BMD, the amount of bone per unit of skeletal area in g/cm^2, which follows a similar pattern. As well as differences with gender and age, low levels of physical activity, smoking, alcohol, and hormonal status (postmenopausal women, testosterone deficient men) are also known be associated with reduced BMD. *(Figure © by Anatomy & Physiology, Connexions website. http://cnx.org/content/col11496/1.6/, June 19, 2013. OpenStax College, CC BY 3.0, https://commons.wikimedia.org/w/index.php?curid=30017602.)*

expressed as a T-score, which reflects the number of standard deviations (SD) above or below the mean peak in healthy young adults (aged 30 years) matched for gender and ethnicity. In pediatric populations, a Z-score may be used, representing the SD above or below the mean of healthy age-matched controls. With each SD decrease in BMD, there is a twofold increased risk of nontraumatic fractures.

The World Health Organization (WHO) [7a] defines osteoporosis as a "progressive systemic skeletal disease characterized by low bone mass and microarchitectural deterioration of bone tissue, with a consequent increase in bone fragility and susceptibility to fracture." Common sites of fragility fracture include the vertebral bodies, distal radius, proximal humerus, pelvis, and proximal femur (hip) [6]. Operationally, osteoporosis is defined as a BMD T-score of less than −2.5 SD. A T-score between −2.5 and − 1 SD is considered osteopenic (also referred to as low bone mass), and > 1 is considered normal. However, the use of BMD alone is not enough to assess fracture risk. This is because despite a high specificity, the sensitivity is low, such that half of fractures will occur in patients not meeting the criteria for a diagnosis of osteoporosis on BMD.

2.2 Vitamin D

Vitamin D is a secosteroid, most of which is synthesized in the skin dependent on sunlight exposure. The primary active metabolite is 1,25-dihydroxyvitamin D, which in addition to its role on bone metabolism, has significant roles in cell proliferation and differentiation, influencing the immune and reproductive systems, and a potential role in a wide range of conditions [8]. Hypovitaminosis D is an independent risk factor for fracture, and in addition to its role in bone health, may have other relevant consequences, including muscle weakness and an increased liability to falls [9]. The cutaneous production of Vitamin D is also affected by age (increasing age reduces the effects of sun exposure), skin pigmentation (pigmented skin requires more sun), and cultural factors (e.g., clothing, use of sunscreen). Thus populations who are housebound/institutionalized or have less sunlight exposure for other reasons will, by default, rely more on dietary sources, and be at risk of deficiency. Serum levels of 25-hydroxyvitamin D are usually measured. Severe vitamin D deficiency (<20 nmol/L) results in defective bone mineralization (rickets in children and osteomalacia in adults), but defining the lower limit of normal and what constitutes mild insufficiency has been a topic of considerable debate over the years. The UK scientific advisory committee on nutrition states that a mean level over the year of 30 nmol/L (12.5 microg/L), never falling below 25 nmol/L, is sufficient to maintain bone health for most people. However this doesn't consider serum levels in the presence of additional bone health insults, and many [10, 11], including the U.S. authorities [12] advocate a target of above 50 nmol/L to optimize protection for at least 97.5% of the population. The lack of consensus about what constitutes deficiency makes it difficult to establish its true prevalence beyond the fact that it is clearly not uncommon. Recent data has suggested an increasing proportion of the U.S. general population, potentially up to 32% [13], have vitamin D insufficiency. In the UK in winter 30%–40% of all age groups in the general population are classed as vitamin D deficient, and even towards the end of summer 8% of adults and 13% of adolescents remain deficient [14], such that consideration to routine fortification of foods is under consideration. Others argue this is an over interpretation and misunderstanding of the data [15] and that overscreening and overtreatment puts those at other end of the spectrum with serum levels >150 nmol/L at risk of adverse effects. While serum levels of up to 600 nmol/L (with intakes of up to 10,000 IU/day) are generally asymptomatic, an association between even modestly raised levels and all-cause mortality is recognized, including cardiovascular events and some types of cancer [12]. We shall return to this issue later on when considering supplementation for people with epilepsy.

2.3 Other markers of bone turnover

Additional traditional markers relating to bone health include serum levels of calcium, phosphate, parathyroid hormone, and bone-specific alkaline phosphatase.

Numerous other markers have also been shown to correlate with bone turnover, including serum or urine levels of osteocalcin, N- and C-terminal polypeptides of type 1 procollagen, tartrate resistant acid phosphatase (TRACP), and deoxypyridinoline or hydroxyproline. While these are often measured in research studies and may have the potential to aid in risk assessment or in monitoring response to treatment [6], none have been prospectively validated against fracture risk of other clinically meaningful endpoints.

3. Fracture risk in people with epilepsy

Following the early signals of concern, the first study demonstrating an increased risk of fracture in people with epilepsy was published [16] in 1977. This and many other early studies, showing up to a sixfold increased risk, were carried out in institutionalized patients in whom low activity levels and poor sunlight exposure were important confounders. However, a large body of evidence now supports that the risk of fractures is at least doubled in people with epilepsy compared to matched controls, including in ambulatory community-based populations. One of the largest studies came from the UK general practice database [17]; although retrospective, this included over 40,000 epilepsy patients and 80,000 controls and reported an overall twofold increase risk of fractures in epilepsy patients compared to age- and sex-matched controls. The relative risk was highest for hip, and neck of femur fracture in particular, which was increased threefold in patients over the age of 50, as might be expected if the risk is bone health related. This was also the conclusion from a meta-analysis of published work reported around the same time [18]. Some of this, of course, may not be related to drug treatment, as people with epilepsy also have significantly increased rates of accidental injury per se [19]. This is true for almost all types of injury ranging from minor to severe and life-threatening, even when comorbidities are taken into account. Studies suggest that around 25%–37% of fractures in people with epilepsy are due to seizure-associated falls [20–22], with tonic-clonic seizures, unsurprisingly, carrying the highest risk, including in the absence of a fall due to the strength of muscular contractions. Aside from the impact of seizures and bone health, other contributory factors to increased fracture risk include impaired motor function due to comorbid cognitive or physical disabilities [23, 24] and the sometimes subtle effects AEDs can have on balance and postural control, although to date, there have been relatively few studies done regarding this [25–27]. Thus, while optimizing seizure control, especially where there are seizure-related falls and/or convulsive seizures, remains a priority, avoiding drug toxicity, and being aware of general fall prevention strategies (e.g., good lighting, appropriate correction of refractive errors, identification and modification of environmental hazards) is also important.

4. AEDs and fracture risk

All that said, the main concern in recent years has been establishing whether AEDs themselves confer additional risks to bone health. If they do, it is clearly important we know this in order that we can properly advise patients with mild or infrequent seizures and those in remission on the risks/benefits of continued AED treatment. Also, it is important to ensure that those who need or choose to stay on AEDs are aware of the potential risks and to implement any strategies that might mitigate or reduce individual risks. As with epilepsy, while an association between AED use and increased fracture risk was readily identifiable in large population-based studies of ambulatory patients over 20 years ago [28], separating out the effects of AEDs on bone health from the many potential confounders has been a difficult job. A considerable number of cross-sectional, case-control, and prospective cohort studies in ambulatory patients addressing this question have now been published, varying in size and population under study and methodology and sometimes with contradictory conclusions. Taken together, however, they suggest a robust association between use of AEDs and fracture risks, as summarized in a systematic review and random-effects meta-analysis published in 2014 [29]. This covered 22 original epidemiological studies that provided a risk estimate for fracture (any site) related to AED exposure, whether for epilepsy or other conditions, such as pain, anxiety, or migraine, which controlled for at least some confounders. Of these, data was extractable from 15 studies encompassing almost 1.3 million patients and demonstrated a significant increase in fracture risk among AED users: Relative Risk (RR) 1.86, 95% Confidence Interval (CI) 1.62–2.12. In further support of this being a drug effect, some of the larger, better-controlled studies, such as that by Vestergaard [21], which included almost 125,000 fractures and did adjust for confounders such as steroid use, comorbidities, social variables, and prior fractures, demonstrated a dose-response effect for carbamazepine, phenobarbitone, oxcarbazepine, and valproate. The risk appears higher with liver enzyme-inducing AEDs (LEI-AEDs) than non-LEI-AEDs ([29] RR 1.18, 95CI 1.11–125), but it is not confined to LEI-AEDs, given that valproate, an enzyme inhibitor, is also clearly implicated. Beyond those already mentioned, including other LEI-AEDs (phenytoin, topiramate), there is insufficient data on any of the other newer AEDs in relation to fracture risk to draw firm conclusions as yet. At least, in part, this may reflect the impact of duration of exposure (i.e., a cumulative dose effect). According to the UK general practice database study [30], which also attempted to control for disease severity (using a number of drugs and medical contacts as surrogate markers), each year of exposure to AEDs was associated with a 9% increase in fracture risk. The clinical significance of this depends on the starting point of absolute risk for that individual. For those on LEI-AEDs, with the highest risks, this means an additional 48 fractures for every 100,000 women treated with LEI-AEDs for 1 year, including 10 hip fractures, and 4 additional hip fractures in every 10,000 men [31]. Thus, it does appear that at least the older AEDs, including all enzyme inducers and valproate, are themselves associated with a modest increase in risk of fractures, and evidence is accumulating to support cause and effect. This becomes more significant the longer individuals are on AEDs, due both to advancing age and the cumulative dose effect.

5. How might AEDs affect bone health?

There are a number of biologically plausible, and in some cases well-established, mechanisms by which AEDs might directly or indirectly influence bone health. LEI-AEDs are known to increase vitamin D catabolism. Notwithstanding the aforementioned debate about what constitutes deficiency, vitamin D insufficiency appears worryingly prevalent (often 40%–80%) in adult and pediatric epilepsy populations, both in the developed [32–34] and the developing world [35], and may develop very quickly (within months) of starting AEDs [36, 37]. In cross-sectional studies, use of LEI-AEDs [34, 38–40], polytherapy and cumulative duration [32, 35] have all been reported as independently associated. Other typical findings in parallel include increased bone alkaline phosphatase, reduced calcitonin levels and reduced serum calcium [40–45] associated with LEI-AED use compared to matched controls. Enzyme inducers may also result in decreased levels of bioavailable endogenous sex hormones, specifically estradiol and testosterone, which are also associated with increased rates of bone loss [46]. Of note in this context, women with epilepsy have an increased risk for developing premature ovarian failure and early menopause, similarly an independent risk factor for osteoporosis and fractures. Enzyme induction is also associated with vitamin K deficiency, in turn contributing to undercarboxylation of osteocalcin and accelerated bone loss [47]. There are clearly additional mechanisms, however, given the clear association with non-LEI-AEDs, valproate in particular, and that low BMD is often identified in the presence of normal or even above-average vitamin D levels [39, 41]. Furthermore, in the large population-based fracture study cited previously by Vestergaard [21], the risk of fracture was higher than predicted based on BMD changes alone. Numerous other markers of increased bone turnover have also been identified in association with use of both older and newer AEDs, though often with contradictory and inconsistent results in cross-sectional studies, with many methodological issues and confounders, the results of which are thus not summarized here. Prospective clinical studies, some with an attempt to control for confounders, are summarized in Table 2 but are again mostly underpowered and of relatively short duration and with sometimes conflicting results.

Other potential mechanisms implicated in bone loss, largely from animal and in vitro studies, include direct effects cation (calcium) transport in the intestine and via direct effects on bone turnover on proliferation of osteoblasts [38, 43]. Sodium channel blockers, specifically carbamazepine and phenytoin, have recently been shown to also inhibit sodium currents in osteoblasts [56] influencing function. Valproate and phentyoin

Table 2 Prospective clinical studies assessing bone health markers in relation to antiepileptic drug exposure

Population (age in years)	Drugs (n)	Evaluation time (relative to AED initiation)	Controlled for confounders[a]	BMD, site	Main biochemical findings
Children (range 6–19) [48]	CBZ (60)	0 and 2 y	BMI, exercise, Vit D	ND	↑ turnover
Adult men (mean 45, range 25–54) [39]	Any AED (81, most CBZ, PHT, or VPA)	Variable and +mean 19 m (range 12–29)	BMI, smoking, alcohol, diet, exercise, other drugs	↓ femur 1.8%/yr	↔ all
Adults (mean 28.9 +/− 5) (mean 30.4 +/− 5.6y) [49]	VPA (50) Control (60)	Mean 6.7 +/− 4y and +6 m	BMI, alcohol, smoking, coffee, diet, exercise	↓ lumbar & femur ∝ duration	ND
Children (mean 7.4 +/− 3.3 y) [50]	CBZ/VPA (51) Control (80)	0 and >1 y	BMI, diet, exercise, season	ND	↔ most, ↓ Vit D ↔ all
Children (mean 7.8 +/− 3.7 y, range 3–15.5) [51]	VPA (15), CBZ (11), PB(4)	0 and 2 y	BMI	↔ lumbar	↔ all
Adults (range 18–50 y) [52]	CBZ (10) VPA (15) LTG (8)	0 and 6 m	BMI, diet, exercise	↓ calcaneus ↔ ↔	↔ most ↓ Vit D ↔ incl Vit D, ↑ calcitonin ↔ incl Vit D, ↑ calcitonin
Adults (mean 31.0 ±13.1) [53]	LEV (61)	0 and 14 ±3 m	BMI, diet, exercise	↑ lumbar ↔ others	↔ all incl Vit D
Adults (mean 28.2 +/− 8.4) [54]	OXC (41)	0 and 11.6 ±6 m	BMI, diet, exercise	↓ lumbar	↔ most, ↓ Ca & Alk Phos
Adults (mean 44 +/− 15 AED users, 50 +/− 16 non) [55]	CBZ (11) VPA (13), LEV (13) Control (57)	Mean 3.5 and 27.6 m	BMI, diet, exercise, other drugs, smoking	↓ hip ↔ ↔	ND

[a] All controlled for gender and age and excluded or controlled for other comorbidities known to independently effect bone health. y, years; m, months; n, number; CBZ, carbamazepine; LEV, levetiracetam; LTG, lamotrigine; VPA, valproate; PB, phenobarbital; BMI, body mass index; ND, not done; Vit, vitamin. ↔ no significant change.

have also been shown to reduce the amount of two key proteins, collagen 1, the major bone matrix protein, and osteonectin in cultured osteoblast like cells, both crucial to bone formation and mineralization [57, 58]. "AED bone disease" is thus likely not a single entity and should probably not be considered synonymous with osteoporosis. This is also supported by histomorphometric data, albeit limited, illustrating increased bone remodeling [59] and not necessarily decreased cortical bone mass. Other than vitamin D, BMD is the only measurement consistently associated with the key clinical endpoint of increased fracture risk; therefore, from a practical perspective at least on current evidence, assessing the effects of AEDs by looking at BMD remains the best approach.

6. AEDs and BMD in people with epilepsy

After the first report of osteomalacia associated with phenytoin use [1], others quickly followed [60, 61], though also from institutionalized patients, thus likely confounded by poor nutrition, reduced physical activity, and sunlight exposure. Since then, however, a large number of studies, mostly cross-sectional or retrospective case-control in design have been reported on BMD in people with epilepsy. Some not cited here used non-validated methods or sites, so are difficult to interpret. However, using the recommended standard of DEXA at the spine or hip, also taking adequate care to control for confounders, most support that AED use, at least in adults taking any of the older AEDs (carbamazepine, valproate, phenytoin, phenobarbitone) is independently associated with reduced BMD in ambulatory patients [39, 41, 62–64]. These studies show that up to 59% of patients are osteopenic and 23% are osteoporotic by WHO definitions and that significant reductions in BMD may be apparent as early as 1 year into treatment [65], though the size of any AED effect and the extent of correlation with different drug classes or duration of therapy were inconsistent. Studies in children and adolescents are less consistent, with an inevitably larger data spread reflecting that this is anyway a time of considerable change and skeletal development. Several well-controlled earlier studies have not found any significant reduction in DEXA Z-scores in children taking CBZ [66–70] or lamotrigine [71, 72]. Others have found BMD reductions associated with treatment, especially polytherapy and long duration, though often without adequate controls for potential confounders [73–75]. Similarly, there are conflicting reports for valproate [40, 66–70, 73, 76]. Whether this reflects methodological difficulties and shorter duration of AED therapy, whether younger skeletons are better able to tolerate metabolic changes or problems will become apparent in later life remains unclear. As for hypovitaminosis D, that cumulative drug burden may be significant is supported by one cross-sectional study from a tertiary population, all with established osteoporosis, in whom a surrogate marker of cumulative drug burden (total duration of epilepsy multiplied by number of AEDs) was the dominant factor in predicting fracture risk [77]. Prospective longitudinal studies, as summarized previously in Table 1, show a similar picture supporting a reduction in BMD associated with at least older AEDs in adults but less consistent findings in children, though almost all are underpowered and control for only some confounders.

7. AEDs, fracture risk, and BMD in the general population

AEDs have long been used for conditions other than epilepsy, so if this is a drug effect, AED exposure should be an independent risk factor in the general population, not just in people with epilepsy. AED use has been shown to be associated with increased fracture rates among intensive treatment unit patients [78], hypovitaminosis D in medical inpatients [79], increased hip fracture rates in Caucasian women in the community [28], and lower extremity fracture in young men with spinal cord injuries [80]. Two large prospective community-based studies from the same group have now systematically addressed this. In the first, over 9000 women over 65 underwent DEXA at the hip and calcaneous with an average of 5.7 years between scans [81]. With careful adjustment for confounders, the average rate of decline in total hip BMD increased from -0.7%/year in non-AED users (ever) to -0.87%/year in partial users (AEDs at some time during the study, but not throughout) and to -1.16%/year in continuous users (p for trend 0.015). While these numbers sound small, such is the importance of BMD, this translates to a nearly 30% increase in the risk of hip fracture over 5 years, associated with AED use in this population. Phenytoin looked like the worst offender but was also the most commonly used AED, and the smaller numbers on other AEDs may have hidden any effect. Hormone replacement therapy (HRT) and exercise also came through as protective factors, independent of AED usage. In a subsequent similar study in over 4200 men over 65 [82], a mean 4.6-year interval between scans showed, as expected, that all rates of decline were lower compared to women, but again showed significantly greater rates of loss associated with non-LEI-AEDs use (-0.53%/year, $p = 0.04$), though, perhaps surprisingly, not LEI-AED use (-0.46%/year, $p = 0.31$) compared to controls (0.35%/year). As might be expected, AED users in the large community studies [81, 82] were also different in other respects (e.g., as a group having less good general health, being thinner and more depressed). Of note in this context, depression is a well-established risk factor for bone health and fractures, perhaps even more so than in epilepsy confounded by reduced rates of exercise, nutritional factors, and sun exposure, with an emerging debate about whether antidepressants might also confer additional risks [83].

Across populations, age, gender, and hormonal status certainly have the largest influence on BMD, and AED use has been estimated to contribute to only 5% of the total variation in BMD at the femoral neck [62]. Attempting to control even more tightly for age, gender, and associated genetic factors, a recent study of 48 same-sex twin/age-matched sibling pairs [84], well-matched for potential confounders but discordant for AED use, reported significantly reduced BMD in the hip areas associated with

AED use, and repeated assessments two years later. Forty of the 48 were female pairs, and of the AED users, 20 were on LEI-AEDS, 16 on non-LEI-AEDs, and the remaining 12 on a combination. Although across the whole cohort the annual rate of change in all regions didn't differ between the pairs, LEI-AEDs were associated with significantly greater BMD loss compared to non-users (1.7 vs 0.3% in total hip and 0.7 vs 0.1% whole body, $p = 0.013$), and AED use (any) over 20 years or more was also a predictor. So, however you look at the data, there is a clear and consistent message supporting a causal relationship between AED use and reduced BMD to an extent that is likely to be clinically significant in some populations. The risks are greater with LEI-AEDs but still present with older non-LEI AEDs, such as valproate.

8. Are newer AEDs safer?

Given the difficulties in determining individual drug risks when almost everyone was on one of only a small number of drugs and that inevitably fewer people have been exposed to the newer AEDs, and for less time, unsurprisingly, there isn't yet a definitive answer to this question. All the newer agents are initially licensed as adjunctive therapies, and good prospective monotherapy studies of sufficient size and duration have yet to be published and would be expensive to do well. It's reasonable to assume that any LEI-AEDs, including oxcarbazepine, eslicarbazepine, topiramate, perampanel, and rufinamide are likely to carry risks similar to those of carbamazepine. Of these there is sufficient clinical data only for topiramate thus far, with a 39% increased risk of fracture in the large meta-analysis study [29]. In gonadally intact rats [85], although there was no reduction in BMD after 12 weeks of treatment, osteoblast surface and bone mineralizing surface were significantly lowered, suggesting topiramate at best isn't bone-neutral.

With regard to non-LEI AEDs, lamotrigine has been put forward as a potentially safer alternative [86]. A cross-sectional study of premenopausal women on monotherapy found those on lamotrigine ($n = 19$) had no significant increases in markers of bone turnover or calcium in contrast to women on carbamazepine ($n = 37$), valproate ($n = 18$), or phenytoin ($n = 19$), though, notably, they had also been on AEDs for a significantly shorter time (under 2 years, compared to five or more), and there were no differences between the groups with respect to BMD or vitamin D status [44]. Another short-term prospective monotherapy study [52] comparing lamotrigine with carbamazepine and valproate found reductions in BMD and vitamin D only in the carbamazepine group at 6 months. In pediatric populations there is limited data, but 13 children on monotherapy for a mean of $3.9 +/- 3.3$ years [71] were indistinguishable from controls on BMD. Finally, in animal studies, at least in gonadally intact rats over 3 months [85], lamotrigine, in contrast to topiramate, did not affect BMD, bone strength, or bone turnover. Thus, overall, lamotrigine is certainly promising, but lack of evidence of harm is not, of course, equivalent to evidence of safety, and longer larger clinical studies are still needed.

The jury is also very much still out with respect to levetiracetam. A cross-sectional study reported reduced BMD in monotherapy patients on levetiracetam compared to those on topiramate, lamotrigine, and carbamazepine [87]. All patients had been on AEDs for at least two years (mean 14), which might account for why no such reduction was found in a study of drug naïve patients after just one year of levetiracetam treatment [53]. A recent open study [88] compared patients who had previously failed initial monotherapy and were then randomized to treatment with levetiracetam ($n = 42$) or an older AED (carbamazepine or valproate, n = 42). In those who completed the assessments at 3 and 15 months (40 on levetiracetam, 30 on other AEDs), both groups had accelerated bone loss at clinically relevant sites as well as reduced bone turnover [88]. In contrast, patients who switch from phenytoin to levetiracetam show improvements in BMD and vitamin D at 2 years compared to those who continue, as did those stopping treatment completely, although this may reflect the particular risks of phenytoin as much as anything [89]. Studies in mice [90] and gonadally intact rats [91] also suggest levetiracetam has limited effects, at least compared to older drugs.

Conflicting data has also been reported for oxcarbazepine [45, 54, 87, 92], and there is even more limited data on any of the other newer AEDs. The reality is it is reasonable to conclude that non-LEI-AEDs, or at least those with weaker LEI effects, such as oxcarbazepine, are likely less harmful to bone health than strong inducers, such as phenytoin, but we can't say for certain that they are safe, especially in the longer term.

9. So what should we do?

By now it should be clear that at least some people with epilepsy on AEDs are at increased risk of bone health problems, including reduced BMD, hypovitaminosis D, and, ultimately, fractures, compared to the general population. For many if not most, stopping AEDs isn't an option, and switching to newer AEDs that might have lower risks is also not without difficulties, with no guarantee of better outcomes in the long term. As a minimum, in line with standard guidance for the general population [6], clinicians should be actively thinking about bone health for people with epilepsy and including bone health risks in discussions about the benefits and risks of treatment, particularly where these are more finely balanced with respect to seizure risks. Particularly in an older seizure-free patient whose absolute risk of fracture may already be approaching 10% over 10 years, a realization that ongoing treatment with AEDs might almost double this risk is surely something they need to know to inform their decision about whether to continue treatment or not. Ensuring all patients are aware of lifestyle measures to improve bone health include increasing the level of physical activity, stopping smoking, reducing alcohol intake to ≤ 2 units/day, reducing the risk of falls, and ensuring adequate dietary calcium intake and vitamin D also seems reasonable. Widespread screening and primary prevention for osteoporosis/reduced BMD are not, however, recommended on the grounds that most fractures will occur not in the small numbers at very high risk, but in the larger numbers at moderate risk. Instead, a selected case finding or targeted risk assessment approach has been consistently recommended since the 1990s.

9.1 Case finding and targeted risk assessment

Essentially, this means identifying those most likely to be at risk and then offering screening with BMD only to those groups within those populations where it is appropriate to inform decisions about treatment. In the UK, the National Institute for Health and Care Excellence (NICE) [93] recommends assessment of fracture risk in all women >65 and men >70 years, as well as those over 50 years in the presence of specific additional risk factors for fracture or osteoporosis. Two web-based tools, FRAX (http://www.shef.ac.uk/FRAX) and QFracture (http://www.qfracture.org/) have been externally validated in independent cohorts and are the recommended first step in the UK. Both ask for basic demographics and additional clinical information on proven risks (low body mass index; prior characteristic fracture; parental hip fracture; alcohol intake; smoking; rheumatoid arthritis, glucocorticoid treatment; other known cause secondary osteoporosis) and give an 10-year probability of major osteoporotic fracture (%), as recommended by international consensus, plotted on a chart with associated thresholds for interventions (treat, measure BMD, or give lifestyle advice and reassure). FRAX can be used in patients >40 years, can include BMD results if these are known, has been developed from studying population-based cohorts from Europe, North America, Asia, and Australia, and is preferred by the UK guideline group, at least [6]. However, neither AED use nor epilepsy are among the many selectable risk factors listed within FRAX, whereas both have been recognized as secondary risks within the QFracture tool since 2012 [94]. QFracture can be used for patients >30 and produces a helpful Cates plot showing 10-year probabilities of any osteoporotic fracture, and separately hip fracture, to facilitate shared decision-making, but is only strictly applicable to UK populations. For those identified as being at risk using such tools, BMD measurement DEXA is the next step, from which a definite diagnosis of osteoporosis or osteopenia can be confirmed or excluded, and treatment decisions then made based on this. The bottom line is that treatment, beyond lifestyle advice, is rarely indicated unless the fracture risk is approaching 10% in younger patients, or 10%–20% in older patients. In patients with risks above that, arguably, treatment should be offered anyway, irrespective of BMD results. In other countries, including the United States [95], specific guidance on the use of risk assessment tools is less prescriptive, suggesting instead that DEXA to measure BMD should be offered by default to all women over 65, men over 70, as well as any postmenopausal women or men over 50 years who have already sustained a fragility fracture and other groups with additional risk factors. A full list of national and international guidelines is available via the International Osteoporosis Foundation https://www.iofbonehealth.org/guideline-references.

Given the weight of evidence now supporting that AED use is an independent risk factor, that this is still not included in most consensus guidelines may reflect that the risk, while genuine, is almost certainly substantially lower than that associated with, for example, long-term glucocorticoid use, which in all guidelines triggers active assessment and monitoring of bone health. For example, the odds ratio (OR) for fracture risk in patients on long-term glucocorticoid treatment [96] ranges from around 2 (hip) to over 5 (spine) after as little as six months of treatment, compared to the ~1.4 OR that might be attributable to AEDs (excluding seizure-related fractures) after many years. Importantly, the cost, clinical effectiveness and service implications of including epilepsy patients as a high-risk group have also barely been evaluated, though perhaps are deserving of further research to inform future practice and guidelines. On this basis, it makes sense to ensure that people with epilepsy are proactively offered at least the access to risk assessment and DEXA as the general population, and many will have additional risk factors, such as reduced mobility and increased risk of falls, aside from their AEDs. Some have argued that BMD screening should be considered for people with symptomatic epilepsy, post-menopausal women with epilepsy, or even all patients who have been on AEDs for at least 3–5 years [86]. However, it is important to remember that the absolute risk is very low in younger patients, thus the assessment tools have only been developed for adults. In the UK, NICE specifically cautions against even undertaking risk assessments (FRAX or QFracture) in those under 40 [93], where the absolute risk never reaches a minimum threshold for treatment (1% over 10 years). The utility of BMD and screening in younger patients, including whether such a strategy would be cost-effective, or indeed safe, in the longer term has not been established. Similarly, there is really no evidence base to support serial assessments of biochemical markers of bone turnover in people with epilepsy, which has been suggested [59], beyond a standard bone profile, including serum vitamin D every 2–5 years [97].

9.2 Vitamin D and calcium supplementation

As discussed previously, hypovitaminosis D is a well-established independent risk factor for fracture, prevalent in the general population, even more so in people with epilepsy, and a readily modified one. The United States recommends a dietary allowance for adults of 600 IU/day (12 µg) [12], whereas in the UK the defined threshold is 400 IU/Day (10 µg). However, both also acknowledge that while this refers to intakes from all sources, it is difficult to achieve the recommended nutritional intake from natural food sources alone, such that the latest UK report [14] has recommend that the government consider population-wide strategies to address this. Supplements are most commonly available as 400 IU vitamin D3 (cholecalciferol), usually with calcium at this dose, or higher doses (2000–5000 IU, either tablet or spray) without calcium. Vitamin D is cheap, well-tolerated, and supplementation is of proven efficacy in reducing fracture risk in community-based studies of high-risk groups (principally the elderly), both with calcium [98] and alone [99], irrespective of vitamin D status. Recommending supplements by default to some high-risk groups is already standard practice in some settings, including in the UK for infants and children under four, pregnant and breastfeeding women, people over 65 years, those with low sun exposure or darker skins, and those on vegan, halal, or kosher diets [100]. Modeling supports that this would likely be cost-effective, as a result of reduced fractures, and potentially reduced serum testing as well [101]. In the United States, many foods and milk are already fortified, and supplements are recommended for the same groups, as well as obese patients and those with inflammatory bowel disease or following gastric bypass surgery [12]. However, people with epilepsy, particularly those on LEI-AEDs, or with severe (<25 nmol/sL) deficiency may require higher doses in order to achieve satisfactory serum levels (>50 nmols/L) [37, 102]. The value of vitamin D supplementation in ambulatory people with epilepsy has also now been demonstrated in two randomized controlled trials, in children and adults on AEDs reported together [103]. In adults, the baseline BMD was lower than in control populations consistent with other studies. After 1 year of supplementation, only high-dose (4000 IU/day) and not low-dose (400 IU/day), vitamin D was effective as assessed by BMD increases. In children, baseline BMD was normal but increased in both low- and high-dose treatment groups, though this would be expected in this age group without treatment. Reflecting this, the UK issued guidance in 2009 recommending that vitamin D supplementation should be considered for at-risk patients taking long-term enzyme-inducing AEDs or valproate [104]. "At risk" and "long-term" were, however, not defined, nor was there guidance on dose or what levels to aim for in this population, and the exclusion of those on newer non-enzyme-inducing AEDs may well reflect absence of evidence rather than evidence of safety as discussed earlier. Our own practice is not only to ensure that at least a standard (400 IU/day) supplement is discussed with all patients early on in treatment (400 IU/Day) but also to test serum levels early on to guide dosage. For those with levels in the 30–50 nmol/L range, a standard supplement (one or two tablets of 400 IU/Day with calcium) is often sufficient, with those below 30 nmol/L sometimes requiring doses of up to 4000 IU/day for at least a few months before then transferring to a standard supplement [11].

9.3 Treatment of identified cases

For anyone in whom osteoporosis is confirmed, including people with epilepsy, other than ensuring adequate vitamin D, a broad range treatment options are now available. A comprehensive osteoporosis treatment program includes a focus on proper nutrition, exercise, and safety issues to prevent falls that may result in fractures, as well as medication to improve or at least slow deterioration of BMD. Currently recommended treatments of proven efficacy include bisphosphonates, HRT (estrogen in postmenopausal women, testosterone in men), recombinant parathyroid hormone, estrogen receptor modulators, calcitriol and monoclonal antibodies with effects on bone turnover [6, 7]. Low-cost generic bisphosphonates that have a broad spectrum of effects are usually the first line in the absence of contraindications and are typically continued for up to 3 years in the first instance, with regular monitoring [105]. There has only been one trial of osteoporosis treatment (a bisphosphonate) in people with epilepsy on AED, which as in the general population, improved BMD and reduced fracture risk [106]. Ensuring access to more than minimal advice, selecting the correct treatment, and determining the frequency and nature of outcome monitoring is not within the scope of any epilepsy service, so referral and cooperation with local osteoporosis services is recommended. Giving consideration to the possibility of switching AEDs to those that might be less deleterious on bone health in parallel is not unreasonable, but in practice it is often not achievable without other risks, and it should be remembered that it is only a small part of the overall bone health profile for that individual.

10. Conclusions and implementation

It is now 50 years since the first reports linking AED use to bone health concerns. There is now clear evidence of an approximately twofold risk of fracture in people with epilepsy, including in ambulatory patients in the community of all ages. Around two-thirds of the increased risk is likely due to the effects of AEDs on bone metabolism, through a range of biologically plausible direct and indirect mechanisms. LEI-AEDs appear to have a higher risk than non-LEI-AEDs, but valproate is also implicated. Newer non-LEI AEDs, such as lamotrigine and levetiracetam, may be associated with lower risks, but this is not yet certain, and longer-term studies are needed. Low levels of vitamin D and reduced BMD are independent risk factors for fracture, treatable, and more prevalent in people with epilepsy than in the general population. Since at least 2012, UK epilepsy guidelines have recommended "high-level vigilance" [97] or "counseling," including dietary and lifestyle advice [107] to minimize the risk of treatment emergent adverse effects on bone health with respect to bone epilepsy. This should include advice to stop smoking, with access to support to facilitate this, limiting alcohol (<2 units per day), promoting a health body mass index and weight-bearing exercises, together with adequate vitamin D and calcium. We aim to consider at least a standard vitamin D supplement (400 IU/day) in all patients early on, guided by serum levels checked every 2–5 years, and recommend a higher dose in those with levels below 30 nmol/L. Bone health should also be a standard component of any discussion about the risks and benefits of discontinuing treatment in seizure-free patients. For those aged 50 or above continuing on treatment, and in some younger patients with multiple additional risk factors, our own practice is to also undertake, or at least recommend, a risk assessment (FRAX or QFracture). While it could be argued that the onus of responsibility for bone health falls to the family practitioner, as for the general population, AEDs recommended by epilepsy specialists are a contributor. Furthermore patients with epilepsy have been shown to be less well-informed on bone health issues than the general population [108], with highly variable clinical practice in this area [109]. Whether this reflects poor knowledge among those managing epilepsy, the higher prevalence of learning, memory, and psychosocial problems in patients with epilepsy, or that for the general physician or indeed the epileptologist managing a patient with epilepsy, bone health simply falls down the list of priorities is not known, but surely supports that this is at least a shared responsibility. All of above can be efficiently achieved with a "bone health in epilepsy" leaflet, even in a busy clinic, or pointing the patient to one of the epilepsy societies supporting patients, most of which also now include information about bone health on their websites, together with a statement about vitamin D in the clinic letter. That said, from our own experience even in a center with a local "champion," embedding this in practice is difficult but can be facilitated by the use of automated prompts associated with, for example, electronic prescribing [110]. Any who suffer a fragility fracture are identified as high risk on formal assessment, with or without confirmed low BMD and should be referred to specialist services for advice on fall prevention, determination of any additional treatment needs, and monitoring. Managing epilepsy well is increasingly about far more than reducing the risk of seizures [111].

References

[1] Kruse R. Osteopathien bei antiepileptishcer Langzeittherapie. Monatsschr Kinderhelikd 1968;116: 378–81.
[2] Petty SJ, O'Brien TJ, Wark JD. Anti-epileptic medication and bone health. Osteoporos Int 2007;18 (2):129–42.
[3] Ioannidis G, Papaioannou A, Hopman WM, Akhtar-Danesh N, Anastassiades T, Pickard L, et al. Relation between fractures and mortality: results from the Canadian multicentre osteoporosis study. Can Med Assoc J 2009;181(5):265–71.
[4] Hernlund E, Svedbom A, Ivergård M, Compston J, Cooper C, Stenmark J, et al. Osteoporosis in the European Union: medical management, epidemiology and economic burden. Arch Osteoporos 2013;8(1):136.
[5] Svedbom A, Hernlund E, Ivergård M, Compston J, Cooper C, Stenmark J, et al. Osteoporosis in the European Union: a compendium of country-specific reports. Arch Osteoporos 2013;8(1):137.
[6] Compston J, Cooper A, Cooper C, Gittoes N, Gregson C, Harvey N, et al. UK clinical guideline for the prevention and treatment of osteoporosis. Arch Osteoporos 2017;12(1).
[7] NIH. Osteoporosis overview. Bethesda, MD: National Institute of Health; 2015. Report No.: Pub. No. 15–AR–8004.
[7a] World Health Organization. Assessment of fracture risk and its application to screening for postmenopausal osteoporosis: report of a WHO study group [meeting held in Rome from 22 to 25 June 1992]. Geneva: World Health Organization; 1994. http://www.who.int/iris/handle/10665/39142.
[8] Pike JW, Christakos S. Biology and mechanisms of action of the vitamin D hormone. Endocrinol Metab Clin N Am 2017;46(4):815.
[9] Rosen CJ, Adams JS, Bikle DD, Black DM, Demay MB, Manson JE, et al. The nonskeletal effects of vitamin D: an endocrine society scientific statement. Endocr Rev 2012;33(3):456–92.
[10] Francis R, Aspray T, Fraser W, Gittoes N, Javaid K, MacDonald H, et al. Vitamin D and bone health: a practical clinical guideline for patient management. Bath, UK: National Osteoporosis Society; 2013.

[11] Dobson R, Cock HR, Brex P, Giovannoni G. Vitamin D supplementation. Pract Neurol 2018;18(1): 35–42.

[12] NIH. Vitamin D: Fact sheet for health professionals. Bethesda, MD: National Institute for Health; 2018.

[13] Ganji V, Zhang X, Tangpricha V. Serum 25-hydroxyvitamin D concentrations and prevalence esti- mates of hypovitaminosis D in the US population based on assay-adjusted data. J Nutr 2012;142 (3):498–507.

[14] Scientific Advisory Committee on Nutrition. Vitamin D and health. London, UK: Crown Copyright; 2016.

[15] Manson JE, Brannon PM, Rosen CJ, Taylor CL. Vitamin D deficiency—is there really a pandemic? N Engl J Med 2016;375(19):1817–20.

[16] Lidgren L, Wallöe A. Incidence of fracture in epileptics. Acta Orthop Scand 1977;48(4):356–61.

[17] Souverein PC, Webb DJ, Petri H, Weil J, Van Staa TP, Egberts T. Incidence of fractures among epi- lepsy patients: a population-based retrospective cohort study in the general practice research database. Epilepsia 2005;46(2):304–10.

[18] Vestergaard P. Epilepsy, osteoporosis and fracture risk—a meta-analysis. Acta Neurol Scand 2005;112 (5):277–86.

[19] Kwon CS, Liu MF, Quan HD, Wiebe S, McChesney J, Wirrell E, et al. The incidence of injuries in persons with and without epilepsy—a population-based study. Epilepsia 2010;51(11):2247–53.

[20] Persson HBI, Alberts KA, Farahmand BY, Tomson T. Risk of extremity fractures in adult outpatients with epilepsy. Epilepsia 2002;43(7):768–72.

[21] Vestergaard P, Rejnmark L, Mosekilde L. Fracture risk associated with use of antiepileptic drugs. Epilepsia 2004;45(11):1330–7.

[22] Koppel BS, Harden CL, Nikolov BG, Labar DR. An analysis of lifetime fractures in women with epilepsy. Acta Neurol Scand 2005;111(4):225–8.

[23] Wirrell EC. Epilepsy-related injuries. Epilepsia 2006;47(Suppl. 1):79–86.

[24] Ahmad BS, Hill KD, O'Brien TJ, Gorelik A, Habib N, Wark JD. Falls and fractures in patients chron- ically treated with antiepileptic drugs. Neurology 2012;79(2):145–51.

[25] Zaccara G, Cincotta M, Borgheresi A, Balestrieri F. Adverse motor effects induced by antiepileptic drugs. Epileptic Disord 2004;6(3):153–68.

[26] Pomeroy VM, Hiscock A, Cock HR, Tallis RC. Impact of carbamazepine on postural control in older adults: an exploratory study. Physiotherapy 2008;94:230–5.

[27] Zaccara G, Giovannelli F, Maratea D, Fadda V, Verrotti A. Neurological adverse events of new gen- eration sodium blocker antiepileptic drugs. Meta-analysis of randomized, double-blinded studies with eslicarbazepine acetate, lacosamide and oxcarbazepine. Seizure Eur J Epilepsy 2013;22(7):528–36.

[28] Cummings SR, Nevitt MC, Browner WS, Stone K, Fox KM, Ensrud KE, et al. Risk factors for hip fracture in white women. N Engl J Med 1995;332(12):767–73.

[29] Shen CH, Chen F, Zhang YX, Guo Y, Ding MP. Association between use of antiepileptic drugs and fracture risk: a systematic review and meta-analysis. Bone 2014;64:246–53.

[30] Souverein PC, Webb DJ, Weil JG, Van Staa P, Egberts ACG. Use of antiepileptic drugs and risk of fractures—case-control study among patients with epilepsy. Neurology 2006;66(9):1318–24.

[31] Nicholas JM, Ridsdale L, Richardson MP, Grieve AP, Gulliford MC. Fracture risk with use of liver enzyme inducing antiepileptic drugs in people with active epilepsy: cohort study using the general practice research database. Seizure 2013;22(1):37–42.

[32] Nettekoven S, Strohle A, Trunz B, Wolters M, Hoffmann S, Horn R, et al. Effects of antiepileptic drug therapy on vitamin D status and biochemical markers of bone turnover in children with epilepsy. Eur J Pediatr 2008;167(12):1369–77.

[33] Shellhaas RA, Barks AK, Joshi SM. Prevalence and risk factors for vitamin D insufficiency among children with epilepsy. Pediatr Neurol 2010;42(6):422–6.

[34] Teagarden DL, Meador KJ, Loring DW. Low vitamin D levels are common in patients with epilepsy. Epilepsy Res 2014;108(8):1352–6.

[35] Lee YJ, Park KM, Kim YM, Yeon GM, Nam SO. Longitudinal change of vitamin D status in children with epilepsy on antiepileptic drugs: Prevalence and risk factors. Pediatr Neurol 2015;52(2):153–9.

[36] Menon B, Harinarayan CV, Raj MN, Vemuri S, Himabindu G, Afsana TK. Prevalence of low dietary calcium intake in patients with epilepsy: a study from South India. NeurolIndia 2010;58(2):209–12.

[37] Krishnamoorthy G, Nair R, Sundar U, Kini P, Shrivastava M. Early predisposition to osteomalacia in Indian adults on phenytoin or valproate monotherapy and effective prophylaxis by simultaneous supplementation with calcium and 25-hydroxy vitamin D at recommended daily allowance dosage: a prospective study. NeurolIndia 2010;58(2):213–9.

[38] Feldkamp J, Becker A, Witte OW, Scharff D, Scherbaum WA. Long-term anticonvulsant therapy leads to low bone mineral density—evidence for direct drug effects of phenytoin and carbamazepine on human osteoblast-like cells. Exp Clin Endocrinol Diabetes 2000;108(1):37–43.

[39] Andress DL, Ozuna J, Tirschwell D, Grande L, Johnson M, Jacobson AF, et al. Antiepileptic drug-induced bone loss in young male patients who have seizures. Arch Neurol 2002;59(5):781–6.

[40] Kumandas S, Koklu E, Gumus H, Koklu S, Kurtoglu S, Karakukcu M, et al. Effect of carbamezapine and valproic acid on bone mineral density, IGF-I and IGFBP-3. J Pediatr Endocrinol Metab 2006;19(4):529–34.

[41] Valimaki MJ, Tiihonen M, Laitinen K, Tahtela R, Karkkainen M, Lambergallardt C, et al. Bone mineral density measured by dual-energy X-ray absorptiometry and novel markers of bone-formation and resorption in patients on antiepileptic drugs. J Bone Miner Res 1994;9(5):631–7.

[42] Sato Y, Kondo I, Ishida S, Motooka H, Takayama K, Tomita Y, et al. Decreased bone mass and increased bone turnover with valproate therapy in adults with epilepsy. Neurology 2001;57(3):445–9.

[43] Fitzpatrick LA. Pathophysiology of bone loss in patients receiving anticonvulsant therapy. Epilepsy Behav 2004;5:S3–S15.

[44] Pack AM, Morrell MJ, Marcus R, Holloway L, Flaster E, Done S, et al. Bone mass and turnover in women with epilepsy on antiepileptic drug monotherapy. Ann Neurol 2005;57(2):252–7.

[45] Mintzer S, Boppana P, Toguri J, DeSantis A. Vitamin D levels and bone turnover in epilepsy patients taking carbamazepine or oxcarbazepine. Epilepsia 2006;47(3):510–5.

[46] Hamed SA. The effect of epilepsy and antiepileptic drugs on sexual, reproductive and gonadal health of adults with epilepsy. Exp Rev Clin Pharmacol 2016;9(6):807–19.

[47] Ali II, Schuh L, Barkley GL, Gates JR. Antiepileptic drugs and reduced bone mineral density. Epilepsy Behav 2004;5(3):296–300.

[48] Verrotti A, Greco R, et al. Increased bone turnover in prepubertal, pubertal, and postpubertal patients receiving carbamazepine. Epilepsia 2002;43(12):1488–92.

[49] Boluk A, Guzelipek M, et al. The effect of valproate on bone mineral density in adult epileptic patients. Pharmacol Res 2004;50(1):93–7.

[50] Nicolaidou P, Georgouli H, et al. Effects of anticonvulsant therapy on vitamin D status in children: prospective monitoring study. J Child Neurol 2006;21(3):205–9.

[51] Tekgul H, Serdaroglu G, et al. Bone mineral status in pediatric outpatients on antiepileptic drug monotherapy. J Child Neurol 2006;21(5):411–4.

[52] Kim SH, Lee JW, Choi KG, Chung HW, Lee HW. A 6-month longitudinal study of bone mineral density with antiepileptic drug monotherapy. Epilepsy Behav 2007;10(2):291–5.

[53] Koo DL, Joo EY, Kim D, Hong SB. Effects of levetiracetam as a monotherapy on bone mineral density and biochemical markers of bone metabolism in patients with epilepsy. Epilepsy Res 2013;104(1–2):134–9.

[54] Koo DL, Hwang KJ, Han SW, Kim JY, Joo EY, Shin WC, et al. Effect of oxcarbazepine on bone mineral density and biochemical markers of bone metabolism in patients with epilepsy. Epilepsy Res 2014;108(3):442–7.

[55] Ahmad BS, O'Brien TJ, et al. Bone mineral changes in epilepsy patients during initial years of antiepileptic drug therapy. J Clin Densit 2016;19(4):450–6.

[56] Petty SJ, Milligan CJ, Todaro M, Richards KL, Kularathna PK, Pagel CN, et al. The antiepileptic medications carbamazepine and phenytoin inhibit native sodium currents in murine osteoblasts. Epilepsia 2016;57(9):1398–405.

[57] Humphrey EL, Morris GE, Fuller HR. Valproate reduces collagen and osteonectin in cultured bone cells. Epilepsy Res 2013;106(3):446–50.

[58] Wilson EL, Garton M, Fuller HR. Anti-epileptic drugs and bone loss: phenytoin reduces pro-collagen I and alters the electrophoretic mobility of osteonectin in cultured bone cells. Epilepsy Res 2016;122:97–101.

[59] Drezner MK. Treatment of anticonvulsant drug-induced bone disease. Epilepsy Behav 2004;5(Suppl 2): S41–7.

[60] Dent CE, Richens A, Rowe DJF, Stamp TCB. Osteomalacia with long-term anticonvulsant therapy in epilepsy. Br Med J 1970;4(5727):69–72.

[61] Hahn TJ, Birge SJ, Scharp CR, Avioli AV. Phenobarbital-induced alterations in vitamin D metabolism. J Clin Investig 1972;51:741–8.

[62] Stephen LJ, McLellan AR, Harrison JH, Shapiro D, Dominiczak MH, Sills GJ, et al. Bone density and antiepileptic drugs: a case-controlled study. Seizure Eur J Epilepsy 1999;8(6):339–42.

[63] Farhat G, Yamout B, Mikati MA, Demirjian S, Sawaya R, Fuleihan GEH. Effect of antiepileptic drugs on bone density in ambulatory patients. Neurology 2002;58(9):1348–53.

[64] Pack AM, Olarte LS, Morrell MJ, Flaster E, Resor SR, Shane E. Bone mineral density in an outpatient population receiving enzyme-inducing antiepileptic drugs. Epilepsy Behav 2003;4(2):169–74.

[65] Pack AM, Morrell MJ, Randall A, McMahon DJ, Shane E. Bone health in young women with epilepsy after one year of antiepileptic drug monotherapy. Neurology 2008;70(18):1586–93.

[66] Sheth RD, Wesolowski CA, Jacob JC, Penney S, Hobbs GR, Riggs JE, et al. Effect of carbamazepine and valproate on bone-mineral density. J Pediatr 1995;127(2):256–62.

[67] Akin R, Okutan V, Sarici U, Altunbas A, Gokcay E. Evaluation of bone mineral density in children receiving antiepileptic drugs. Pediatr Neurol 1998;19(2):129–31.

[68] Kafali G, Erselcan T, Tanzer F. Effect of antiepileptic drugs on bone mineral density in children between ages 6 and 12 years. Clin Pediatr 1999;38(2):93–8.

[69] Altay EE, Serdaroglu A, Tumer L, Gucuyener K, Hasanoglu A. Evaluation of bone mineral metabolism in children receiving carbamazepine and valproic acid. J Pediatr Endocrinol Metab 2000;13 (7):933–9.

[70] Ecevit CG, Aydogan A, Kavakli T, Altinoz S. Effect of carbamazepine and valproate on bone mineral density. Pediatr Neurol 2004;31(4):279–82.

[71] Sheth RD, Hermann BP. Bone mineral density with lamotrigine monotherapy for epilepsy. Pediatr Neurol 2007;37(4):250–4.

[72] Dimic MD, Dimic NA. Bone mineral density in epileptic adolescents treated with antiepileptic monotherapy. Eur J Neurol 2014;21:500.

[73] Babayigit A, Dirik E, Bober E, Cakmakci H. Adverse effects of antiepileptic drugs on bone mineral density. Pediatr Neurol 2006;35(3):177–81.

[74] Sheth RD, Binkley N, Hermann BP. Progressive bone deficit in epilepsy. Neurology 2008;70(3): 170–6.

[75] Sheth RD, Binkley N, Hermann BP. Gender differences in bone mineral density in epilepsy. Epilepsia 2008;49(1):125–31.

[76] Tsukahara H, Kimura K, Todoroki Y, Ohshima Y, Hiraoka M, Shigematsu Y, et al. Bone mineral status in ambulatory pediatric patients on long-term anti-epileptic drug therapy. Pediatr Int 2002;44 (3):247–53.

[77] Beerhorst K, Schouwenaars FM, Tan IY, Aldenkamp AP. Epilepsy: fractures and the role of cumulative antiepileptic drug load. Acta Neurol Scand 2012;125(1):54–9.

[78] Desai TK, Carlson RW, Geheb MA. Prevalence and clinical implications of hypocalcaemia in acutely ill patients in a medical intensive care setting R. Am J Med 1988;84(2):209–14.

[79] Thomas MK, Lloyd-Jones DM, Thadhani RI, Shaw AC, Deraska DJ, Kitch BT, et al. Hypovitaminosis D in medical inpatients. N Engl J Med 1998;338(12):777–83.

[80] Carbone L, Chin AS, Lee TA, Burns SP, Svircev JN, Hoenig H, et al. The association of anticonvulsant use with fractures in spinal cord injury. Am J Phys Med Rehabil 2013;92(12):1037–46.

[81] Ensrud KE, Walczak TS, Blackwell T, Ensrud ER, Bowman PJ, Stone KL. Antiepileptic drug use increases rates of bone loss in older women—a prospective study. Neurology 2004;62(11): 2051–7.

[82] Ensrud KE, Walczak TS, Blackwell TL, Ensrud ER, Barrett-Connor E, Orwoll ES. Antiepileptic drug use and rates of hip bone loss in older men—a prospective study. Neurology 2008;71 (10):723–30.

[83] Warden SJ, Fuchs RK. Do selective serotonin reuptake inhibitors (SSRIs) cause fractures? Curr Osteoporos Rep 2016;14(5):211–8.

[84] Ahmad BS, Petty SJ, Gorelik A, O'Brien TJ, Hill KD, Christie JJ, et al. Bone loss with antiepileptic drug therapy: a twin and sibling study. Osteoporos Int 2017;28(9):2591–600.

[85] Kanda J, Izumo N, Kobayashi Y, Onodera K, Shimakura T, Yamamoto N, et al. Effects of the antiepileptic drugs topiramate and lamotrigine on bone metabolism in rats. Biomed Res Tokyo 2017;38 (5):297–305.

[86] Pack AM. Treatment of epilepsy to optimize bone health. Curr Treat Options Neurol 2011;13 (4):346–54.

[87] Beniczky SA, Viken J, Jensen LT, Andersen NB. Bone mineral density in adult patients treated with various antiepileptic drugs. Seizure Eur J Epilepsy 2012;21(6):471–2.

[88] Hakami T, O'Brien TJ, Petty SJ, Sakellarides M, Christie J, Kantor S, et al. Monotherapy with Levetiracetam versus older AEDs: a randomized comparative trial of effects on bone health. Calcif Tissue Int 2016;98(6):556–65.

[89] Phabphal K, Geater A, Limapichat K, Sathirapanya P, Setthawatcharawanich S, Leelawattana R. Effect of switching hepatic enzyme-inducer antiepileptic drug to levetiracetam on bone mineral density, 25 hydroxyvitamin D, and parathyroid hormone in young adult patients with epilepsy. Epilepsia 2013;54(6):e94–8.

[90] Anwar MJ, Radhakrishna KV, Vohora D. Phenytoin and sodium valproate but not levetiracetam induce bone alterations in female mice. Can J Physiol Pharmacol 2014;92(6):507–11.

[91] Karesova I, Simko J, Fekete S, Zimcikova E, Malakova J, Zivna H, et al. The effect of levetiracetam on rat bone mineral density, bone structure and biochemical markers of bone metabolism. Eur J Pharmacol 2018;824:115–9.

[92] Cetinkaya Y, Kurtulmus YS, Tutkavul K, Tireli H. The effect of oxcarbazepine on bone metabolism. Acta Neurol Scand 2009;120(3):170–5.

[93] NICE. Osteoporosis: Assessing the risk of fragility fracture. London, UK, 2012.

[94] Hippisley-Cox J, Coupland C. Derivation and validation of updated QFracture algorithm to predict risk of osteoporotic fracture in primary care in the United Kingdom: prospective open cohort study. Br Med J 2012;344(e3427):1–16.

[95] Cosman F, de Beur SJ, LeBoff MS, Lewiecki EM, Tanner B, Randall S, et al. Clinician's guide to prevention and treatment of osteoporosis. Osteoporos Int 2014;25(10):2359–81.

[96] Royal College of Physicians Consensus Group. Glucocorticoid-induced osteoporosis: A concise guide to prevention and treatment. London: Royal College of Physicians; 2003.

[97] NICE. The epilepsies: The diagnosis and management of the epilepsies in adults and children in primary and secondary care: Pharmacological update. London updated (Last update February 2016). Available from: https://www.nice.org.uk/guidance/cg137; 2012.

[98] Compston JE. Vitamin D deficiency: time for action. Br Med J 1998;317(7171):1466–7.

[99] Trivedi DP, Doll RD, Khaw KT. Effect of four monthly oral vitamin D3 (cholecalciferol) supplementation on fractures and mortality in men and women living in the community: randomised double blind controlled trial. BMJ 2003;326:469–72.

[100] NICE. Vitamin D: Supplement use in specific population groups. London, UK: National Institute for Health and Care Excellence; 2014. Guideline PH; (Updated 2017).

[101] NICE. Costing statement: Vitamin D increasing supplement use among at-risk groups (PH56). London, UK: National Institute of Health and Care Excellence; 2014.

[102] Collins N, Maher J, Cole M, Baker M, Callaghan N. A prospective study to evaluate the dose of vitamin-D required to correct low 25-hydroxyvitamin D levels, calcium and alkaline phosphatase in patients at risk of developing antiepiletpic drug induced osteomalacia. Q J Med 1991;78 (286):113–22.

[103] Mikati MA, Dib L, Yamout B, Sawaya R, Rahi AC, Fuleihan GEH. Two randomized vitamin D trials in ambulatory patients on anticonvulsants—impact on bone. Neurology 2006;67(11):2005–14.

[104] MHRA. Antiepileptics: adverse effects on bone. Drug Safety Update 2009;2(9):2.

[105] NICE. Bisphosphonates for treating osteoporosis. London, UK: National Institute for Health and Care Excellence; 2017. Report No.: TA 464.

[106] Lazzari AA, Dussault PM, Thakore-James M, Gagnon D, Baker E, Davis SA, et al. Prevention of bone loss and vertebral fractures in patients with chronic epilepsy—antiepileptic drug and osteoporosis prevention trial. Epilepsia 2013;54(11):1997–2004.

[107] SIGN. Diagnosis and management of epilepsy in adults. A natonal clinical guideline. Edinburgh, UK: Scottish Intercollegiate Guidelines Network; 2015. Report No.: 70.

[108] Elliott JO, Jacobson MP. Bone loss in epilepsy: Barriers to prevention, diagnosis, and treatment. Epilepsy Behav 2006;8(1):169–75.

[109] Wasade VS, Spanaki M, Iyengar R, Barkley GL, Schultz L. AAN epilepsy quality measures in clinical practice: a survey of neurologists. Epilepsy Behav 2012;24(4):468–73.

[110] Minshall I, Mahon M, Neligan A. Bone protection and anti-epileptic drugs: the effect of audit and computer messaging on supplementation prescribing practices. Seizure Eur J Epilepsy 2013;22(9): 757–9.

[111] Mula M, Cock HR. More than seizures: Improving the lives of people with refractory epilepsy. Eur J Neurol 2014;22(1):24–30.

CHAPTER 4

Epilepsy and sexual dysfunction

Mahinda Yogarajah

Atkinson Morley Regional Neuroscience Centre, St George's University Hospitals NHS Foundation Trust, London, United Kingdom
Institute of Medical and Biomedical Education, St George's University of London, London, United Kingdom

Contents

The Comorbidities of Epilepsy
https://doi.org/10.1016/B978-0-12-814877-8.00004-0

1. Introduction

Epilepsy is one of the most common, serious, chronic neurological conditions in the world, and it is increasingly evident that a number of different factors affect quality of life and well-being in men and women with epilepsy beyond seizure control [1]. Among these factors, there is increasing awareness of the impact of epilepsy and antiepileptic drug (AED) treatment on sexual function in both men and women [1] and that sexual well-being is critical for a good quality of life in patients with epilepsy [2]. The cause of sexual dysfunction in patients with epilepsy is multifactorial and involves several factors, including the epilepsy itself, the AEDs used to treat it, and psychosocial factors.

In exploring sexual dysfunction in epilepsy in this chapter, the first step is to define both normal and abnormal sexual function (sexual dysfunction). Given the central role played by sex hormones in sexual dysfunction, a familiarity of the basic metabolism and regulation of sex hormones is also needed. This chapter will then discuss the prevalence and types of sexual dysfunction that occur in patients with epilepsy before discussing the mechanisms that give rise to this problem. The chapter will conclude by discussing individual AEDs and strategies for the management of sexual dysfunction in patients with epilepsy. For information about how epilepsy and AEDs may affect fertility and reproductive endocrine functions, the reader is referred to Chapter 5

2. Definition and classification of sexual dysfunction

Sexual dysfunction can be defined as a chronic inability to respond sexually in a way that is satisfying [3]. Any discussion of sexual dysfunction demands oversight of the normal physiology of sexual function, and an understanding of the classification of sexual dysfunction.

The sequence of events that characterizes the progression from the sexually unaroused to the aroused state, and the resolution of these changes, has been described as the human sexual response cycle. At a basic level, it can be divided into several phases: desire, excitement, orgasm, and resolution [4]. Sexual desire can be defined as a object-focused, willingness to engage in sexual behavior and can come about spontaneously (proceptive desire) or by activation through sexual excitation (responsive desire) in response to appropriate sexual stimuli [4]. Androgens are thought to be essential to support sexual desire in both men and women [5–8]. Sexual excitement (the subjective awareness of arousal) and sexual or genital arousal (its physiological counterpart) can be defined as the capacity to respond to appropriate sexual stimuli. These stimuli can be "psychogenic," arising in the brain and triggered by input from the special senses or by conscious sexual fantasies, or "reflexogenic," arising from stimulation of genital and/or erotogenic sites (e.g., breasts, nipples, inner thighs, perineum) [4]. It is mediated by androgens and estrogens in men and women, respectively [5–8], although testosterone is also important in women and there is laboratory evidence that it increases vaginal blood flow [9]. It should be noted that sexual desire can occur without sexual arousal, and the opposite is also true. Genital arousal consists of penile erection in men and clitoral tumescence, genital vasocongestion, and increased vaginal lubrication in women. In men erection is, therefore, normally an index of subjective arousal or sexual desire, although immediately after ejaculation, arousal may persist for a short period without sexual desire. In women, genital arousal is not always commensurate with subjective arousal, and genital arousal can result from physical stimulation without corresponding subjective arousal [4]. The increase in heart rate and blood pressure that occur during sexual arousal ensure there is increased blood flow to the genitals. Orgasm represents the brief, ecstatic pleasure of the sexual climax, and in males is typically related to ejaculation. In women it may be accompanied by pelvic musculature contractions and uterine/vaginal contractions, which facilitate sperm transport. The resolution phase occurs after orgasm, during which muscles relax and physiological changes revert to normal. The changes described above represent the sexual response, whose biological purpose in men is to allow the introduction of sperm into the vagina, while in women the changes enable painless penile penetration and thrusting and encourage sperm survival and transport [4].

Problems at any stage of the cycle previously described can lead to sexual dysfunction. A robust classification system of sexual dysfunction in patients with epilepsy is critical, therefore, not only for the diagnosis and management but also for research in these patients. However, many published studies in patients with epilepsy do not use any well-recognized classification systems. Given the multifactorial and often unknown basis of sexual dysfunction, a descriptive rather than an etiologically based organization has been commonly used in defining sexual dysfunction. The most commonly used classification systems are the International Classification of Diseases, 10th edition (ICD-10) [3] and the Diagnostic and Statistical Manual of Mental Disorders, 5th edition (DSM-V) [10] (Table 1). One of the major problems associated with these classification systems is the assumption of mind versus body dualism, whereby the disorder is either psychiatric or medical in etiology, when in fact sexual dysfunction can often arise due to peripheral and central mechanisms [11]. DSM-V [10] separates out sexual dysfunction according to sex for the first time and is no longer based on the sexual response cycle as proposed by Masters and Johnson [4].

3. Neuroanatomy of sexual function

Sexual functioning involves an integrated series of physiological processes with complicated peripheral and central control systems. While understanding of the physiology of the peripheral mechanisms is well understood, central mechanisms remains poorly understood. The advent of noninvasive functional imaging with positron emission tomography and magnetic resonance has started to highlight those regions of the brain

Table 1 Major classification systems of sexual dysfunction

ICD-10 definitions of sexual dysfunction not caused by an organic disorder or disease[a]

Lack or loss of sexual desire	Loss of sexual desire is the principal problem and not secondary to other sexual problems such as erectile failure or dyspareunia. Lack of sexual desire does not preclude sexual enjoyment or arousal but makes initiation of sexual activity less likely
Sexual aversion	Strong negative feelings associated with the prospect of sexual interaction resulting in avoidance of sexual activity
Lack of sexual enjoyment	Sexual responses and orgasm occur normally, but there is lack of appropriate pleasure
Failure of sexual response	In men the principal problem is difficulty in getting and/or maintaining an erection (erectile dysfunction). Provided there is no organic etiology to erectile dysfunction (e.g., diabetes or hypertension), erections may occur normally in certain situations, such as masturbation or sleeping with a different partner In women the primary problem is vaginal dryness or failure of lubrication
Orgasmic dysfunction	Orgasm does not occur or is markedly delayed
Premature ejaculation	The inability to control ejaculation sufficiently for both partners to enjoy sexual interaction. In severe cases, ejaculation might occur before vaginal entry or in the absence of an erection
Nonorganic vaginismus	Spasm of the muscles that surround the vagina, causing occlusion of the vaginal opening and resulting in painful or impossible penile entry. Can often be due to local cause of pain in which case that should be coded
Dyspareunia	Pain in women (or men) during sexual intercourse. Can often be due to local pathology in which case that condition should be coded. Category should only be used when there is no other primary sexual dysfunction (e.g., vaginal dryness)
Excessive sexual drive	When excessive sexual drive is secondary to another disorder, such as dementia or an affective disorder, the underlying disorder should be coded

---

DSM-5 definitions of sexual dysfunction[b]

Female sexual interest–arousal disorder	Lack of, or significantly reduced sexual interest or arousal is manifested by at least three of the following characteristics: - absent or decreased interest in sexual activity - absent or decreased sexual or erotic thoughts or fantasies - no or decreased initiation of sexual activity - absent or decreased sexual excitement or pleasure during sexual activity in at least 75% of sexual encounters

Table 1 Major classification systems of sexual dysfunction—cont'd

	- absent or decreased sexual interest or arousal in response to any internal or external sexual or erotic cues - absent or decreased genital or non-genital sensations during sexual activity in at least 75% of sexual encounters
Female orgasmic disorder	Marked delay/infrequent/absent orgasms during at least 75% of sexual activity or decreased intensity of orgasmic sensations during at least 75% of sexual activity
Female genito-pelvic pain-penetration disorder	Persistent or recurrent difficulties with at least one of the following: - vaginal penetration during intercourse - vulvovaginal or pelvic pain during vaginal intercourse or penetration attempts - marked fear or anxiety about vulvovaginal or pelvic pain in anticipation, during, or as a result of vaginal penetration - marked tensing or tightening of pelvic floor muscles during attempted vaginal penetration
Male hypoactive sexual desire disorder	Persistent or recurrent deficient (or absent) sexual or erotic thoughts or fantasies and desire for sexual activity
Male erectile disorder	Experience during at least 75% of sexual activity of at least one of the following: - difficulty in obtaining an erection - difficulty in maintaining an erection until completion of sexual activity - marked decrease in erectile rigidity
Male premature (early) ejaculation	Persistent or recurrent pattern of ejaculation within approximately 1 min of vaginal penetration and before an individual wishes it
Male delayed ejaculation	Either marked delay in ejaculation or infrequent/absent ejaculation during at least 75% of sexual activity.

[a]ICD-10 organic sexual dysfunction codes include erectile dysfunction, vaginismus, and dyspareunia of organic etiology.
[b]DSM-V specifies that problems should have persisted for at least 6 months, have occurred on approximately 75% or more of sexual occasions, and cause clinically significant distress in order to be classified as sexual dysfunction. Symptoms should not be the consequence of a nonsexual mental disorder, severe relationship distress, or attributable to the effect of a medication or illness.
Adapted from McCabe MP, Sharlip ID, Atalla E, Balon R, Fisher AD, Laumann E, et al. Definitions of sexual dysfunctions in women and men: a consensus statement from the fourth international consultation on sexual medicine 2015. J Sex Med 2016;13(2):135–43.

that are thought to be important for sexual function. They include, among others, the limbic and paralimbic regions, which are thought to be important for sexual motivation, and parietal areas that modulate emotional and motor responses [12]. The autonomic nervous system connects the brain and spinal cord to the genitalia and mediates genital engorgement, erections, ejaculation, and climax. Several components of the autonomic system are particularly important. The superior hypogastric plexus is a network of fibers anterior to the lower abdominal aorta and is connected with the pelvic (inferior hypogastric) plexus by the hypogastric nerves. The pelvic plexus itself has connections with sacral roots S2 to S4 through the pelvic splanchnic nerves, while the lumbosacral motor neurons also receive central projections from the ventral tegmental region of the brainstem, which is thought to be important in sexual function [12]. If these regions of the nervous system, which are important for sexual function, are damaged or malfunctioning, sexual dysfunction may arise.

4. Sex hormone synthesis and metabolism

The release of the sex steroid hormones is controlled by the hypothalamic-pituitary-gonadal axis. The major sex steroid hormones are testosterone from the testis, and estrogen and progesterone from the ovaries. The adrenal gland also makes a significant contribution to androgen production. Peripheral conversion to other biologically active steroid forms occurs in the skin and adipose tissue.

The control center of the reproductive system is the nuclei of the medial basal hypothalamus. Regions of the hypothalamus that are involved in the regulation, production, and secretion of gonadotropin-releasing hormone (GnRH) receive direct connections from the cerebral hemispheres including the temporolimbic structures, such as the amygdala [13, 14]. Functionally distinct regions of the amygdala exert opposite modulatory effects on pituitary hormone secretion [15]. As a result of these connections, epileptiform discharges from the temporal lobe may travel via amygdala–hippocampal pathways and disrupt the normal pulsatile secretion of gonadotropic hormones and basal levels of dopamine secretion, resulting in hyperprolactinemia and subsequent hypogonadism [16]. At the pituitary gland GnRH stimulates the release of luteinizing hormone (LH) and follicle-stimulating hormone (FSH) into the blood. LH binds to its target cells, which are the Leydig cells in the testes of the males and theca cells in ovaries of females.

In men testosterone and other androgens, such as dehydroepiandrosterone (DHEA), dehydroepiandrosterone sulfate (DHEAS), and androstenedione, are produced in the zona reticulata/fasciculata of the adrenal cortex, and the Leydig cells adjacent to the seminiferous tubules of the testes. Testosterone itself exists in three different forms in the bloodstream, namely free (2%–3%), albumin bound (53%–55%), and sex hormone-binding globulin (SHBG) bound (43%–45%). While free testosterone and part of the albumin-bound testosterone are available to tissues, the SHBG portion is unavailable to tissues and is not considered biologically active. Testosterone is converted to dihydrotestosterone (DHT) by the action of 5α-reductase in target tissues. Although this steroid is much less abundant than testosterone, it accounts for most of testosterone's biological action. Androgens are also synthesized in females either from circulating precursors in their target tissues, or in the zona reticularis of the adrenal glands and the ovarian stroma.

DHT is also produced in females, but in low quantities and is mainly produced in peripheral target tissues. Testosterone, but not DHT, is converted to estradiol (E2) by the action of aromatase in peripheral tissues and is an important source of estrogens in some women.

In women estrogens are produced in the granulosa and theca cells of the ovaries as well as the corpus luteum. The theca cells are stimulated by LH to produce pregnenolone, which is eventually converted to androstenedione. The androstenedione is converted to estrone (E1) by aromatase in the granulosa cells of the ovary, which is then converted to E2 by 17β-HSD. The expression of aromatase and 17β-HSD is controlled by FSH stimulation. Aromatase is also expressed in non-gonadal tissue and facilitates the peripheral conversion of androgens to E1. Estrogens are, therefore, also made in males in peripheral tissues that express aromatase (e.g., Leydig cells and Sertoli cells in testes), which convert circulating testosterone to E2 and androstenedione to E1. These estrogens act and are metabolized locally, which limits their systemic effects.

5. The epidemiology of sexual dysfunction in men and women with epilepsy

The rates of sexual dysfunction in patients with epilepsy vary from 30% to 66% in men [17] and 14% to 50% in women [17]. This variability is due to several factors. Patients with different types of epilepsy are assessed in different studies and not always compared with control groups. Varying methods of assessment of sexual dysfunction are also used in studies, each with their own problems. Those studies that have used clinical interviews are often nonblinded and opaque in their definitions of sexual dysfunction. Interviews with patients may result in a selection bias for sexually experienced subjects. There is also evidence of gender bias, whereby men may be more likely to overreport, and women to underreport, sexual experiences [18]. However, the use of questionnaires to assess sexual dysfunction also has problems. Although there are a number of questionnaires that have been used in normative populations and applied to epilepsy patients, none have been formally validated in patients with epilepsy. Many studies are also limited by confounding factors, such as concurrent physical or psychiatric disease and the study setting. These tend to be tertiary centers where patients either have refractory epilepsy, or are presurgical candidates. These studies may, therefore, not be representative of the epilepsy population at large. Finally, the cultural background of patients can influence results. For example, a cross-sectional study carried out in Egypt [19] reported no increase in sexual dysfunction, but all types of sexual dysfunction in women with epilepsy in Egypt were less common than in normal control women in the United States, suggesting that cultural factors may play a major role in the willingness to admit to, or even recognize, symptoms of sexual dysfunction.

5.1 Women with epilepsy

Studies suggest that at least 20%–30% of women with epilepsy may suffer from sexual dysfunction [20]. The nature of this sexual dysfunction consists primarily of reduced sexual desire or orgasmic dysfunction. An early study [21] evaluated 50 women with epilepsy in a tertiary epilepsy care center, 32 of whom had focal epilepsy and 28 of whom were taking only one AED. Patients and controls were asked about the frequency of both their desire for sex and sexual intercourse. Though equal numbers of women in both groups had a frequent desire for sex, a greater number of controls had a very frequent desire compared with none in the epilepsy group. In addition, a greater proportion of patients compared to controls had very infrequent sexual desire, and 20% of patients reported that they almost never had sexual desire. These differences were not due to access to a sexual partner, and there was no correlation with age, prescribed anticonvulsants, duration of epilepsy, or seizure type.

In contradiction to this finding, other studies report that the main type of sexual dysfunction in patients with epilepsy is not a reduction in sexual desire but orgasmic dysfunction or other physical symptoms. Morrell et al. [18] conducted a study of 116 women with epilepsy attending a tertiary clinic, using patient self-report questionnaires, which included the Sexual Arousability Inventory—Expanded (SAI-E), Sexual Behavior Inventory (SBI), and Sexual Functioning Inventory (SFI). Compared with historical controls, these women did not have less sexual desire but did report less sexual satisfaction. Specifically, 18% (9%), 28% (7%), 39% (8%), and 42% (14%) of women with focal epilepsy had global anorgasmia, vaginismus, dyspareunia, and arousal insufficiency, respectively (figures in parentheses represent controls). In women with generalized epilepsy, 31% (9%), 13% (7%), 19% (8%), and 33% (14%) had global anorgasmia, vaginismus, dyspareunia, and arousal insufficiency, respectively (figures in parentheses represent controls). Although the women with epilepsy in this study were not less sexually experienced than controls, they reported more sexual anxiety, which may have also exacerbated problems with sexual arousal. In another study of 195 women with epilepsy attending a tertiary clinic who completed the Frenken Sexuality Experience Scale, those with epilepsy reported higher levels of inadequate orgasmic satisfaction compared to healthy controls [22]. They also reported that women with epilepsy desired intercourse as much as healthy controls but were more "moral" and less sexually adventurous. Jensen et al. [23] studied sexuality in 48 women with epilepsy in comparison to patients with diabetes mellitus and healthy controls. Although the authors found no difference in sexual desire between the three groups, 19% of the women with epilepsy had orgasmic dysfunction compared with 11% of the diabetes mellitus group and 8% of the controls. There was no correlation between sexual dysfunction and type and duration of epilepsy or AED use. A more recent, larger study [24] reported both reduced sexual desire and orgasmic dysfunction as well as other physical symptoms in female patients with epilepsy. This study used a study specific questionnaire to assess 171 inpatients and outpatients at a tertiary epilepsy center. The most common form of sexual dysfunction was reduced sexual desire, followed by problems with orgasm, and then vaginal dryness and pain during intercourse. This study also reported that 75% of women compared with 12% of controls had sexual dysfunction, which was associated with a worse quality of life and depression.

Despite the importance of the psychosexual factors previously described in relation to sexual dysfunction, there is also direct support for physiological impairment of sexual function in women with epilepsy, including orgasmic dysfunction. A study measuring genital blood flow in nine women with temporal lobe epilepsy as they watched erotic or neutral videos reported that blood flow was significantly reduced in the patient group compared to healthy controls [25]. There were no mood differences between the two groups, but the patients were less sexually experienced and more anxious when imagining specific sexual activities compared to controls.

5.2 Men with epilepsy

Anywhere between 20% and 70% of men with epilepsy are affected by sexual dysfunction, which can include loss of sexual desire, reduced sexual activity or sexual arousal, anorgasmia, and erectile dysfunction [26–28]. Although the prevalence figures differ between studies [29], erectile dysfunction consistently appears to be more common in patients with epilepsy than in healthy controls and indeed other neurological disorders [30]. In the large study [24] previously described, 63% of men suffered from sexual dysfunction compared with 10% of controls. This manifested as erectile dysfunction, reduced sexual desire, premature ejaculation, and problems with orgasms in order of decreasing incidence. This finding is corroborated by a more recent study, which used the international inventory of erectile function questionnaire in 61 male patients with epilepsy. Thirty-seven percent reported sexual dysfunction, with erectile dysfunction being the most common problem, followed by sexual drive dysfunction, and finally orgasmic dysfunction [31]. Refractory epilepsy syndromes may be associated with higher rates of sexual dysfunction, with up to 80% of male patients reporting hyposexuality and erectile dysfunction in some studies [32, 33]. In contrast community-based studies of patients with less severe epilepsy [34] have reported that 57% of men with epilepsy and attending their general practitioner's surgery have erectile dysfunction compared with 18% of controls, and 39% had ejaculatory failure compared with 0% of controls. However, it should be noted that it is difficult to separate the direct effects of epilepsy and multiple medications in refractory epilepsy patients because of the difficulty of finding untreated epilepsy patients to serve as a control group.

Although erectile dysfunction appears to be common in men with epilepsy, it is also a common problem in the general population and elderly men. It is associated with a number of variables, including age, smoking, physical activity, and educational level in individuals without coexisting medical conditions, in addition to common medical conditions such as diabetes mellitus and hypertension [35]. This might explain why some studies report conflicting results in men with epilepsy suggesting no differences in sexual dysfunction between patients with epilepsy and healthy controls [23, 29]. In an attempt to resolve this problem, a population-based case control approach has been taken by some groups [36]. This study looked at 6427 patients with erectile dysfunction and 32,135 age-matched controls. After adjusting for other conditions, such as hypertension, diabetes mellitus, dyslipidemia, renal disease, ischemic heart disease, obesity, alcohol abuse/dependence, and socioeconomic status, a conditional logistic regression analysis revealed that patients with erectile dysfunction were more likely to have been diagnosed with prior epilepsy than controls. Compared with controls, the adjusted odds ratios for prior generalized epilepsy and focal epilepsy for cases were 2.13 (95% CI = 1.52–3.00) and 1.64 (95% CI = 1.31–2.06), respectively. The most pronounced associations were detected in patients with erectile dysfunction aged between 30 and 39. These men were three times more likely than controls to have been previously diagnosed with epilepsy. Moreover, these figures may be an underestimate because erectile dysfunction remains a taboo subject in Taiwan where the study was based.

As was the case for women, despite the clear importance of psychosexual factors in sexual dysfunction, there is also direct evidence for physiological factors causing the impairment of sexual function in men with epilepsy, including erectile dysfunction. In addition to the nine women previously described [25], reduced genital blood flow compared to controls was reported in eight men with epilepsy as they watched erotic or neutral videos.

6. Etiology of sexual dysfunction in epilepsy

There is a significant body of evidence that demonstrates that sex hormone levels are variable in patients with epilepsy and that patients have higher levels of endocrine reproductive disorders. In exploring the link between these observations and sexual dysfunction in epilepsy, two issues arise. Firstly, it is unclear how much of the alteration in sex hormones is due to AEDs [37] and how much is due to the ictal/interictal discharges or underlying structural abnormalities, both of which can cause reproductive endocrine disorders [15, 28]. On the one hand, studies have demonstrated sexual dysfunction and reproductive endocrine abnormalities in drug naive patients highlighting the fact that epileptiform discharges or underlying structural abnormalities may give rise to sexual dysfunction in patients with epilepsy [16, 38, 39]. Indeed, epileptic discharges can be associated with abnormal testosterone and gonadotropin levels, altered LH response to GnRH stimulation and increased serum prolactin concentrations [40]. On the other hand, studies have also shown no difference in sex hormone levels between patients having seizures and those off AEDs with no seizures [41], suggesting that ictal and interictal discharges in epilepsy may only partly explain sex hormone abnormalities. Other studies highlight the role of AEDs and abnormal hormone levels in patients with epilepsy. For example, one study prospectively measured hormone levels after enzyme-inducing AED withdrawal in seizure-free patients and demonstrated increases in biologically active testosterone levels four months after drug withdrawal compared to baseline [42].

The second issue that arises is that despite the number of studies that independently demonstrate high levels of sexual dysfunction and reproductive endocrine disorders in patients with epilepsy, there is not a consistent correlation between the two observations [43, 44]. Indeed, it is clear that reproductive endocrine disorders do not always lead to sexual dysfunction in people without epilepsy [5–8]. In patients with epilepsy, although some studies show a clear relationship between sex hormone levels and sexuality in patients with epilepsy [43, 45, 46], other studies have failed to show such a concordance [23, 44, 47]. The reason for this discrepancy is likely to be the multifactorial basis of sexual dysfunction in epilepsy, which includes not only changes in sex hormone levels caused by the epilepsy (ictal/interictal discharges +/− structural basis) itself and AEDs but also psychosocial factors, and disturbances in neurotransmission, not all of which are mediated by changes in sex hormones (Fig. 1).

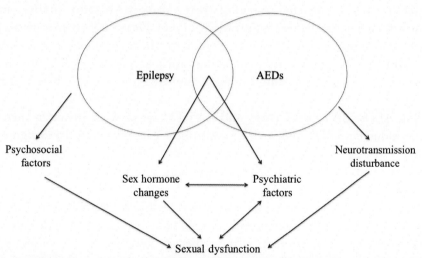

Fig. 1 The multifactorial nature of sexual dysfunction in epilepsy. Both epilepsy (which includes ictal/interictal discharges +/− any structural cause of epilepsy) and AEDs can give rise to sexual dysfunction, which is mediated by changes in sex hormones. However, both epilepsy and AEDs can also cause mood disturbances, which can lead to sexual dysfunction and may also be mediated by changes in sex hormones. Conversely, sexual dysfunction and hypogonadism may lead to mood disturbance. AEDs can also cause sexual dysfunction directly by affecting neural transmission in those pathways that are important for the sexual response. Finally, social factors caused by epilepsy can also lead to sexual dysfunction. *From Yogarajah M, Mula M. Sexual dysfunction in epilepsy and the role of antiepileptic drugs. Curr Pharm Des 2017;23(37):5649–61.*

6.1 Effect of antiepileptic drugs on hormone levels

Evidence for a correlation between sexual dysfunction and hormonal changes in patients with epilepsy comes primarily from the multiple studies that have shown that changes in SHBG are associated with sexual dysfunction [48]. A consistent finding is that patients treated with older AEDs (carbamazepine, phenytoin, and barbiturates) which are inducers of the cytochrome P450 enzyme system, typically have lower levels of free and bioactive testosterone than those treated with noninducing AEDs, such as lamotrigine or levetiracetam [37, 44, 49–51]. While total testosterone levels do not differ between patient groups, SHBG is significantly elevated among patients taking enzyme-inducing AEDs. This leads to lower levels of unbound, biologically active testosterone, which may contribute to sexual dysfunction seen in this patient group [50, 52–55]. Enzyme-inducing drugs may also induce aromatase, which converts testosterone to E2, which inhibits LH secretion and may contribute to a drop in testosterone levels and sexual dysfunction [27]. In a landmark study, Herzog et al. [43] studied 85 men with a focal epilepsy syndrome (25 on carbamazepine, 25 on phenytoin, 25 on lamotrigine, and 10 on no AEDs), and a controls group of men without epilepsy. Sexual function scores were obtained using a self-reported questionnaire (S-score questionnaire), and serum measurements included bioactive testosterone (BAT), bioactive estradiol (BAE), BAT:BAE ratio, SHBG, and LH. Gonadal efficiency was defined as the ratio BAT:LH. Nearly 25% of men with epilepsy had sexual dysfunction, and S-scores were lower in men taking enzyme-inducing AEDs, which in this study were men taking carbamazepine or phenytoin, compared to men with epilepsy taking lamotrigine or compared to controls. There was a correlation between BAT levels and S-scores for men with epilepsy taking enzyme-inducing AEDs. BAT, BAT:BAE, and BAT:LH ratios were lower in men taking enzyme-inducing AEDs compared to controls or patients taking lamotrigine. More recent, prospective studies confirm the role hormonal changes may play in the development of sexual dysfunction in patients taking enzyme-inducing AEDs, such as carbamazepine [31].

Similar findings are apparent in women with epilepsy. Morrell et al. [56] studied 57 women of reproductive age with either localization related epilepsy (LRE) or primary generalized epilepsy (PGE) on AED monotherapy and 17 controls without epilepsy. They completed several questionnaires assessing sexual experience, arousability, anxiety, and symptoms of depression. An endocrine assessment was also performed. Compared to the controls, women with epilepsy had significantly higher sexual dysfunction scores, lower arousal, and higher depressions scores. Mean arousal scores were also lower in the PGE group. Women on enzyme-inducing AEDs (in this study defined as carbamazepine, Phenobarbital, and phenytoin), when combined into one group, had significantly higher sexual dysfunction and lower sexual arousal compared to controls. This was not the case in women taking enzyme-inhibiting AEDs (sodium valproate) or enzyme neutral AEDs (gabapentin, lamotrigine) Furthermore, E2 levels negatively correlated with sexual anxiety, and DHEAS was negatively correlated with sexual dysfunction and positively correlated with sexual arousal.

Other studies involving AEDs that do not induce cytochrome P-450 enzymes appear to support the concept that these AEDs have little effect on sex hormones [43, 44]. In a randomized prospective study of patients taking non-enzyme-inducing AEDs and randomized to either valproate or lamotrigine monotherapy, there were no reported changes in total testosterone or free testosterone after 6 to 12 months of treatment in either treatment group [57].

6.2 Psychiatric disorders

Despite the aforementioned studies, there are other studies that have failed to demonstrate a correlation between hormonal changes in patients with epilepsy and sexual function [28]. Part of the reason for this may be psychiatric comorbidities, which may also contribute to sexual dysfunction in patients with epilepsy [56, 58]. Talbot et al. [44] evaluated sexual function, anxiety, and depression with the Hospital Anxiety and Depression Scale (HADS) in 60 men with epilepsy receiving AED monotherapy and 60 controls. They reported that while patients taking enzyme-inducing AEDs did have lower levels of free testosterone compared to patients taking newer AEDs, most patients had levels of testosterone appropriate for sexual functioning. Moreover, they found no correlation between testosterone levels and sexual function and no difference in sexual function between men taking enzyme-inducing and non-enzyme-inducing medications. Instead, they reported that sexual function correlated with levels of anxiety and depression, suggesting that reductions in sexual desire and self-belief in being able to behave sexually were related to a patient's mood. Other reports have also highlighted that anxiety and depression can impact sexual desire and erectile function in patients with epilepsy [47]. Conversely, other studies have shown that hypogonadism in epilepsy can lead to an affective disorder with loss of energy and competitive drive [15, 59], and that testosterone treatment in epilepsy patients with hypogonadism can lead to significant improvements in mood [59]. A recent systematic review has confirmed for the first time a bidirectional association between depression and sexual dysfunction [60]. Given that it is well documented that a number of AEDs, including barbiturates, vigabatrin, and topiramate, can cause adverse mood-related side effects [61], this is another potential mechanism by which AEDs can cause sexual dysfunction.

6.3 Epileptic factors

Aside from AEDs and psychiatric factors, structural and physiological factors associated with the epilepsy itself may also contribute to sexual dysfunction in patients with epilepsy.

Patients with focal seizures, especially temporal lobe epilepsy (TLE), appear to be more prone to hypogonadism and sexual dysfunction than patients with generalized epilepsy syndromes [13, 14, 21, 52, 62, 63]. This finding is corroborated by both animal [64], and clinical studies that have shown that a significant proportion of patients develop an improvement in sexual function after temporal, but not extra-temporal, lobe surgery for their epilepsy [65] and that a normalization of serum androgens can occur after surgery even in patients with maintained AEDs [66]. This is perhaps not surprising given the anatomical connections between medial temporal lobe structures like the amygdala and the hypothalamus-pituitary-gonadal axis as described earlier. Fixed lesions or epileptiform discharges affecting these areas may, therefore, predispose to sexual dysfunction. Moreover, some studies suggest that there is a lateralization effect such that patients with right-sided lesions and right TLE are more likely to have sexual dysfunction, and this may relate to lateralization in the central regulation of gonadotropin secretion and its disruption by ictal and interictal discharges [67, 68]. These findings suggest that in addition to seizures and AEDs, structural and physiological factors associated with the epilepsy may also have a role to play in the development of hormonal abnormalities that may mediate sexual dysfunction in patients with epilepsy.

6.4 Neurotransmission changes

Calabro highlights another mechanism by which AEDs might cause sexual dysfunction in patients with epilepsy [27, 69]. He proposes that AEDs might inhibit and disrupt the normal neurotransmission of sexual excitement and arousal, which may lead to sexual dysfunction. These mechanisms, which do not rely on changes in sexual hormone levels, may be particularly relevant to newer, non-enzyme-inducing AEDs. They include enhancement of GABAergic inhibition and unbalancing of the cerebral serotonin/dopamine ratio (carbamazepine, phenobarbital, and phenytoin), AMPA receptor blockade via inhibition of the glutamatergic pathway (topiramate), the impairment of serotonergic and nitrergic pathways (zonisamide), or the reduction of central nervous system excitatory transmission by changing the dopamine/serotonin ratio (oxcarbazepine, levetiracetam) [69, 70].

6.5 Psychosocial factors

Psychosocial factors may also have a role to play in the etiology of sexual dysfunction in patients with epilepsy. Stigmatization, psychological distress, low self-esteem, and fear of rejection may lead to social isolation and feelings of inadequacy that contribute to sexual dysfunction. In a survey of quality of life of patients with epilepsy, many subjects reported low levels of satisfaction with sexual relationships, partly because they felt stigmatized by having epilepsy [71].

7. Specific AEDs and sexual dysfunction in epilepsy

Given the multiple potential mechanisms underlying sexual dysfunction in epilepsy, sexual dysfunction can only reliably be ascribed to AEDs in specific circumstances. These include where randomized clinical trials report sexual dysfunction as a side effect, where sexual dysfunction is reported in a comparative, cross-sectional study between patients on different AEDs, between patients taking AEDs and healthy controls, and in case reports or series where sexual dysfunction arises after commencement of an AED and ceases when the AED is discontinued.

7.1 Carbamazepine

As the archetypal enzyme-inducing AED, carbamazepine is probably the most common AED to cause sexual dysfunction in men and women. In the study by Herzog et al. [43] described earlier, sexual function scores were below the control range in 32%, 24%, 20%, and 4% of patients on carbamazepine phenytoin, no AEDs, and lamotrigine, respectively. These findings are consistently corroborated by other studies. In an observational cross-sectional study of 90 men comparing the effects of valproate, carbamazepine, and oxcarbazepine to healthy controls, 7 of the 18 men (18%) taking carbamazepine had diminished sexual dysfunction [50]. These were the highest rates among the patients studied.

The most commonly reported types of sexual dysfunction reported in patients taking carbamazepine are decreased libido, erectile dysfunction, and orgasmic dysfunction. In two multicenter, randomized, controlled trials [72, 73], 7% of 231 and 13% of 101 patients with epilepsy taking carbamazepine developed decreased libido or impotence, respectively, during a one-year follow-up period. In a controlled cross-sectional study of 63 men receiving carbamazepine for temporal lobe epilepsy, all of whom completed the International Index of Erectile Function (IIEF-5) questionnaire, 41/63 (65.1%) patients with epilepsy had erectile dysfunction compared with 4/55 (7.3%) control subjects, all of which were mild cases [74]. Kuba et al. [75] evaluated the incidence of sexual dysfunction and hormonal profile in men with focal epilepsy. They prospectively analyzed sexual function using the IIEF, but without a control group. The authors reported that all patients with orgasmic dysfunction were taking carbamazepine in monotherapy or combination therapy. In patients with at least one type of sexual dysfunction, they also reported a higher percentage of valproate treatment in monotherapy or combination therapy in comparison with carbamazepine. The other AEDs patients were taking in this study included lamotrigine, levetiracetam, topiramate, and valproate. The other types of sexual dysfunction that have been reported in the use of carbamazepine are rarer and limited to case reports, including ejaculatory failure [76] and hypersexuality [77].

7.2 Oxcarbazepine

Oxcarbazepine is a carbamazepine derivative, but is metabolized by different pathways and unlikely to induce liver enzymes unless used at higher doses (>900 mg/day) [78, 79]. Most studies indicate that it has a low incidence of sexual dysfunction associated with its use, and in some cases can improve sexual function. Rattya et al. [50] observed that in 29 patients with epilepsy taking oxcarbazepine monotherapy for an average of 2.4 years, 5 patients had diminished sexual function, while 1 had enhanced sexual function. Although this study did not use a validated sexual function questionnaire, it also showed that while valproate increased serum androgen concentrations in men with epilepsy, the endocrinological effects of carbamazepine and oxcarbazepine were different. Carbamazepine appeared to decrease the bioactivity of androgens, whereas oxcarbazepine did not have this effect, which is consistent with its relative lack of adverse effect on sexual functioning at conventional doses. Other reports of sexual dysfunction caused by oxcarbazepine are limited to case reports and include anorgasmia [80], anejaculation [81], or a combination of both symptoms [82]. In all of these cases, symptoms resolved on discontinuation of oxcarbazepine, and in two of the three cases, effects were seen only at 1800 mg daily of oxcarbazepine.

Several studies have also suggested that oxcarbazepine can improve sexual function, especially if used in patients who have developed carbamazepine-related sexual dysfunction. Luef et al. [83] conducted a prospective study in 228 male epileptic patients who had preexisting sexual dysfunction and were treated with oxcarbazepine. After 12 weeks, 181 (79.4%) patients had improved sexual function and 23 (10.1%) had no sexual dysfunction. In those patients who had been pretreated with carbamazepine, the improvement was most marked. Smaller case series report identical findings, namely resolution of erectile dysfunction when patients are switched from carbamazepine to oxcarbazepine [84].

7.3 Phenytoin

Phenytoin, like carbamazepine, is associated with high rates of sexual dysfunction. In the blinded, randomized controlled trial previously described [72], 11% of 110 patients with focal or secondarily generalized seizures taking phenytoin experienced impotence during a 12-month treatment period. These findings are replicated in smaller cross-sectional studies. Herzog et al. [43] in the previously described study, reported that after carbamazepine, phenytoin was the most likely drug to be associated with sexual dysfunction developing in 24% of male patients taking the drug, compared to 20% of patients with epilepsy and taking no AEDs. As an enzyme-inducing drug, phenytoin is associated with increased SHBG levels and reduced serum levels of free testosterone. However, it is also associated with an increase in E2 levels [62, 85] suggesting that it may also induce the production of aromatase, which then converts free testosterone to E2. Although E2 only makes up 1% of a male's total steroid sex hormone, it exerts powerful negative feedback on male LH secretion and increases the synthesis of SHBG, all of which contribute to a hypogonadotropic hypogonadism state [86]. There are also case reports that phenytoin may rarely cause retrograde ejaculation in male patients with epilepsy [87].

Similar effects on sexual function are apparent in female patients with epilepsy. One study [56] reported that sexual dysfunction and anxiety were significantly higher, and sexual arousal significantly lower, in 27% of female patients taking phenytoin compared to healthy controls.

7.4 Phenobarbital

As an enzyme-inducing AED, phenobarbital, and its structural analogue primidone, have been shown to increase SHBG levels and decrease free testosterone and E2 levels [88]. Cross-sectional studies have demonstrated prevalence rates of up to 22% patients suffering with decreased libido and impotence [72].

7.5 Sodium valproate

Sodium valproate is a first generation AED that inhibits, rather induces, liver enzymes. It is an inhibitor of the UDP-glucuronosyltransferase (UGT) enzyme system, which is involved in the metabolism of androgens and estrogens [89]. However, its effects on sex hormone levels are complex with some studies reporting increased testosterone and E2 levels, and others reporting unchanged testosterone, E2, and bioactive testosterone/bioactive E2 levels [89]. The effect of valproate on SHBG levels is also mixed, with reports of both no change or increases in SHBG levels. In the randomized, controlled trail reported by Mattson et al. [73], 10% of the 240 patients taking sodium valproate developed impotence or reduced libido during a one-year follow-up period. Cross-sectional, observational studies report similar results. One study [90] reported that a group of 25 male patients treated with sodium valproate reported worse erectile function as measured by a simplified version of the IIEF-5, when compared to healthy controls. Interestingly, however, these patients also reported satisfactory sexual intercourse. This unexpected observation may be consistent with the finding by Rattya et al. [50] that in 21 male patients taking sodium valproate, only 1 (5%) reported diminished sexual function while 4 patients (19%) reported enhanced sexual function. In this study sexual function was considered enhanced if the patient reported increased libido, potency, or satisfaction with erection or orgasms and was diminished if the patient reported decreased libido, potency, or satisfaction with erection and orgasm, or no interest in sex. It is therefore possible that some of the patients reporting enhanced sexual function may also have had erectile difficulties, in addition to increases in other sexual domains. Given that androgen levels were increased as a group in these patients, it is possible that some of these effects may have been mediated by these hormonal changes. In women it is well documented that women can develop hyperandrogenic states and polycystic ovarian syndrome with the use of sodium valproate, but the link between these reproductive endocrine abnormalities and sexual function is not clear [8].

7.6 Lamotrigine

Although there are rare case reports of lamotrigine causing sexual dysfunction [91], there is an increasing body of evidence to suggest that lamotrigine may improve sexual function. Whether this is a direct effect of lamotrigine or an indirect effect mediated by the mood enhancing effects of lamotrigine is less clear. Gil-Nagel et al. [92] conducted a prospective, unblinded study in 141 patients treated with lamotrigine over 8 months using the Changes in Sexual Functioning Questionnaire (CSFQ). Of these patients, 79 patients started treatment with lamotrigine monotherapy, while 62 patients were switched to lamotrigine therapy because of lack of efficacy or adverse events to a previous AED. In women who started treatment with lamotrigine, a significant improvement was observed, both in the total CSFQ score and in the five dimensions of the scale (i.e., desire/frequency, desire/interest, pleasure, arousal/excitement, and orgasm). In men, a significant improvement was only observed in the pleasure dimension. In the group of patients in whom a previous AED was substituted by lamotrigine, significant improvement was recorded in the dimensions of pleasure and orgasm in men and in the desire/frequency dimension in women. However, the results of this study should be interpreted with caution. Indirect factors may also be relevant, including improvement in epilepsy control, changes in the quality of life of the patients, and cessation of side effects from other AEDs. However, the results of this study are also supported by two other important results. Herzog et al. [43] reported sexual dysfunction in 20% of untreated patients, but a lower rate of 4% of patients treated with LTG. In another cross-sectional study [51] the sexual function of 40 women and 37 men receiving lamotrigine monotherapy for 6 months was evaluated using the Arizona Sexual Experience Scale Score (ASEX). The ASEX test assesses five areas of sexual dysfunction: drive, arousal, vaginal lubrication/penile erection, ability to reach orgasm, and satisfaction from orgasm. Sexual function across all categories was significantly better in female, but not male, patients taking lamotrigine compared to healthy controls and those patients taking carbamazepine. The findings of these studies and case reports [93] therefore suggest that lamotrigine may have an effect in improving sexual function, particularly in women switching to it from other AEDs.

7.7 Levetiracetam

Levetiracetam is a relatively new, widely used, broad spectrum AED. In the cross-sectional study described earlier, the effects of levetiracetam on sexual and hormonal function in 30 men and 26 women over 6 months were assessed using the ASEX rating scale [51]. There were no hormonal changes associated with levetiracetam in men or women, but like lamotrigine, it was associated with improved sexual function across almost all categories of the ASEX compared with controls in women only. However, there are also reports of levetiracetam being associated with a decrease in sexual function, such as decreased libido [94], all in men. In another study [90], although hormonal levels were no different in 20 male patients taking levetiracetam compared to controls, the patient group as whole scored worse on IIEF-5.

7.8 Topiramate

Topiramate is an AED used for the treatment of both focal and generalized epilepsy syndromes, in addition to migraine prophylaxis. Holtkamp et al. [95] were one of the first to report 2 cases of erectile dysfunction from their case series of 40 patients who had been treated with topiramate for focal epilepsy. The dosage of topiramate reached ranged from 100 mg/day to 200 mg/day, and symptoms resolved on discontinuation of the medication. A recent review of all case reports of sexual dysfunction caused by topiramate indicate rates of between 7.4% and 12.5% of sexual dysfunction, and rates of libido and orgasmic dysfunction of 9% and 2.6%, respectively [96]. This review also reported orgasmic disorder as the most common reported problem in women, and erectile dysfunction in men [96]. The mechanism by which topiramate exerts these effects are likely to be complex and involve modulation of brain neurotransmitters [97].

7.9 Pregabalin

Pregabalin (PGB) is structurally related to gabapentin and is used for pain and anxiety as well as epilepsy. The incidence of sexual dysfunction appears to be low and is typically related to erectile dysfunction or anorgasmia. Hitiris et al. [98] reviewed the incidence of sexual dysfunction related to PGB in placebo-controlled trials across several of its indicated uses. In the placebo-controlled trials of PGB in epilepsy, 363 males received PGB and 156 males received placebo. Impotence was reported by 11 (3.0%) men taking PGB and 3 (1.9%) taking placebo, which amounted to an insignificant difference between groups [98]. The dose of PGB reached ranged from 150 mg/day to 600 mg/day. Across all placebo-controlled trials for all indications, a total of 2428 males received PGB, of whom 71 (2.9%) reported the adverse event of impotence compared to 8/1009 (0.7%) of participants receiving placebo [98]. Sexual dysfunction was not reported by female patients with epilepsy receiving treatment with PGB during the epilepsy trials and only in 3 patients (0.1%) across the entire population treated with PGB. A small number of case reports appear to support this finding of rare complications of anorgasmia and erectile dysfunction, which are reversible on cessation of PGB [99, 100].

7.10 Gabapentin

Gabapentin is widely used in migraines, paresthesia, neuralgia, bipolar disorder, and epilepsy. Sexual dysfunction is an uncommon side effect of gabapentin, and the published data is limited to case reports despite its multiple indications. The most common symptom is anorgasmia, which can be seen at doses from 900 mg/day to 3600/day in all indications, and may be more common in elderly patients [101, 102]. Symptoms are reversible on cessation of the drug.

7.11 Other AEDs

Both zonisamide and lacosamide are relatively new AEDs. To date there is only one case report for each AED reporting sexual dysfunction [70, 103]. In both cases, male patients reported erectile dysfunction, and a decrease in libido in the case of lacosamide. Symptoms resolved on cessation of the offending AED. To our knowledge no sexual dysfunction has been reported in the use of other newer AEDs (Table 2).

Table 2 Summary of antiepileptic drugs and reported effects on sexual function

Drug	Most commonly reported types of sexual dysfunction	How common?
Carbamazepine	Decreased libido Erectile dysfunction Orgasmic dysfunction	***
Phenytoin	Decreased libido Erectile dysfunction	***
Phenobarbital	Decreased libido Erectile dysfunction	***
Primidone	Decreased libido Erectile dysfunction	***
Sodium valproate	Decreased libido Erectile dysfunction	**
Oxcarbazepine	Increased libido	**
	Anorgasmia/anejaculation	*
	Improved sexual function (especially if switching from carbamazepine)	**
Lamotrigine	Increased libido (especially in women switching to it from other antiepileptic drugs)	**
Levetiracetam	Improved sexual function (especially in women)	**
	Decreased libido (men only) and erectile dysfunction	*
Topiramate	Erectile dysfunction Decreased libido Orgasmic dysfunction	*
Pregabalin	Erectile dysfunction Orgasmic dysfunction	*
Gabapentin	Orgasmic dysfunction	*
Zonisamide	Erectile dysfunction	*
Lacosamide	Erectile dysfunction Decreased libido	*

Asterisks indicate frequency of side effects relative to other AEDs. *, rare; **, common; ***, very common. Note that the relative frequency of side effects noted in the table is based on a qualitative assessment of the literature.

8. Management of sexual dysfunction related to AEDS

The use of AEDs in patients with epilepsy is clearly associated with the frequent occurrence of sexual dysfunction in both men and women. However, the relationship between sexual dysfunction, hormones, seizures, and AEDs remains unclear. In addition, the psychosocial complications of epilepsy may also affect sexual health. Given the multifactorial nature of this problem, it is not surprising that there is little research in this challenging area, and there are no guidelines or expert consensus statement on the management of sexual dysfunction induced by AEDs in patients with epilepsy. Regardless of this, some general principles of management can be applied to this problem.

Firstly, when prescribing an AED to a patient with epilepsy, there should be awareness that any preexisting sexual dysfunction, depression, or anxiety may facilitate the development and progression of sexual dysfunction. In any evaluation of a patient with epilepsy presenting with symptoms of sexual dysfunction, management of the patient should be guided by an awareness of the multifactorial nature of the problem. To this end, any history taking from the patient should also include a thorough medication history, sexual/relationship history, and screening for anxiety and depression. Besides AEDs there are numerous other classes of drugs commonly prescribed in this patient population that can cause sexual side effects, including antidepressants, neuroleptics, sedatives, and beta-blockers. Questionnaires for assessing sexual dysfunction may prove a useful adjunct by allowing quantification of the problem, especially in patients who may be embarrassed to discuss their sexual problems in detail. Two widely used scales are the ASEX and the IIEF. However, it is notable that neither of these instruments has been validated in an epilepsy population. Further assessment of the patient should include a general and urogenital as well as standard neurological examination, particularly as erectile dysfunction can be the first manifestation of cardiovascular disease. Blood tests should include a metabolic and endocrinological screen, including serum levels of testosterone, SHBG, DHEAS, E2, LH, FSH, prolactin, and thyroid function.

In those patients in whom sexual dysfunction is thought to be due to the AED, switching to an alternative AED should be considered. As previously discussed, the most commonly reported positive switch is from carbamazepine to oxcarbazepine, although there is also some evidence to suggest that switching to lamotrigine may also be helpful. Phosphodiesterase type 5 inhibitors (PDE5 inhibitors) may also have a role in those patients with erectile dysfunction where a switch in AEDs is not possible or useful [26, 84, 104]. However, caution is also needed because tonic-clonic seizures have been reported in patients taking PDE5 inhibitors [105].

Ultimately, improvements in the management of sexual dysfunction secondary to AEDs in patients with epilepsy are contingent on improving our understanding of this topic. Further research into the incidence and specific nature of sexual dysfunction for individual AEDs, and the dosages at which they occur, would enable better counseling of patients when they commence AEDs. A better understanding of the mechanisms that cause AEDs, especially non-enzyme-inducing AEDs, to give rise to sexual dysfunction would help to improve treatment of these patients.

References

[1] Taubøll E, Luef G. Gender issues in epilepsy—the science of why it is special. Seizure 2008 Mar;17(2): 99–100.

[2] Jacoby A, Snape D, Baker GA. Determinants of quality of life in people with epilepsy. Neurol Clin 2009;27(4):843–63.

[3] World Health Organization. International statistical classification of diseases and related health problems. World Health Organization; 1992.

[4] Levin R, Riley A. The physiology of human sexual function. Psychiatry 2007;6(3):90–4.

[5] Corona G, Isidori AM, Aversa A, Burnett AL, Maggi M. Endocrinologic control of men's sexual desire and arousal/erection. J Sex Med 2016;13(3):317–37.

[6] Davis SR, Worsley R, Miller KK, Parish SJ, Santoro N. Androgens and female sexual function and dysfunction—findings from the fourth international consultation of sexual medicine. J Sex Med 2016;13(2):168–78.

[7] Santoro N, Worsley R, Miller KK, Parish SJ, Davis SR. Role of estrogens and estrogen-like compounds in female sexual function and dysfunction. J Sex Med 2016;13(3):305–16.

[8] Worsley R, Santoro N, Miller KK, Parish SJ, Davis SR. Hormones and female sexual dysfunction: beyond estrogens and androgens—findings from the fourth international consultation on sexual medicine. J Sex Med 2016;13(3):283–90.

[9] Traish AM, Kim SW, Stankovic M, Goldstein I, Kim NN. Testosterone increases blood flow and expression of androgen and estrogen receptors in the rat vagina. J Sex Med 2007;4(3):609–19.

[10] American Psychiatric Association. Diagnostic and statistical manual of mental disorders. 5th ed. Washington, DC.: American Psychiatric Publishing; 2013.

[11] Hatzimouratidis K, Hatzichristou D. Sexual dysfunctions: classifications and definitions. J Sex Med 2007;4(1):241–50.

[12] Rees PM, Fowler CJ, Maas CP. Sexual function in men and women with neurological disorders. Lancet Lond Engl 2007;369(9560):512–25.

[13] Herzog AG. A hypothesis to integrate partial seizures of temporal lobe origin and reproductive endocrine disorders. Epilepsy Res 1989;3(2):151–9.

[14] Herzog AG, Seibel MM, Schomer DL, Vaitukaitis JL, Geschwind N. Reproductive endocrine disorders in women with partial seizures of temporal lobe origin. Arch Neurol 1986;43(4):341–6.

[15] Herzog AG. Disorders of reproduction in patients with epilepsy: primary neurological mechanisms. Seizure 2008;17(2):101–10.

[16] Spark RF, Wills CA, Royal H. Hypogonadism, hyperprolactinaemia, and temporal lobe epilepsy in hyposexual men. Lancet Lond Engl 1984;1(8374):413–7.

[17] Atif M, Sarwar MR, Scahill S. The relationship between epilepsy and sexual dysfunction: a review of the literature. SpringerPlus 2016;5(1):2070.

[18] Morrell MJ, Guldner GT. Self-reported sexual function and sexual arousability in women with epilepsy. Epilepsia 1996;37(12):1204–10.

[19] Demerdash A, Shaalan M, Midani A, Kamel F, Bahri M. Sexual behavior of a sample of females with epilepsy. Epilepsia 1991;32(1):82–5.

[20] Harden CL. Sexual dysfunction in women with epilepsy. Seizure 2008;17(2):131–5.

[21] Bergen D, Daugherty S, Eckenfels E. Reduction of sexual activities in females taking antiepileptic drugs. Psychopathology 1992;25(1):1–4.

[22] Duncan S, Blacklaw J, Beastall GH, Brodie MJ. Sexual function in women with epilepsy. Epilepsia 1997;38(10):1074–81.

[23] Jensen P, Jensen SB, Sørensen PS, Bjerre BD, Rizzi DA, Sørensen AS, et al. Sexual dysfunction in male and female patients with epilepsy: a study of 86 outpatients. Arch Sex Behav 1990;19(1):1–14.

[24] Henning OJ, Nakken KO, Træen B, Mowinckel P, Lossius M. Sexual problems in people with refractory epilepsy. Epilepsy Behav EB 2016;61:174–9.

[25] Morrell MJ, Sperling MR, Stecker M, Dichter MA. Sexual dysfunction in partial epilepsy: a deficit in physiologic sexual arousal. Neurology 1994;44(2):243–7.

[26] Hellmis E. Sexual problems in males with epilepsy—an interdisciplinary challenge! Seizure 2008;17 (2):136–40.

[27] Calabrò RS, Marino S, Bramanti P. Sexual and reproductive dysfunction associated with antiepileptic drug use in men with epilepsy. Expert Rev Neurother 2011 Jun;11(6):887–95.

[28] Sivaraaman K, Mintzer S. Hormonal consequences of epilepsy and its treatment in men. Curr Opin Endocrinol Diabetes Obes 2011;18(3):204–9.

[29] Calabrò RS, Grisolaghi J, Quattrini F, Bramanti P, Magaudda A. Prevalence and clinical features of sexual dysfunction in male with epilepsy: the first southern Italy hospital-based study. Int J Neurosci 2013;123(10):732–7.

[30] Calabrò RS, Gervasi G, Naro A, de Luca R, Marullo M, Bramanti P. Erectile dysfunction in individuals with neurologic disability: a hospital-based cross-sectional study. Innov Clin Neurosci 2016;13 (1–2):10–4.

[31] Pavone C, Giacalone N, Vella M, Urso L, Zummo L, Fierro B. Relation between sexual dysfunctions and epilepsy, type of epilepsy, type of antiepileptic drugs: a prospective study. Urologia 2017;84(2): 88–92.

[32] Nikoobakht M, Motamedi M, Orandi A, Meysamie A, Emamzadeh A. Sexual dysfunction in epileptic men. Urol J 2007;4(2):111–7.

[33] Taylor DC. Sexual behavior and temporal lobe epilepsy. Arch Neurol 1969;21(5):510–6.

[34] Toone BK, Edeh J, Nanjee MN, Wheeler M. Hyposexuality and epilepsy: a community survey of hormonal and behavioural changes in male epileptics. Psychol Med 1989;19(4):937–43.

[35] Nicolosi A, Glasser DB, Moreira ED, Villa M. Erectile dysfunction epidemiology cross National Study Group. Prevalence of erectile dysfunction and associated factors among men without concomitant diseases: a population study. Int J Impot Res 2003;15(4):253–7.

[36] Keller J, Chen Y-K, Lin H-C. Association between epilepsy and erectile dysfunction: evidence from a population-based study. J Sex Med 2012;9(9):2248–55.

[37] Isojärvi J. Disorders of reproduction in patients with epilepsy: antiepileptic drug related mechanisms. Seizure 2008;17(2):111–9.

[38] Gastaut H, Collomb H. Sexual behavior in psychomotor epileptics. Ann Med Psychol (Paris) 1954;112(25):657–96.

[39] Hierons R, Saunders M. Impotence in patients with temporal-lobe lesions. Lancet Lond Engl 1966;2 (7467):761–3.

[40] Montouris G, Morris GL. Reproductive and sexual dysfunction in men with epilepsy. Epilepsy Behav EB 2005;7(Suppl 2):S7–S14.

[41] Bauer J, Blumenthal S, Reuber M, Stoffel-Wagner B. Epilepsy syndrome, focus location, and treatment choice affect testicular function in men with epilepsy. Neurology 2004;62(2):243–6.

[42] Lossius MI, Taubøll E, Mowinckel P, Mørkrid L, Gjerstad L. Reversible effects of antiepileptic drugs on reproductive endocrine function in men and women with epilepsy—a prospective randomized double-blind withdrawal study. Epilepsia 2007;48(10):1875–82.

[43] Herzog AG, Drislane FW, Schomer DL, Pennell PB, Bromfield EB, Dworetzky BA, et al. Differential effects of antiepileptic drugs on sexual function and hormones in men with epilepsy. Neurology 2005;65(7):1016–20.

[44] Talbot JA, Sheldrick R, Caswell H, Duncan S. Sexual function in men with epilepsy: how important is testosterone? Neurology 2008;70(16):1346–52.

[45] Toone BK, Wheeler M, Nanjee M, Fenwick P, Grant R. Sex hormones, sexual activity and plasma anticonvulsant levels in male epileptics. J Neurol Neurosurg Psychiatry 1983;46(9):824–6.

[46] Herzog AG, Klein P, Jacobs AR. Testosterone versus testosterone and testolactone in treating reproductive and sexual dysfunction in men with epilepsy and hypogonadism. Neurology 1998;50(3): 782–4.

[47] Duncan S, Talbot A, Sheldrick R, Caswell H. Erectile function, sexual desire, and psychological well-being in men with epilepsy. Epilepsy Behav EB 2009;15(3):351–7.

The Comorbidities of Epilepsy

[48] Mölleken D, Richter-Appelt H, Stodieck S, Bengner T. Sexual quality of life in epilepsy: correlations with sex hormone blood levels. Epilepsy Behav EB 2009;14(1):226–31.

[49] Herzog AG, Drislane FW, Schomer DL, Pennell PB, Bromfield EB, Kelly KM, et al. Differential effects of antiepileptic drugs on sexual function and reproductive hormones in men with epilepsy: interim analysis of a comparison between lamotrigine and enzyme-inducing antiepileptic drugs. Epilepsia 2004;45(7):764–8.

[50] Rättyä J, Turkka J, Pakarinen AJ, Knip M, Kotila MA, Lukkarinen O, et al. Reproductive effects of valproate, carbamazepine, and oxcarbazepine in men with epilepsy. Neurology 2001;56(1):31–6.

[51] Svalheim S, Taubøll E, Luef G, Lossius A, Rauchenzauner M, Sandvand F, et al. Differential effects of levetiracetam, carbamazepine, and lamotrigine on reproductive endocrine function in adults. Epilepsy Behav EB 2009;16(2):281–7.

[52] Herzog AG, Seibel MM, Schomer DL, Vaitukaitis JL, Geschwind N. Reproductive endocrine disorders in men with partial seizures of temporal lobe origin. Arch Neurol 1986;43(4):347–50.

[53] Isojärvi JI, Repo M, Pakarinen AJ, Lukkarinen O, Myllylä VV. Carbamazepine, phenytoin, sex hormones, and sexual function in men with epilepsy. Epilepsia 1995;36(4):366–70.

[54] Barragry JM, Makin HL, Trafford DJ, Scott DF. Effect of anticonvulsants on plasma testosterone and sex hormone binding globulin levels. J Neurol Neurosurg Psychiatry 1978;41(10):913–4.

[55] Toone BK, Wheeler M, Fenwick PB. Sex hormone changes in male epileptics. Clin Endocrinol (Oxf) 1980;12(4):391–5.

[56] Morrell MJ, Flynn KL, Doñe S, Flaster E, Kalayjian L, Pack AM. Sexual dysfunction, sex steroid hormone abnormalities, and depression in women with epilepsy treated with antiepileptic drugs. Epilepsy Behav EB 2005;6(3):360–5.

[57] Stephen LJ, Sills GJ, Leach JP, Butler E, Parker P, Hitiris N, et al. Sodium valproate versus lamotrigine: a randomised comparison of efficacy, tolerability and effects on circulating androgenic hormones in newly diagnosed epilepsy. Epilepsy Res 2007;75(2–3):122–9.

[58] Gilliam F, Hecimovic H, Sheline Y. Psychiatric comorbidity, health, and function in epilepsy. Epilepsy Behav EB 2003;4(Suppl 4):S26–30.

[59] Herzog AG, Farina EL, Drislane FW, Schomer DL, Smithson SD, Fowler KM, et al. A comparison of anastrozole and testosterone versus placebo and testosterone for treatment of sexual dysfunction in men with epilepsy and hypogonadism. Epilepsy Behav EB 2010;17(2):264–71.

[60] Atlantis E, Sullivan T. Bidirectional association between depression and sexual dysfunction: a systematic review and meta-analysis. J Sex Med 2012;9(6):1497–507.

[61] Mula M, Sander JW. Negative effects of antiepileptic drugs on mood in patients with epilepsy. Drug Saf 2007;30(7):555–67.

[62] Murialdo G, Galimberti CA, Fonzi S, Manni R, Costelli P, Parodi C, et al. Sex hormones and pituitary function in male epileptic patients with altered or normal sexuality. Epilepsia 1995;36(4):360–5.

[63] Fenwick PB, Toone BK, Wheeler MJ, Nanjee MN, Grant R, Brown D. Sexual behaviour in a centre for epilepsy. Acta Neurol Scand 1985;71(6):428–35.

[64] Edwards HE, Burnham WM, MacLusky NJ. Partial and generalized seizures affect reproductive physiology differentially in the male rat. Epilepsia 1999;40(11):1490–8.

[65] Baird AD, Wilson SJ, Bladin PF, Saling MM, Reutens DC. Sexual outcome after epilepsy surgery. Epilepsy Behav EB 2003;4(3):268–78.

[66] Bauer J, Stoffel-Wagner B, Flügel D, Kluge M, Schramm J, Bidlingmaier F, et al. Serum androgens return to normal after temporal lobe epilepsy surgery in men. Neurology 2000;55(6):820–4.

[67] Herzog AG, Drislane FW, Schomer DL, Levesque LA, Ives J, Blume HW, et al. Abnormal pulsatile secretion of luteinizing hormone in men with epilepsy: relationship to laterality and nature of paroxysmal discharges. Neurology 1990;40(10):1557–61.

[68] Daniele A, Azzoni A, Bizzi A, Rossi A, Gainotti G, Mazza S. Sexual behavior and hemispheric laterality of the focus in patients with temporal lobe epilepsy. Biol Psychiatry 1997;42(7):617–24.

[69] Calabrò RS. Sexual disorders related to new antiepileptic drugs: a need for more studies!. Epilepsy Behav 2011;20(4):734–5.

[70] Calabrò RS, Magaudda A, Nibali VC, Bramanti P. Sexual dysfunction induced by lacosamide: an underreported side effect? Epilepsy Behav EB 2015;46:252–3.

[71] Baker GA, Nashef L, van Hout BA. Current issues in the management of epilepsy: the impact of frequent seizures on cost of illness, quality of life, and mortality. Epilepsia 1997;38(Suppl 1):S1–8.

[72] Mattson RH, Cramer JA, Collins JF, Smith DB, Delgado-Escueta AV, Browne TR, et al. Comparison of carbamazepine, phenobarbital, phenytoin, and primidone in partial and secondarily generalized tonic-clonic seizures. N Engl J Med 1985;313(3):145–51.

[73] Mattson RH, Cramer JA, Collins JF. A comparison of valproate with carbamazepine for the treatment of complex partial seizures and secondarily generalized tonic-clonic seizures in adults. The Department of Veterans Affairs Epilepsy Cooperative Study No. 264 Group. N Engl J Med 1992;327(11):765–71.

[74] Reis RM, de Angelo AG, Sakamoto AC, Ferriani RA, Lara LAS. Altered sexual and reproductive functions in epileptic men taking carbamazepine. J Sex Med 2013;10(2):493–9.

[75] Kuba R, Pohanka M, Zákopcan J, Novotná I, Rektor I. Sexual dysfunctions and blood hormonal profile in men with focal epilepsy. Epilepsia 2006;47(12):2135–40.

[76] Leris AC, Stephens J, Hines JE, McNicholas TA. Carbamazepine-related ejaculatory failure. Br J Urol 1997;79(3):485.

[77] Myers WC, Carrera F. Carbamazepine-induced mania with hypersexuality in a 9-year-old boy. Am J Psychiatry 1989;146(3):400.

[78] Larkin JG, McKee PJ, Forrest G, Beastall GH, Park BK, Lowrie JI, et al. Lack of enzyme induction with oxcarbazepine (600 mg daily) in healthy subjects. Br J Clin Pharmacol 1991;31(1):65–71.

[79] Patsalos PN, Zakrzewska JM, Elyas AA. Dose dependent enzyme induction by oxcarbazepine? Eur J Clin Pharmacol 1990;39(2):187–8.

[80] Calabrò RS, Ferlazzo E, Italiano D, Bramanti P. Dose-dependent oxcarbazepine-related anorgasmia. Epilepsy Behav EB 2010;17(2):287–8.

[81] Calabrò RS, Italiano D, Pollicino P, Bramanti P. Oxcarbazepine-related retrograde ejaculation. Epilepsy Behav EB 2012;25(2):174–5.

[82] Boora K, Chiappone K, Dubovsky SL. Oxcarbazepine-induced reversible anorgasmia and ejaculatory failure: a case report. Prim Care Companion J Clin Psychiatry 2009;11(4):173–4.

[83] Luef G, Krämer G, Stefan H. Oxcarbazepine treatment in male epilepsy patients improves pre-existing sexual dysfunction. Acta Neurol Scand 2009;119(2):94–9.

[84] Sachdeo R, Sathyan RR. Amelioration of erectile dysfunction following a switch from carbamazepine to oxcarbazepine: recent clinical experience. Curr Med Res Opin 2005;21(7):1065–8.

[85] Herzog AG, Levesque LA, Drislane FW, Ronthal M, Schomer DL. Phenytoin-induced elevation of serum estradiol and reproductive dysfunction in men with epilepsy. Epilepsia 1991;32(4):550–3.

[86] Smaldone M, Sukkarieh T, Reda A, Khan A. Epilepsy and erectile dysfunction: a review. Seizure 2004;13(7):453–9.

[87] Elia J, Imbrogno N, Delfino M, Mazzilli F. Retrograde ejaculation and abnormal hormonal profile in a subject under treatment with valproate and phenytoin. Arch Ital Urol Androl Organo Uff Soc Ital Ecogr Urol E Nefrol 2010;82(4):193–4.

[88] Luef G, Madersbacher H. Sexual dysfunction in patients with epilepsy. Handb Clin Neurol 2015;130:383–94.

[89] Ocek L, Tarhan H, Uludağ FI, Sarıteke A, Köse C, Colak A, et al. Evaluation of sex hormones and sperm parameters in male epileptic patients. Acta Neurol Scand 2018;137(4):409–16.

[90] Xiaotian X, Hengzhong Z, Yao X, Zhipan Z, Daoliang X, Yumei W. Effects of antiepileptic drugs on reproductive endocrine function, sexual function and sperm parameters in Chinese Han men with epilepsy. J Clin Neurosci Off J Neurosurg Soc Australas 2013;20(11):1492–7.

[91] Kaufman KR, Coluccio M, Sivaraaman K, Campeas M. Lamotrigine-induced sexual dysfunction and non-adherence: case analysis with literature review. BJPsych Open 2017;3(5):249–53.

[92] Gil-Nagel A, López-Muñoz F, Serratosa JM, Moncada I, García-García P, Alamo C. Effect of lamotrigine on sexual function in patients with epilepsy. Seizure 2006;15(3):142–9.

[93] Husain AM, Carwile ST, Miller PP, Radtke RA. Improved sexual function in three men taking lamotrigine for epilepsy. South Med J 2000;93(3):335–6.

[94] Calabrò RS, Italiano D, Militi D, Bramanti P. Levetiracetam-associated loss of libido and anhedonia. Epilepsy Behav EB 2012;24(2):283–4.

[95] Holtkamp M, Weissinger F, Meierkord H. Erectile dysfunction with topiramate. Epilepsia 2005;46 (1):166–7.

[96] Chen LW-H, Chen MY-S, Chen K-Y, Lin H-S, Chien C-C, Yin H-L. Topiramate-associated sexual dysfunction: a systematic review. Epilepsy Behav EB 2017;73:10–7.

[97] Calabrò RS. Sexual dysfunction and topiramate: what does lie beneath the tip of the iceberg? Epilepsy Behav EB 2017;73:281–2.

[98] Hitiris N, Barrett JA, Brodie MJ. Erectile dysfunction associated with pregabalin add-on treatment in patients with partial seizures: five case reports. Epilepsy Behav EB 2006;8(2):418–21.

[99] Calabrò RS, De Luca R, Pollicino P, Bramanti P. Anorgasmia during pregabalin add-on therapy for partial seizures. Epileptic Disord Int Epilepsy J Videotape 2013;15(3):358–61.

[100] Calabrò RS, Bramanti P. Pregabalin-induced severe delayed ejaculation. Epilepsy Behav EB 2010;19 (3):543.

[101] Calabrò RS. Gabapentin and sexual dysfunction: an overlooked and underreported problem? Epilepsy Behav EB 2011;22(4):818.

[102] Perloff MD, Thaler DE, Otis JA. Anorgasmia with gabapentin may be common in older patients. Am J Geriatr Pharmacother 2011;9(3):199–203.

[103] Maschio M, Saveriano F, Dinapoli L, Jandolo B. Reversible erectile dysfunction in a patient with brain tumor-related epilepsy in therapy with zonisamide in add-on. J Sex Med 2011;8(12):3515–7.

[104] Civardi C, Collini A, Gontero P, Monaco F. Vasogenic erectile dysfunction Topiramate-induced. Clin Neurol Neurosurg 2012;114(1):70–1.

[105] Gilad R, Lampl Y, Eshel Y, Sadeh M. Tonic-clonic seizures in patients taking sildenafil. BMJ 2002;325(7369):869.

Further reading

[106] McCabe MP, Sharlip ID, Atalla E, Balon R, Fisher AD, Laumann E, et al. Definitions of sexual dysfunctions in women and men: a consensus statement from the fourth international consultation on sexual medicine 2015. J Sex Med 2016;13(2):135–43.

[107] Yogarajah M, Mula M. Sexual dysfunction in epilepsy and the role of anti-epileptic drugs. Curr Pharm Des 2017;23(37):5649–61.

CHAPTER 5

Epilepsy, diabetes, and other endocrinological disorders

Bastien Rioux, Mark Keezer
Research Centre of the University of Montreal Hospital Centre (CRCHUM), Montreal, QC, Canada
Department of Neurosciences, University of Montreal, Montreal, QC, Canada

Contents

Abbreviations

AED	antiepileptic drug
ATP	adenosine triphosphate
C1	first pattern of catamenial epilepsy
C2	second pattern of catamenial epilepsy
C3	third pattern of catamenial epilepsy
CNS	central nervous system
CSF	cerebrospinal fluid
DEND	developmental delay, epilepsy and neonatal diabetes
DKA	diabetic ketoacidosis

The Comorbidities of Epilepsy
https://doi.org/10.1016/B978-0-12-814877-8.00005-2

DM	diabetes mellitus
EEG	electroencephalogram
FSE	focal status epilepticus
GABA	gamma-aminobutyric acid
GAD	glutamic acid decarboxylase
HHS	hyperosmolar hyperglycemic state
IGE	idiopathic generalized epilepsy
KD	ketogenic diet
LT4	levothyroxine
mg/dL	milligram per deciliter
mM	millimolar
mOsm/L	milliosmole per liter
MRI	magnetic resonance imaging
MTS	mesial temporal sclerosis
PNDM	permanent neonatal diabetes mellitus
PRL	prolactin
SPS	stiff-person syndrome
SUR1	sulfonylurea receptor 1
T1DM	type 1 diabetes mellitus
T2DM	type 2 diabetes mellitus
T3	triiodothyronine
T4	thyroxine
TRH	thyrotropin-releasing hormone
TSH	thyroid-stimulating hormone

Since the first report of a possible link between diabetes mellitus (DM) and epilepsy in a series of two children with diabetes and epilepsy in 1952 [1], multiple cohort studies have supported an association between these two conditions. Over the past decades, further investigations on epilepsy with comorbid DM focused on its descriptive epidemiology, its underlying mechanisms, and its specific therapeutic implications. Several hypotheses that include gene defects, autoimmunity, and brain damage have shed light on the causes of epilepsy associated with DM, resulting in important therapeutic advances. This example illustrates how people with epilepsy can present with comorbid endocrine disorders that may affect the clinical manifestations and management of epilepsy. Therapies used in epilepsy can also disrupt endocrine homeostasis. Health care professionals working with individuals with epilepsy can only improve their practice by knowing how to recognize and handle these issues. In this chapter, selected endocrine disorders and hormone abnormalities will be discussed with an emphasis on descriptive epidemiology, pathophysiology, diagnosis, and management. These conditions include DM, thyroid disease, prolactin abnormalities, and sex steroid hormone fluctuations.

1. Diabetes and epilepsy: General considerations

Diabetes mellitus represents a spectrum of metabolic disorders that are characterized by chronic hyperglycemia resulting from impairment in insulin secretion, function, or both.

Type 2 diabetes mellitus (T2DM) is the most often encountered in clinical practice as it accounts for 90%–95% of all cases and has a global prevalence of 8.3% [2]. Type 1 diabetes mellitus (T1DM) is the cause of 5%–10% of DM and is most often incident in children and adolescents, in whom it accounts for 80%–90% of cases [2].

The pathogenesis of T1DM and T2DM is different and mainly involves insulin depletion and resistance, respectively. While T1DM results from an autoimmune process that attacks the pancreatic beta cells that are responsible for the production of insulin, T2DM is the consequence of an increased insulin demand by insulin-dependent tissues, owing mostly to obesity [2, 3].

Most current research defines epilepsy in people with DM as two or more unprovoked euglycemic seizures with or without supporting electroencephalogram (EEG) abnormalities [4]. This distinction should be kept in mind when referring to epilepsy with comorbid DM and seizures associated with acute glycemic disturbances.

2. Metabolic abnormalities leading to epileptic seizures in diabetes mellitus

Epileptic seizures may occur in acute glycemic abnormalities of both T1DM and T2DM. Hyperglycemia, ketoacidosis, and hypoglycemia have all been linked to seizures and abnormal EEG patterns.

2.1 Hyperglycemia

Hyperglycemia in DM is a frequent complication that presents along a spectrum of metabolic decompensation, with most serious forms consisting of either a hyperosmolar hyperglycemic state (HHS) or diabetic ketoacidosis (DKA). HHS is a syndrome seen most frequently in elderly individuals with T2DM that combines severe hyperglycemia (>33.3 mM), effective serum hyperosmolality (>320 mOsm/L), and dehydration in the absence of ketoacidosis [3, 5]. DKA presents most often in T1DM individuals as a triad of hyperglycemia (>13.9 mM), hyperketonemia, and metabolic acidosis [3]. DKA remains the leading cause of mortality among children and young adults with T1DM, while HHS is fatal in 5%–16% of people, a proportion tenfold higher than that seen in DKA [3, 5].

Epileptic seizures as a manifestation of hyperglycemia were first described in a series of seven individuals with HHS, in 1965 [6]. Epileptic seizures related to hyperglycemia are rare in general clinical practice [7] but may be encountered in up to 25% of people with HHS [8, 9]. Epileptic seizures are less frequently seen in DKA than in HHS. A report of children admitted to a pediatric intensive care unit for DKA found that only 5.4% of children had seizures at the time of presentation [10].

Hyperglycemia typically produces focal seizures rather than generalized seizures, which are more often associated with hypoglycemia. In a review of 80 individuals with HHS and seizures, the vast majority had focal motor seizures (86%), while 11% had generalized seizures, and 3% had focal sensory seizures characterized by visual phenomena [9]. Focal status epilepticus (FSE) is the most frequent initial seizure type in hyperglycemia, even in the absence of severe hyperosmolality or magnetic resonance imaging (MRI) abnormalities [11, 12]. In a report of HHS-induced seizures, FSE was seen in 14 of the 22 (64%) individuals with focal seizures, while 6 (27%) evolved to bilateral tonic-clonic seizures, and 2 (9%) were focal seizures with impaired awareness features [13]. Focal status epilepticus may also be encountered in children with diabetes who present with nonketotic hyperglycemia [14]. Diabetic ketoacidosis can present with FSE, but this remains rare and less frequent than in HHS [15, 16]. Occipital seizures presenting as bright lights, flickering objects or complex visual hallucinations with or without secondary visual field deficits may occur in HHS, but such descriptions are scant [12, 17].

Investigators have described reflex seizures in HHS, but are much less frequent. For example, proprioceptive-induced reflex seizures can present as a result of unstable blood glucose [18]. Individuals with nonketotic hyperglycemia can exhibit posture-induced focal seizures and interictal focal neurological findings that resolve with control of the hyperglycemia [19]. Since these manifestations are specific to hyperglycemia, some authors suggested that reflex seizures in the setting of nonketotic hyperglycemia constitute a neuroendocrine syndrome [18, 19]. Descriptions of twitching and myoclonus are reported, but are likely related to neurophysiologic alterations along the whole neuraxis since they do not correlate with EEG findings [20].

The mechanisms that lead to seizures in HHS and DKA remain speculative. In HHS, a depression of the inhibitor neurotransmitter gamma-aminobutyric acid (GABA) caused by its increased metabolism presumably lowers the seizure threshold [18]. A disruption of the Krebs cycle in HHS is observed in vivo, which may force the utilization of an alternate metabolic pathway to generate energy, known as the GABA shunt. In this process, cells consume GABA to form succinic acid and bypass the usual pathway that requires alpha-ketoglutarate (see Fig. 1) [20, 21].

A reversible blood–brain barrier disruption may also play a role in hyperglycemia-induced seizures, as proposed by MRI studies. Delayed gadolinium enhancement of the cerebrospinal fluid (CSF) space on fluid-attenuated inversion recovery imaging, seen with increased blood–brain barrier permeability, has been found in HHS-induced seizures and resolves in parallel to clinical improvement [22]. In the course of hyperglycemia, an osmotic gradient is also generated between the hypertonic extracellular and the isotonic intracellular compartments and leads to subsequent brain cell dehydration [8]. This phenomenon is associated with a depressed sensorium and seizures, and is seen in both HHS and DKA as it occurs as a result of hyperglycemia rather than hyperosmolality [8, 20]. Only rapid hyperglycemia induction, however, leads to a hyperosmotic transcellular water shift. A slower glycemic disturbance triggers the intracellular production and accumulation of idiogenic osmoles and solutes (e.g., sorbitol, myoinositol) to compensate and equilibrate with extracellular tonicity [20].

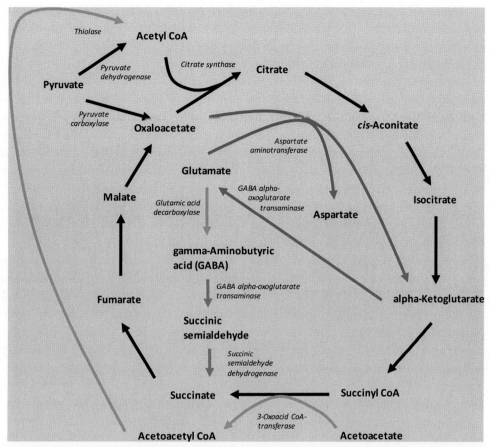

Fig. 1 The Krebs cycle in acute glycemic disturbances leading to epileptic seizures. In hyperglycemic hyperosmolar state *(green arrows)*, a disruption of the Krebs cycle forces the utilization of the gamma-aminobutyric acid (GABA) shunt, in which cells consume GABA to form succinate and bypass the usual pathway that requires alpha-ketoglutarate. In ketosis, the GABA shunt is compensated by the use of ketone bodies available to the brain that lead to GABA production *(yellow arrows)*. The ketone body acetoacetate is used to generate acetyl CoA, which enters the Krebs cycle via the citrate synthase pathway and leads to the consumption of oxaloacetate. The lower level of oxaloacetate reduces the activity of the aspartate aminotransferase pathway and creates an accumulation of glutamate, which in turn becomes more available to form GABA. In hypoglycemia *(blue arrows)*, unavailable glucose-derived pyruvate creates a bypass in the Krebs cycle to favor the use of oxaloacetate to form aspartate and alpha-ketoglutarate to form glutamate. This excess of glutamate and aspartate creates an overstimulation of glutamate receptors. *(Adapted from Olsen RWDT. GABA synthesis, uptake and release. In: Siegel GJ AB, Albers RW, et al., eds. Basic neurochemistry: Molecular, cellular and medical aspects. 6th ed. Philadelphia: Lippincott-Raven; 1999; Neil WPH, Hemmen TM. Neurologic manifestations of hypoglycemia. In: Rigobelo E, ed. Diabetes—damages and treatments. InTech; 2011; Masino SARJ. Mechanisms of ketogenic diet action. In: Noebels JLAM, Rogawski MA, et al., ed. Jasper's basic mechanisms of the epilepsies. Bethesda: National Center for Biotechnology Information; 2012.)*

The reason why a systemic condition like HHS unexpectedly results in focal neurological features (such as focal seizures) is unknown. The most likely explanation is that certain areas of vascular insufficiency are more vulnerable to the metabolic changes seen in HHS and are preferentially disrupted [20, 23].

The explanation for the lower rate of epileptic seizures in DKA compared to HHS is speculative but could relate to the anticonvulsant action of ketosis [24]. As opposed to the decreased brain concentration of GABA found in HHS, a normal level of the neurotransmitter is observed in DKA and may lead to a higher seizure threshold. In ketosis, the GABA shunt is compensated by the use of ketone bodies available to the brain that lead to GABA production. The ketone body acetoacetate is used to generate acetyl CoA, which enters the Krebs cycle via the citrate synthase pathway and leads to the consumption of oxaloacetate. The lower level of oxaloacetate reduces the activity of the aspartate aminotransferase pathway and creates an accumulation of glutamate, which in turn becomes more available to form GABA (see Fig. 1) [20, 25].

The level of blood glucose associated with seizure onset is variable. Values at the time of a seizure can be as low as 16 mM and as high as 61 mM, but are usually in the range of 30–35 mM [13]. The International League Against Epilepsy recommends the use of an operational definition for acute symptomatic seizures induced by hyperglycemia [26]. Hyperglycemia should be considered the cause of a seizure if blood glucose is over 25 mM (450 mg/dL) on a blood sample taken within 24 h of the seizure and is associated with ketoacidosis, whether or not there is long-standing diabetes. Unsurprisingly, since central nervous system (CNS) osmotic changes correlate with hyperglycemia rather than hyperosmolality, the vast majority of people who present with seizures and hyperglycemia have osmolality values below the usual diagnostic level of 320 mOsm/L [13].

EEG abnormalities in HHS are well associated with ictal semiology and consist of paroxysmal bursts of high-amplitude activity or spike and wave activity with generalized slowing of background frequencies [20, 27]. The most frequent locations of EEG changes in hyperglycemia among T1DM are fronto-central followed by temporal/temporo-central and occipital (see Fig. 2) [28].

Usually, HHS-induced seizures are refractory to antiepileptic drugs (AEDs) and respond to hydration and insulin therapy [27]. This may explain why such seizures are more protracted and can last 15–30 min [4]. Epileptic seizures in HHS are reported to stop at an average blood glucose of 11 mM, but their cessation has been observed in a wide range of values as low as 4 mM and as high as 22 mM [13].

Since diagnostic and treatment delays are frequent in hyperglycemia-induced seizures, it is crucial for clinicians to search for high blood glucose in people with focal seizures. Even among those with diagnosed epilepsy, the new onset of focal seizures can be the initial presentation of DM. For example, in a report of three adolescents with previously well-controlled epilepsy, the onset of intractable focal seizures lead to a new

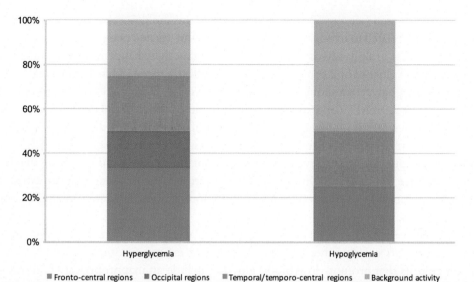

Fig. 2 The most frequent locations of electroencephalogram changes observed in glycemic disturbances with type 1 diabetes mellitus. Changes in fronto-central regions are most often encountered in hyperglycemia, while abnormal background activity is most often seen in hypoglycemia. *(Adapted from Verrotti A, Scaparrotta A, Olivieri C, Chiarelli F. Seizures and type 1 diabetes mellitus: current state of knowledge. Eur J Endocrinol. 2012;167(6):749–758.).*

diagnosis of T1DM as well as prompt cessation of seizures upon institution of insulin therapy and correction of hyperglycemia [24].

2.2 Hypoglycemia

Limited epidemiological data is available to characterize seizures secondary to hypoglycemia. The true incidence of seizures induced by hypoglycemia is unknown. Metabolic factors account for a small proportion of status epilepticus with estimates of 4% in children and 11% in adults, and the proportion of abnormal blood glucose in these groups is not known [29, 30]. Published data suggest that coma is the leading neurological manifestation of hypoglycemia and that seizures are rare. A prospective study in an emergency department collected data from 125 individuals who presented with symptomatic hypoglycemia and found that seizures only accounted for 7.2% of the observed neurological manifestations. More frequent symptoms were depressed sensorium in 52%, behavioral changes in 30%, and dizziness or tremor in 8%. The majority of the seizures were generalized tonic-clonic seizures as compared to the focal seizures most often seen in hyperglycemia [31]. When focal seizures do occur, they may involve the temporal region, which is felt to be more sensitive to hypoglycemia-induced dysfunction [32].

The most frequent locations for EEG changes in hypoglycemia among T1DM are the temporal and fronto-central regions, although slowing of the background activity is most often encountered (see Fig. 2) [28]. The glycemic threshold necessary to trigger an epileptic seizure related to hypoglycemia varies. In insulin-treated people, a symmetrical and diffuse decrease in alpha activity and increase in theta activity happens abruptly on EEG at a mean blood glucose of 2.0 mM, which could reflect a threshold for neuronal dysfunction [33]. Hypoglycemia should be considered the cause of a seizure if the blood glucose level is below 2.0 mM (36 mg/dL) on a blood sample taken within 24 h of the seizure [26]. The risk of seizures is higher with a faster onset of the metabolic disturbance [26].

Cerebral metabolism depends on a continuous supply of its key source of energy: glucose. A disruption in glucose availability to the brain initiates a cascade of events that leads to progressive neurological symptoms. The spectrum of these manifestations correlates with the duration and severity of hypoglycemia and includes behavioral changes, confusion, seizures, and coma.

Hypoglycemia in diabetic people results from an excessive consumption of glucose compared to its supply either from endogenous or exogenous sources. In T1DM, the main culprits that promote low blood glucose include an inappropriately high insulin intake that exceeds metabolic needs and a defect in the proper counterregulatory mechanisms in response to hypoglycemia, such as impaired glucagon release from the pancreatic alpha cells. In T2DM, hypoglycemia is produced in most people as a result of excessive insulin intake or oral hypoglycemic agents side effects [34]. Among these drugs, sulfonylureas account for the majority of hypoglycemic episodes as their mechanism of action includes an increased endogenous insulin secretion by the pancreatic beta cells.

People living with DM may experience frequent and severe episodes of hypoglycemia. Ninety percent of people with DM receiving insulin therapy experience hypoglycemia at some point in their life [34]. In T1DM, about two episodes of symptomatic hypoglycemia occur every week on average. Each year, 30% to 40% of T1DM people experience a severe hypoglycemic episode (i.e., seizures or coma) that requires an external intervention [35]. Among people with T2DM, the risk of hypoglycemia in the first 2 years of insulin therapy is similar to the risk related to sulfonylureas, with severe episodes experienced by about 7% of them [36].

Investigators have described perturbations in the neurotransmitters serotonin, dopamine, and excitatory amino acid pathways that may explain the occurrence of seizures in the setting of hypoglycemia, rather than the hypoglycemia itself [37]. In the case of parenchymal glucopenia, unavailable glucose-derived pyruvate creates a bypass in the Krebs cycle to favor the use of oxaloacetate to form aspartate and alpha-ketoglutarate to form glutamate (see Fig. 1) [38]. This excess of glutamate and aspartate creates an overstimulation of glutamate receptors (mostly N-methyl-D-aspartate receptors) to cause excitotoxicity [39]. This pathologic event initially creates an influx of sodium and water, followed by cellular edema and calcium entrance into the cell before triggering neuronal dysfunction [38].

The reduction of the burden of hypoglycemia-related seizures in diabetic people, whether they represent comorbid epilepsy or not, should be viewed as an important therapeutic endpoint by clinicians and kept in mind when attempting to achieve optimal glycemic control. The prevention of low blood glucose, prompt recognition, and its adequate correction remain the primary approach to reduce the incidence and consequences of such events. Self-management education programs promoting patient empowerment and informing patients on the symptoms, risks, prevention, and treatment of hypoglycemia lead to better glycemic outcomes [40]. An adequate blood glucose monitoring helps to recognize hypoglycemia and guide the therapeutic regimen [41]. The goals of glycemic control should be individualized according to age, comorbidities, disease duration, and the risk of severe hypoglycemia [34]. Thus, physicians caring for patients with epilepsy and comorbid DM should evaluate the risk of severe hypoglycemia in their patients and ensure that appropriate measures to reduce their incidence have been proposed.

3. Type 1 diabetes mellitus and epilepsy

There are strong associations between epilepsy and numerous autoimmune diseases among children and young adults. In the largest population-based retrospective cohort study of epilepsy in autoimmune diseases, the likelihood of being diagnosed with epilepsy among people with T1DM under 65 years old is increased by more than five times when compared to people without DM [42]. Health care professionals working with people with epilepsy could only improve their practice by recognizing the interplays between T1DM and epilepsy.

3.1 Descriptive epidemiology

A possible association between DM and epilepsy was first reported in a series of two children with DM and epilepsy in 1952 [1]. Since then, multiple retrospective and prospective cohort studies have shown a positive association between T1DM and epilepsy, especially in children [42–46]. The burden, however, of DM in people with epilepsy remains inconsistent, in part because of methodological issues. Few studies distinguish between T1DM and T2DM in spite of their different pathophysiology, entangling their respective associations with epilepsy. Since people with T1DM often present with seizures provoked by glycemic disturbances, the diagnosis of unprovoked seizures can be challenging and may be underrecognized. Nevertheless, an increasing number of population-based studies report incidences of epilepsy among people with T1DM that are higher than expected, as compared to people without DM.

Two of the largest population-based cohort studies recently reported that people with T1DM were 2.8 to 3.0 times more likely to be diagnosed with epilepsy than those without T1DM [43, 44]. In the UK, this represents an increased incidence of epilepsy of 132 per 100,000 person-years in T1DM compared to the 44 per 100,000 person-years observed in people without DM [43]. A secondary-care pediatric diabetes clinic in the UK reported a prevalence of epilepsy of 2.1%, six times greater than the prevalence in the general pediatric population in the country [45]. Most people are diagnosed with T1DM prior to epilepsy, with a median onset interval of 1.5 years [46].

3.2 Pathophysiology of epilepsy in type 1 diabetes mellitus

Numerous hypotheses have been proposed to explain the association between epilepsy and T1DM (see Fig. 3). Specific genetic defects are recognized to result in both diseases, but the prevalence of these diseases is fairly low and they are therefore unlikely to explain the majority of this association. Genetic factors not yet identified could constitute a shared risk factor for both epilepsy and T1DM, as supported by the observed varying temporal relationship between these two conditions (i.e., epilepsy occurs first in some individuals, DM occurs first in others). The hypothesis of a shared underlying autoimmune process has a strong pathophysiological basis and likely explains a portion of the association. T1DM may also indirectly lead to epilepsy through cerebrovascular disease.

3.2.1 Genetic entities causing epilepsy and diabetes

Two specific but rare syndromes are described that lead to epilepsy and DM: permanent neonatal diabetes mellitus (PNDM) with developmental delay, epilepsy, and neonatal

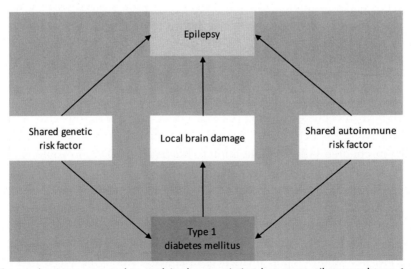

Fig. 3 The mechanisms proposed to explain the association between epilepsy and type 1 diabetes mellitus (T1DM). Genetic factors not yet identified may constitute a shared risk factor for both epilepsy and T1DM. A shared underlying autoimmune process may also contribute to this association. Diabetes mellitus could indirectly lead to epilepsy through the production of local brain damage.

diabetes syndrome, as well as PNDM, microcephaly with simplified gyration and infantile epileptic encephalopathy. Although these monogenic entities are infrequent and account for only a small proportion of the association observed between epilepsy and T1DM in population-based studies, they shed light on the possibility that more prevalent but less pathogenic mutations may be involved in the disruption of the cellular physiology of both pancreatic beta cells and neurons. Such genes remain to be identified.

PNDM is commonly defined as DM diagnosed within the first 6 months of life and has an incidence of at least 1 in 260,000 live births [47]. Neurological manifestations are found in about 20% of people with PNDM. They range from mild psychomotor retardation to a more severe condition termed developmental delay, epilepsy, and neonatal diabetes (DEND) syndrome. Milder forms of the latter condition are identified as intermediate DEND syndrome. In addition to DM, this condition is associated with severe developmental delay, hypotonia, and drug-resistant epilepsy. These individuals also present with mild dysmorphic features such as a prominent metopic suture and manifestations of muscle weakness like bilateral ptosis and a downturned mouth. Most individuals will develop generalized epilepsy before the age of 1 year. Their EEG most often shows bilateral sharp waves and may present hypsarrhythmia.

PNDM is mainly caused by activating heterozygous mutations in the *KCNJ11* and *ABCC8* genes, which respectively encode the Kir6.2 and the sulfonylurea receptor 1 (SUR1) subunits of the adenosine triphosphate-sensitive potassium (K_{ATP}) channel in the pancreatic beta cells [48, 49]. Investigators have identified mutations of both genes in people with DEND syndrome, which are likely responsible for its neurological features [50]. The abnormal function of the Kir6.2 and SUR1 subunits leads to an increased permeability of the K_{ATP} channels expressed by inhibitory neurons. This may lead to an efflux of potassium with subsequent hyperpolarization of inhibitory neurons, reducing their inhibitory tone on target neurons and decreasing seizure threshold [51, 52]. Three groups of gain-of-function mutations affecting the Kir6.2 subunit have been identified based on the decremental sensitivity of the K_{ATP} channel and the consequent incremental neurological symptoms (see Fig. 4) [52].

Mutations in the gene *IER3IP1* are described in a small number of individuals who presented with a syndrome consisting of PNDM, microcephaly with simplified gyration, and infantile epileptic encephalopathy [53]. These individuals present with drug-resistant focal with secondary generalization, generalized tonic–clonic, and myoclonic seizures.

IER3IP1 is a protein found in cells of both developing cortex and beta cells of the pancreas that mediates the transport between the endoplasmic reticulum and the Golgi complex [53]. The protein is also thought to be involved in cell differentiation and death processes [54]. Its abnormal function could dysregulate physiological cell death pathways and lead to an increased level of apoptosis in the brain and pancreas to produce congenital microcephaly and insulin-dependent diabetes [53]. Further research remains necessary to better understand the complex genetic associations of infantile epilepsy and diabetes.

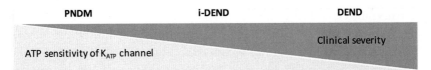

Fig. 4 The three groups of gain-of-function mutations affecting the Kir6.2 subunit have been identified based on the decremental sensitivity of the K_{ATP} channel and the consequent incremental neurological symptoms. PNDM, permanent neonatal diabetes mellitus; DEND, developmental delay, epilepsy, and neonatal diabetes; i-DEND, intermediate DEND. *(Adapted from Hattersley AT, Ashcroft FM. Activating mutations in Kir6.2 and neonatal diabetes: new clinical syndromes, new scientific insights, and new therapy. Diabetes. 2005;54(9):2503–13.)*

3.2.2 Autoimmunity

Anti-glutamic acid decarboxylase (GAD) antibodies may play a role in the pathophysiology of epilepsy. The main means by which anti-GAD antibodies may lead to seizures is thought to involve an alteration of GABA transmission, leading to an increased excitability of neurons and a lowered seizure threshold. Glutamic acid decarboxylase is an enzyme involved in the synthesis of GABA, and laboratory studies show that anti-GAD antibodies interfere with adequate GABA function when applied to hippocampal neurons in culture [55]. Intrathecal production of GAD-antibodies has been described and appears essential to its pathogenesis, since these antibodies are unable to cross the blood-brain barrier [56]. Although GAD is located inside the neuron and is not readily exposed to the plasma, the internalization of circulating antibodies by neurons is a well-described phenomenon providing intracellular access to antibodies [57].

Positive titers of anti-GAD antibodies have been described in many neurological disorders such as stiff-person syndrome (SPS), cerebellar ataxia, limbic encephalitis, and epilepsy [58]. The diverse array of neurological presentations in people with anti-GAD has its roots in the different epitopes the antibody can recognize [57]. Descriptive data on the association between epilepsy and anti-GAD antibodies are diverse and relate to seizure severity, type, and treatment response.

Epilepsy with positive anti-GAD titers may present in two forms: chronic epilepsy without active encephalitis, or limbic encephalitis. These two clinical presentations could respectively represent the chronic and acute stages of the same disorder characterized by temporal lobe hyperexcitability [58]. In epilepsy without encephalitis, positive titers are associated with temporal lobe epilepsy both clinically and on EEG, and higher titers do not seem to correlate with seizure severity. High anti-GAD titers are found in 2.8% of people with epilepsy, of which 86% have temporal lobe epilepsy [59]. They tend to have normal brain imaging and refractory epilepsy, further supporting the pathogenic role of these antibodies. In the light of these observations, some authors advocate that the search for anti-GAD antibodies should be considered in patients with cryptogenic temporal lobe epilepsy, even in the absence of T1DM [60].

Anti-GAD antibodies, formerly known as the "64k autoantigen in insulin-dependent diabetes," were first identified among people with T1DM in 1990 [61]. These antibodies are still widely recognized as markers of T1DM since 60%–70% of these individuals have positive serum titers, as compared to 0.4%–1% in the general population [56, 60, 61]. The first description of anti-GAD antibodies in drug-resistant epilepsy came in 1998 and has led to numerous case reports [62]. In contrast to T1DM without a neurological comorbidity, individuals presenting with a neurological disorder have higher anti-GAD serum titers, CSF oligoclonal bands, and positive CSF anti-GAD titers [58]. The antibodies found in T1DM recognize conformational epitopes of the middle and C-terminus of the protein, a pattern that is different from that which is seen in SPS [56]. This may explain the different neurologic manifestations and the absence of SPS features seen in T1DM with anti-GAD antibodies [56]. Thus, the mechanism of association of epilepsy with comorbid T1DM may include a shared autoimmune process. This hypothesis is supported by the observation that individuals with comorbid T1DM are more likely to have epilepsy of unknown etiology, when compared to individuals without DM, while structural and genetic causes are less frequent [46].

3.2.3 Local brain damage

Central nervous system changes have been observed in people with T1DM through studies that are mostly limited to EEG and brain imaging [63]. One study demonstrated mesial temporal sclerosis (MTS) on MRI in 16% of 62 individuals with early-onset T1DM, with comparable results in those with and without previous DKA or severe hypoglycemia [64]. This high prevalence of MTS suggests preferential hippocampal damage in early-onset T1DM that could be explained by its greater vulnerability to unrecognized nonsevere hypoglycemic episodes. The MTS seen in T1DM individuals may, in part, be attributed to anti-GAD antibodies rather than glycemic abnormalities. In adults, permanent CNS damage may be seen, following profound episodes of hypoglycemia with particular injuries to glucose-deprivation vulnerable areas, such as the hippocampus, the basal ganglia, and the neocortex [65]. These lesions could be the primary result of hypoxia and hypotension caused by persistent hypoglycemia [66].

Local brain damage caused by cerebral infarctions may contribute to epilepsy in people with both T1DM and T2DM. Cerebrovascular disease is a major cause of epilepsy in elderly people, and DM increases the risk of both seizures and cerebrovascular disease in the elderly population [67]. Fifteen percent of individuals with DM and seizures also have local brain damage on imaging [4]. These observations taken together make it likely that for some individuals with epilepsy, the metabolic abnormalities found in T1DM can have a deleterious effect on the CNS and lead to epilepsy. The mechanism leading to epilepsy in people with DM would, in this instance, be an indirect causal association by which local brain damage mediates the relationship between the initial DM and the subsequent development of epilepsy. The greater risk of epilepsy in T1DM with previous hypogly-cemic episodes as compared to those without and the onset of T1DM before epilepsy in a majority of people support the hypothesis of local brain damage as an indirect causal mechanism.

3.3 Clinical aspects specific to type 1 diabetes mellitus

Numerous cohort studies have reported an association between T1DM without acute glycemic disturbances and various epilepsy etiologies and types. One of the largest cohorts of drug-resistant epilepsy with comorbid T1DM reported more cryptogenic eti-ology (85%) in T1DM when compared to nondiabetic people (49%), as well as fewer structural (15% vs. 45%) and genetic/idiopathic causes (0% vs. 6%) [46]. Some reports suggest that T1DM may also be found in idiopathic generalized epilepsy (IGE) more often than expected by chance [68, 69]. In a cohort of 518 individuals, IGE was associated with a fourfold increased risk of T1DM when compared to the general population [69]. Some subdivisions of IGE may be less likely to be associated with T1DM. Absence epilepsy was not found among individuals with comorbid T1DM, though accounting for almost a third of the cohort [69]. FSE can manifest in the setting of T1DM without glycemic disturbances as reported in a few case reports [15].

People with epilepsy and comorbid T1DM may present cognitive impairment and learning interferences as a result of both epilepsy and DM. Mild cognitive impairments are apparent in children with T1DM, especially in boys, and affect attention, processing speed, long-term memory, and executive skills [63]. The mechanism for these difficulties is thought to involve compromises in brain areas that are sensitive to blood glucose variations, such as frontal and mesial temporal regions. In addition, neuroglycopenic cognitive deterioration can happen in learning situations and disrupt skill acquisition. Although most children with T1DM undergo normal skill acquisition and score within the average or low-average ranges in neurocognitive tests, learning difficulties should be recognized so that proper resources can be offered to support development [63].

4. Therapeutic considerations and implications in diabetes mellitus

There are no standard AEDs recommended to treat epilepsy with comorbid DM. Relevant observational studies are scarce. Phenytoin should be used with caution in people with proven or at risk of DM, as it is known to precipitate DKA and HHS [24, 70, 71]. On serial parenteral glucose challenges in normoglycemic subjects, a brief exposure to phenytoin increased blood glucose by 19% and reduced early insulin secretion by 60% compared to baseline [72]. Phenytoin-induced hyperglycemia results from decreased insulin secretion due to its electrophysiological properties on the pancreas [73]. Carbamazepine has been reported to precipitate DM in children [74]. Moreover, hyperglycemia is found in 60% of children intoxicated with carbamazepine, in which blood glucose correlates with serum carbamazepine levels [75]. Many antiepileptic medications are associated with a significant body weight gain and an increased risk of DM. Valproate carries a particular risk, but other drugs such as gabapentin, pregabalin, vigabatrin, retigabine, and carbamazepine are reported to lead to body weight gain [76]. The underlying mechanism for this side effect seems to differ between AEDs and is still a matter of debate.

Clinicians have used the ketogenic diet (KD) for decades as an anticonvulsant therapy in various forms of drug-resistant epilepsy. It is based on a high fat, low carbohydrate, and moderate protein intake and aims to achieve ketone body production from the oxidation of lipid stores [77]. The mechanisms that lead to its anticonvulsant properties remain uncertain but are associated with increased levels of ketone bodies. Specific pathways have been proposed and include neuroprotective effects, a modulation of biogenic monoamine levels, and a modulation of neurotransmitters that primarily involve GABA and glutamate [77]. Significant reductions in interictal epileptiform discharges and improved seizure control are well established in refractory epilepsy among people without DM [78].

The use of the KD is infrequently reported in people with T1DM, however, and quality evidence is lacking on its efficacy and safety. Considerations with regards to the latter have halted its use in this population. It could be considered hazardous to induce a state of ketosis in individuals predisposed to develop life-threatening ketoacidosis [79]. The KD makes it difficult to differentiate between the desired starvation-induced ketones and those that result from insulin deficiency [80]. Nonetheless, T1DM does not preclude the use of the KD providing frequent measurement of capillary glucose are carried out and prompt correction of hyperglycemia with rapid insulin and strict monitoring of blood ketones are undertaken [79]. Several cases of successful and safe management of refractory epilepsy with comorbid T1DM are reported [78, 80]. None of these individuals had DKA or severe hypoglycemia over the course of their treatment. The targeted ketone levels during ketogenic therapy should be tailored based on the risk of DKA and the benefits on seizure control associated with higher ketone levels. An intermediate ketonuria may suffice in some instances [79].

The management of DM in the setting of DEND syndrome can constitute a greater challenge given the inherent communication limitations and dramatic consequences of hypoglycemia on seizure occurrence in such patients. Individuals with PNDM show insulin dependence and are initially managed by insulin therapy. In cases of *KCNJ11* and *ABCC8* mutations, sulfonylurea drugs may be an alternative to exogenous insulin since they stimulate its endogenous secretion by closing the K_{ATP} channels in the pancreatic beta cells [81]. Moreover, sulfonylureas are thought to close SUR1-type K_{ATP} channels found in the brain and may theoretically improve neurological symptoms [81]. Glibenclamide, a sulfonylurea that blocks both SUR1 and SUR2-type channels with high affinity, is most often used [51]. DEND syndrome is caused by mutations that are less sensitive to sulfonylureas and often requires higher doses [52, 82]. Successful transfers to sulfonylurea drugs have been reported in many individuals with PNDM, among those without neurological symptoms and those with intermediate DEND syndrome [83, 84]. Data supporting the transfer to sulfonylureas in severe forms of DEND syndrome are more limited [51, 82].

Immunotherapy is an interesting option in the management of anti-GAD-associated epilepsy. The potential benefits of immunosuppressive treatment and plasma exchange arise from case reports [58]. Marked seizure control improvement, for example, was observed after pulse therapy with cytostatic cyclophosphamide in an individual with refractory status epilepticus and intrathecal anti-GAD antibody [85]. In a report of autoimmune-related drug-resistant epilepsy, three out of five individuals with anti-GAD antibodies who were offered immunotherapy (intravenous immunoglobulin and/or mycophenolate mofetil and/or corticosteroids) reported seizure freedom at follow-up (ranging from 6 to 18 months). Whether these results can be applied in people with T1DM, epilepsy, and anti-GAD antibodies is unknown since reports in this population are lacking.

5. Thyroid hormones and epilepsy

5.1 Descriptive epidemiology, pathophysiology, and clinical manifestations

The tyrosine-based hormones triiodothyronine (T3) and thyroxine (T4) are synthesized by the thyroid gland. The hypothalamic-pituitary-thyroid axis is a three-level endocrine regulation system in which the hypothalamus produces thyrotropin-releasing hormone (TRH) that acts on the pituitary gland to promote secretion of thyroid-stimulating hormone (TSH), which binds to its receptors on the thyroid gland to release thyroid hormones in the blood [86].

Studies evaluating thyroid function in epilepsy have failed to demonstrate a direct alteration in thyroid hormones caused by seizures [87, 88]. Several thyroid disorders, however, are associated with the occurrence of seizures, including thyrotoxicosis and levothyroxine (LT4) treatment. First-time seizures can be seen in a very small proportion (<1%) of individuals with hyperthyroidism [89, 90]. In a review of individuals without a known history of epilepsy but admitted for thyrotoxicosis (high T3 and free T4 with suppressed TSH), 0.2% had seizures at presentation [90]. Primary generalized tonic-clonic seizures were most frequent (57%) while focal seizures were uncommon (14%). Generalized slowing was seen on EEG in more than half of individuals. After treatment of their thyroid dysfunction, all individuals remained seizure-free [90].

The pathway that leads thyrotoxicosis to epileptic seizures is uncertain. Animal models have shown that thyroid hormones may alter neuronal excitability in several ways, but these mechanisms remain speculative. Thyroid hormones alter sodium exchange in neurons and create an increased neuronal excitability in vitro [91]. The anticonvulsant effects of TRH on hippocampal tissue have also been hypothesized and could be reduced by thyroid hormones as they were found to decrease the level of TRH in various regions of the limbic system [90, 92].

The treatment of hypothyroidism with LT4 may also be associated with seizure deterioration, though such reports are rare. Levothyroxine may precipitate absence seizures in juvenile myoclonic epilepsy even after small doses that do not impact thyroid hormone levels, presumably mediated by changes in the pharmacokinetics and bioavailability of AEDs [93]. Investigators have also observed hyperkinetic seizures induced by LT4, with a strong association between LT4 initiation and dosage [94]. The mechanism for such LT4-induced seizures is unclear but may result from a reduced number of cortical benzodiazepine receptors, observed in models of neuronal cultures exposed to the medication [94]. Limited data are available regarding the prognosis of people with epilepsy and comorbid thyroid disorders.

5.2 Therapeutic considerations and implications

Antiepileptic drugs may alter thyroid hormone plasma levels, although clinically relevant consequences of such alterations remain the exception. Frequently cited AEDs are those with enzyme-inducing properties, such as phenytoin [95, 96] and carbamazepine [96–100], which consistently alter thyroid hormone levels across studies [88]. Phenobarbital [100], oxcarbazepine [98], and sodium valproate [100] may also affect thyroid hormone concentrations, although some results are conflicting [96, 99, 101]. Most commonly found biochemical consequences of these drugs include decreases in both total and free portions of T3 and T4. Parallel increases in TSH levels are rarely seen and remain clinically insignificant. Aforementioned hormonal changes are completely reversible upon discontinuation of the medication [98]. Independent risk factors for low free T4 during AED therapy include female gender, older age, and three or more AEDs [102].

Although clinically irrelevant biochemical abnormalities are most often encountered, other presentations such as subclinical hypothyroidism, mildly symptomatic hypothyroidism, and profound hypothyroidism can be seen. Severe primary hypothyroidism has been described with the combination of phenytoin and carbamazepine [103]. Three major mechanisms are involved in thyroid hormone alterations caused by AEDs. First, phenytoin and carbamazepine have three-dimensional structural similarities with T4 and can bind competitively to circulating thyroxine-binding globulin, thereby displacing the protein-bound T4 and reducing its total plasma concentration [96]. Second, enzyme-inducing AEDs increase hepatic microsomal activity, leading to both greater conversion of T4 to T3 and increased metabolic clearance of thyroid hormones [95, 96]. Earlier reported effects on the hypothalamic-pituitary axis of carbamazepine and sodium valproate have not been found in more recent work, showing that TSH response to TRH was unaffected in people treated with these drugs [99]. In conclusion, since clinically significant thyroid disorders are rare in the course of AED therapy, routine evaluation of thyroid hormone levels in asymptomatic patients on AEDs is generally unwarranted [87].

The treatment of refractory epilepsy with the KD in children has been associated with significant thyroid hormone alterations. The exact mechanisms involved in these changes remain unknown, but may include a reduction of peripheral conversion of T4 to T3 known to occur in fasting state, hypoproteinemia, and selenium deficiency [104]. A six-month follow-up of children with drug-resistant epilepsy treated with the KD revealed that 16.7% of individuals developed subclinical hypothyroidism, defined as an elevated TSH with normal free T4 on two occasions for at least 1 month [104]. Although the treatment of subclinical hypothyroidism in children remains controversial, as the benefits are inconsistent, thyroxine replacement was deemed reasonable considering their burden of comorbidities. Thyroxine replacement normalized TSH values in all treated individuals.

6. Prolactin and epilepsy

Prolactin (PRL) is a polypeptide hormone synthesized and secreted by the lactotrophs of the anterior pituitary. These specialized cells demonstrate a high endogenous secretory activity that requires a tonic inhibitory control exerted by the hypothalamus through PRL inhibitory factors. Dopamine is the most important and potent of these inhibitors, but other peptides such as somatostatin and GABA also play a role in the nondopaminergic inhibitory activity of the hypothalamus [105]. On the other hand, TRH and oxytocin are major PRL-releasing factors [105]. The physiologic roles of PRL include the promotion of growth and development of the mammary gland during pregnancy, the synthesis and maintenance of milk secretion, and the modulation of the immunoneuroendocrine network [105].

Serum PRL has been studied in various settings of seizures over the past few decades to become one of the most extensively described biomarkers in epilepsy. An increase in serum PRL associated with epileptics seizures was first reported following electroconvulsive therapy in 1976 [106], prior to descriptions in spontaneous epileptic seizures [107]. The hypothesized mechanism for seizure-induced serum PRL increase is thought to involve that propagation of epileptic discharges to the hypothalamus from mesial temporal structures, which may lead to a transient decrease in dopamine concentration in the tuberoinfundibular tract and a release of its tonic inhibition on PRL secretion [108, 109].

Based on observational data, serum PRL peaks between 10 and 20 min after an epileptic seizure and returns to baseline within 2–6 h [110]. The normal range of PRL and the threshold for a relevant PRL increase are difficult to define. In addition to its surge prior to awakening from sleep, serum PRL levels are influenced by age, gender, commonly used medications, pregnancy, and physiological stress [110]. In people with epilepsy, higher serum PRL levels are reported compared to controls during interictal episodes, suggesting that epileptiform discharges may interfere with PRL secretion [111]. Most studies use either a twofold relative increase from a previous baseline level or an absolute cut-off level ranging from 16.5 to 45 ng/mL [112].

The validity of elevated serum PRL to differentiate epileptic seizures from psychogenic nonepileptic seizures was first reported in a pooled data analysis of 10 studies [112]. Elevated PRL levels showed a high specificity for the diagnosis of generalized tonic-clonic seizures (95.9%) and focal seizures with impaired awareness (96.3%), and a moderate sensitivity that was better for the former (60%) than the latter (46.1%). These results led to a level B recommendation reaffirmed in 2016 by the American Academy of Neurology stating that elevated serum PRL is a useful adjunct for the differentiation of generalized tonic-clonic and focal seizures with impaired awareness from psychogenic nonepileptic seizures in adults and older children when measured in the proper clinical setting within 10–20 min of a suspected event [112].

These findings taken together suggest that an acute rise in PRL level indicates an epileptic seizure, although a normal level cannot be used to exclude an epileptic seizure nor to diagnose a psychogenic nonepileptic seizure [110]. Serum PRL measurement is of limited help to distinguish syncope from epileptic seizures, since reports of tilt-table-induced syncope show an elevation of serum PRL level in 60%–80% of subjects [110]. The use of serum PRL in other convulsive conditions, such as focal aware seizures, status epilepticus, repetitive seizures, and neonatal seizures, has not been established [112].

7. Catamenial epilepsy

7.1 Descriptive epidemiology, pathophysiology, and clinical manifestations

Sex steroid hormones affect epilepsy control through their neuroactive properties and their cyclic variation. Women are prone to manifest the effects of sex hormones on seizure severity and frequency because of the physiological shifting of their circulating levels throughout the menstrual cycle [87]. Estradiol is the main circulating estrogen during reproductive years and is largely produced by the ovarian follicles [87]. Estradiol shows proconvulsant and epileptogenic properties in both animal models and humans. It increases neuronal excitability by stimulating glutamate receptor activity, regulating neuronal plasticity to promote excitatory synapses, and reducing GABA synthesis [113]. Progesterone is mostly produced in the luteal phase and secreted by the oocyte-derived corpus luteum. It presents consistent anticonvulsant and antiepileptic properties in animal studies that are primarily due to allopregnanolone, a progesterone-derived neurosteroid produced in the peripheral tissue and the brain [87]. Allopregnanolone increases

$GABA_A$-mediated neuronal inhibition, while progesterone modulates the synthesis and release of numerous neurotransmitters [114].

Since the first published description of perimenstrual worsening of epileptic seizures in 1881, the propensity of epileptic seizures to cluster during particular phases of the menstrual cycle is increasingly recognized. It is only recently, however, that a more accurate description and a uniform definition of the phenomenon were reported [115]. Catamenial epilepsy commonly refers to a recurrent cyclical increase in epileptic seizure frequency during specific phases of the menstrual cycle. Three phenotypes of catamenial epilepsy may be encountered and are linked to circulating levels of sex hormones (see Fig. 5) [116].

The first pattern of catamenial epilepsy (C1) is characterized by an increase in epileptic seizure frequency in the perimenstrual phase (days −3 to 3, where day 1 represents the first day of the menstrual flow). The second pattern (C2) involves an increased frequency during the preovulatory phase (days 10 to −13). These two forms of catamenial epilepsy occur in women with ovulatory cycles, which involve an appropriate surge of estrogen and progesterone prior to ovulation with subsequent decrease at the end of the luteal phase. The peak in circulating estrogen-to-progesterone ratio seen in the perimenstrual and preovulatory phases may decrease the seizure threshold and explain these phenotypes [113]. Progesterone withdrawal at the time of menses may also independently contribute to C1 seizure susceptibility [114]. The third pattern (C3) is seen in anovulatory cycles where progesterone remains low in an inadequate luteal phase. The mechanism underlying this form of catamenial epilepsy likely involves a midcycle surge of proconvulsant estrogen that is insufficiently opposed due to low-circulating progesterone [113].

Earlier reports on catamenial epilepsy prevalence in women of reproductive age ranged from about 10% to >70%, owing to discrepancies in the definition [117]. A cut-off corresponding to a twofold increase of epileptic seizure frequency in at least one of the three catamenial phenotypes as compared to the average daily frequency was more recently proposed [116]. Using this definition, about one third of women presenting with drug-resistant focal epilepsy with impaired awareness are classified as having catamenial epilepsy [116]. The highest frequency of catamenial seizures involves the inadequate luteal phase or C3 pattern [118]. The clinical manifestations of catamenial epilepsy may vary with changes in hormonal status. The transition period of perimenopause may lead to an increase in seizure frequency due to higher estrogen levels, while menopause may decrease seizure frequency as a consequence of decreased estrogen levels [119].

7.2 Therapeutic considerations and implications

Investigators have proposed multiple nonhormonal and hormonal therapeutic approaches to manage catamenial epilepsy (see Table 1). The use of an increased dose of AEDs at days of catamenial exacerbation has been advocated by some

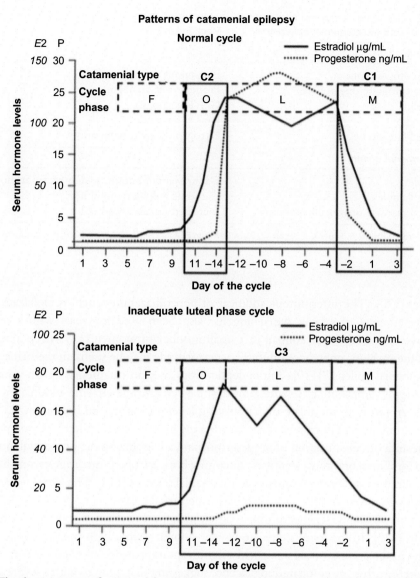

Fig. 5 The three patterns of catamenial epilepsy as proposed by Herzog, 1997. Day 1 is the first day of the menstrual flow and day −14 is the day of ovulation. The first pattern of catamenial epilepsy (C1) involves an increase in epileptic seizure frequency during the perimenstrual phase (days −3 to 3) among women with ovulatory cycles. The second pattern (C2) shows an increased frequency during the preovulatory phase (days 10 to −13). The third pattern (C3) is seen in inadequate luteal phase cycles and involves an exacerbation through the second half of the luteal phase (days 10–3). *(From Pennell PB. Hormonal aspects of epilepsy. Neurol Clin. 2009;27(4):941–965.)*

Table 1 A list of hormonal and nonhormonal agents tested in catamenial epilepsy

Agents tested in catamenial epilepsy	Mechanism
Hormonal agents	
Natural progesterone	Exogenous progesterone
Medroxyprogesterone acetate	Progesterone analogue
Goserelin	GnRH analogue
Triptorelin	GnRH analogue
Clomiphene citrate	Estrogen receptor antagonist
Nonhormonal agents	
Clobazam	Gamma-aminobutyric acid-A receptor modulator
Acetazolamide	Carbonic anhydrase inhibitor
Cyclical increase of antiepileptic drug	Increased seizure threshold

Adapted from Verrotti A, Laus M, Coppola G, Parisi P, Mohn A, Chiarelli F. Catamenial epilepsy: hormonal aspects. Gynecol Endocrinol. 2010;26(11):783–790.

authors [120]. The intermittent addition of benzodiazepines such as clobazam at the anticipated time of seizure worsening has also been used for years with a reported improvement of epilepsy control in a small number of women [119, 121]. The cyclic use of the carbonic anhydrase inhibitor acetazolamide may be useful in the management of catamenial epilepsy [119]. Antiepileptic drugs used in catamenial epilepsy may also theoretically contribute to seizure control since cytochrome enzyme-modulating AEDs have been found to modulate the circulating levels of sex steroid hormones [113].

The principles of hormonal pharmacotherapy in catamenial epilepsy rely on promoting the anticonvulsant action of progesterone and antagonizing the proconvulsant estrogens. Combined oral contraceptives containing both estrogen and progesterone have not been found to modify the frequency of catamenial seizures [119]. The cyclic use of exogenous progesterone in the second half of the menstrual cycle does not lead to a significant reduction of epileptic seizures among women with focal catamenial epilepsy compared to placebo [122]. In the same study, however, women with a high burden of catamenial seizures in the perimenstrual phase had a significant improvement of seizure control with progesterone therapy compared to placebo, suggesting that women with a severe form of catamenial epilepsy caused by end-cycle progesterone withdrawal may benefit from exogenous progesterone [118].

Other hormonal therapies that modulate estrogen production and action have been found to have benefits on seizure control in small studies, including gonadotropin-releasing hormone analogs, such as triptorelin and goserelin, and the estrogen receptor antagonist clomiphene citrate [113]. The progesterone analogue medroxyprogesterone acetate may also improve seizure control in catamenial epilepsy through suppression of menstrual cycling and, to a lesser extent, its conversion to neuroactive steroids [113].

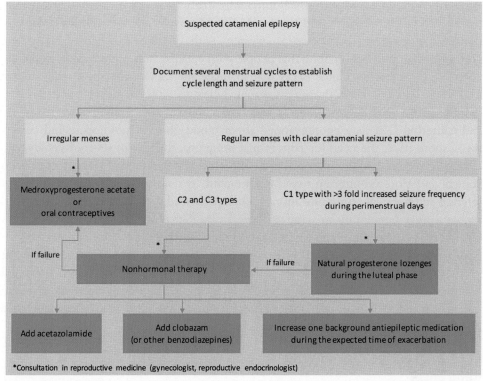

Fig. 6 A basic algorithm for the treatment of suspected catamenial epilepsy. Health care professionals should keep in mind that no treatment is effective for all women with catamenial epilepsy and that therapy should be tailored to a woman's needs. *(Adapted from Navis A, Harden C. A treatment approach to catamenial epilepsy. Curr Treat Options Neurol. 2016;18(7):30.)*

Along with the women's preferences, a multidisciplinary team involving a gynecologist or a reproductive endocrinologist may help to choose the most appropriate hormonal therapy. Some authors have recently proposed a basic algorithm that can be used by health care professionals to assist treatment decision-making, while keeping in mind that no treatment is effective for all women with catamenial epilepsy and that therapy should be tailored to a woman's needs (see Fig. 6) [123].

8. Conclusion

The tridirectional relationship between epilepsy, comorbid endocrine conditions, and therapies used in epilepsy is complex. Diabetes mellitus is one such comorbidity that has a great impact on the management of epilepsy. Glycemic disturbances can lead to seizures with specific treatment considerations, and DM may be associated with epilepsy by multiple mechanisms. Some diseases of the thyroid present with epileptic seizures, and

AEDs can disrupt thyroid hormone homeostasis. Prolactin abnormalities are also encountered after epileptic seizures, and sex steroid hormones may affect the clinical manifestations and the control of seizures in women with catamenial epilepsy. Health care professional should keep in mind that people with epilepsy may present comorbid endocrine disorders and hormonal issues that mandate special considerations. The routine evaluation of individuals with epilepsy may include screening for selected endocrine conditions, such as DM, thyroid diseases, and catamenial epilepsy. Individuals with epilepsy and comorbid DM may be questioned about blood glucose monitoring and control, medications used, the need for educational programs, the risk of severe hypoglycemia or hyperglycemia, and the approach to their correction. Some AEDs can affect glycemic control and close monitoring may be warranted. A collaborative approach involving referrals and frequent communications with experienced professionals, such as endocrinologists, may be relevant to achieve optimal care. Screening for symptoms of thyroid disorders among people taking AEDs and considerations for the clinical impact of thyroid disorders in epilepsy may also be integrated in routine practice. Finally, health care professionals may seek for features of catamenial epilepsy to identify the need for specific treatments. The choice of an appropriate nonhormonal or hormonal therapy in such instances may be made in collaboration with a multidisciplinary team that includes sex hormone professionals.

References

[1] Engel R, Halberg F, Ziegler M, Mc QI. Observations on two children with diabetes mellitus and epilepsy. J Lancet 1952;72(5):242–8.

[2] Kharroubi AT, Darwish HM. Diabetes mellitus: the epidemic of the century. World J Diabetes 2015; 6(6):850–67.

[3] Umpierrez G, Korytkowski M. Diabetic emergencies—ketoacidosis, hyperglycaemic hyperosmolar state and hypoglycaemia. Nat Rev Endocrinol 2016;12(4):222–32.

[4] Yun C, Xuefeng W. Association between seizures and diabetes mellitus: a comprehensive review of literature. Curr Diabetes Rev 2013;9(4):350–4.

[5] Pasquel FJ, Umpierrez GE. Hyperosmolar hyperglycemic state: a historic review of the clinical presentation, diagnosis, and treatment. Diabetes Care 2014;37(11):3124–31.

[6] Maccario M, Messis CP, Vastola EF. Focal seizures as a manifestation of hyperglycemia without ketoacidosis. A report of seven cases with review of the literature. Neurology 1965;15:195–206.

[7] Wang X, Yu H, Cai Z, Wang Z, Ma B, Zhang Y. Nonketotic hyperglycemia-related epileptic seizures. Epilepsy Behav Case Rep 2013;1:77–8.

[8] Singh BM, Gupta DR, Strobos RJ. Nonketotic hyperglycemia and epilepsia partialis continua. Arch Neurol 1973;29(3):187–90.

[9] Harden CL, Rosenbaum DH, Daras M. Hyperglycemia presenting with occipital seizures. Epilepsia 1991;32(2):215–20.

[10] Kanwal SK, Bando A, Kumar V. Clinical profile of diabetic ketoacidosis in Indian children. Indian J Pediatr 2012;79(7):901–4.

[11] Cochin JP, Hannequin D, Delangre T, Guegan-Massardier E, Augustin P. Continuous partial epilepsy disclosing diabetes mellitus. Rev Neurol (Paris) 1994;150(3):239–41.

[12] Moien-Afshari F, Tellez-Zenteno JF. Occipital seizures induced by hyperglycemia: a case report and review of literature. Seizure 2009;18(5):382–5.

[13] Tiamkao S, Pratipanawatr T, Tiamkao S, Nitinavakarn B, Chotmongkol V, Jitpimolmard S. Seizures in nonketotic hyperglycaemia. Seizure 2003;12(6):409–10.

[14] Sabharwal RK, Gupta M, Sharma D, Puri V. Juvenile diabetes manifesting as epilepsia partialis continua. J Assoc Physicians India 1989;37(9):603–4.

[15] Baglietto MG, Mancardi MM, Giannattasio A, Minuto N, Rossi A, Capovilla G, et al. Epilepsia partialis continua in type 1 diabetes: evolution into epileptic encephalopathy with continuous spike-waves during slow sleep. Neurol Sci 2009;30(6):509–12.

[16] Placidi F, Floris R, Bozzao A, Romigi A, Baviera ME, Tombini M, et al. Ketotic hyperglycemia and epilepsia partialis continua. Neurology 2001;57(3):534–7.

[17] Lavin PJ. Hyperglycemic hemianopia: a reversible complication of non-ketotic hyperglycemia. Neurology 2005;65(4):616–9.

[18] Ozer F, Mutlu A, Ozkayran T. Reflex epilepsy and non-ketotic hyperglycemia. Epileptic Disord 2003;5(3):165–8.

[19] Brick JF, Gutrecht JA, Ringel RA. Reflex epilepsy and nonketotic hyperglycemia in the elderly: a specific neuroendocrine syndrome. Neurology 1989;39(3):394–9.

[20] Guisado R, Arieff AI. Neurologic manifestations of diabetic comas: correlation with biochemical alterations in the brain. Metabolism 1975;24(5):665–79.

[21] RWDT O. GABA synthesis, uptake and release. In: Siegel GJAB, Albers RW, et al., editors. Basic neurochemistry: Molecular, cellular and medical aspects. 6th ed. Philadelphia: Lippincott-Raven; 1999.

[22] Kim DW, Moon Y, Gee Noh H, Choi JW, Oh J. Blood-brain barrier disruption is involved in seizure and hemianopsia in nonketotic hyperglycemia. Neurologist 2011;17(3):164–6.

[23] Espinas OE, Poser CM. Blood hyperosmolality and neurologic deficit. An experimental study. Arch Neurol 1969;20(2):182–6.

[24] Whiting S, Camfield P, Arab D, Salisbury S. Insulin-dependent diabetes mellitus presenting in children as frequent, medically unresponsive, partial seizures. J Child Neurol 1997;12(3):178–80.

[25] Masino SARJ. Mechanisms of ketogenic diet action. In: Noebels JLAM, Rogawski MA, et al., editors. Jasper's basic mechanisms of the epilepsies. Bethesda: National Center for Biotechnology Information; 2012.

[26] Beghi E, Carpio A, Forsgren L, Hesdorffer DC, Malmgren K, Sander JW, et al. Recommendation for a definition of acute symptomatic seizure. Epilepsia 2010;51(4):671–5.

[27] Raghavendra S, Ashalatha R, Thomas SV, Kesavadas C. Focal neuronal loss, reversible subcortical focal T2 hypointensity in seizures with a nonketotic hyperglycemic hyperosmolar state. Neuroradiology 2007;49(4):299–305.

[28] Verrotti A, Scaparrotta A, Olivieri C, Chiarelli F. Seizures and type 1 diabetes mellitus: current state of knowledge. Eur J Endocrinol 2012;167(6):749–58.

[29] Chin RF, Neville BG, Peckham C, Bedford H, Wade A, Scott RC, et al. Incidence, cause, and short-term outcome of convulsive status epilepticus in childhood: prospective population-based study. Lancet 2006;368(9531):222–9.

[30] Towne AR, Pellock JM, Ko D, DeLorenzo RJ. Determinants of mortality in status epilepticus. Epilepsia 1994;35(1):27–34.

[31] Malouf R, Brust JC. Hypoglycemia: causes, neurological manifestations, and outcome. Ann Neurol 1985;17(5):421–30.

[32] Lapenta L, Di Bonaventura C, Fattouch J, Bonini F, Petrucci S, Gagliardi S, et al. Focal epileptic seizure induced by transient hypoglycaemia in insulin-treated diabetes. Epileptic Disord 2010;12 (1):84–7.

[33] Pramming S, Thorsteinsson B, Stigsby B, Binder C. Glycaemic threshold for changes in electroencephalograms during hypoglycaemia in patients with insulin dependent diabetes. Br Med J (Clin Res Ed) 1988;296(6623):665–7.

[34] Shafiee G, Mohajeri-Tehrani M, Pajouhi M, Larijani B. The importance of hypoglycemia in diabetic patients. J Diabetes Metab Disord 2012;11(1):17.

[35] McCrimmon RJ, Sherwin RS. Hypoglycemia in type 1 diabetes. Diabetes 2010;59(10):2333–9.

[36] Group UKHS. Risk of hypoglycaemia in types 1 and 2 diabetes: effects of treatment modalities and their duration. Diabetologia 2007;50(6):1140–7.

[37] Anuradha K, Hota D, Pandhi P. Investigation of central mechanism of insulin induced hypoglycemic convulsions in mice. Indian J Exp Biol 2004;42(4):368–72.

[38] Neil WPH, Hemmen TM. Neurologic manifestations of hypoglycemia. In: Rigobelo E, editor. Diabetes—Damages and Treatments. InTech; 2011.

[39] Auer RN. Progress review: hypoglycemic brain damage. Stroke 1986;17(4):699–708.

[40] Norris SL, Lau J, Smith SJ, Schmid CH, Engelgau MM. Self-management education for adults with type 2 diabetes: a meta-analysis of the effect on glycemic control. Diabetes Care 2002;25(7):1159–71.

[41] Khamseh ME, Ansari M, Malek M, Shafiee G, Baradaran H. Effects of a structured self-monitoring of blood glucose method on patient self-management behavior and metabolic outcomes in type 2 diabetes mellitus. J Diabetes Sci Technol 2011;5(2):388–93.

[42] Ong MS, Kohane IS, Cai T, Gorman MP, Mandl KD. Population-level evidence for an autoimmune etiology of epilepsy. JAMA Neurol 2014;71(5):569–74.

[43] Dafoulas GE, Toulis KA, McCorry D, Kumarendran B, Thomas GN, Willis BH, et al. Type 1 diabetes mellitus and risk of incident epilepsy: a population-based, open-cohort study. Diabetologia 2017;60(2):258–61.

[44] Chou IC, Wang CH, Lin WD, Tsai FJ, Lin CC, Kao CH. Risk of epilepsy in type 1 diabetes mellitus: a population-based cohort study. Diabetologia 2016;59(6):1196–203.

[45] Ramakrishnan R, Appleton R. Study of prevalence of epilepsy in children with type 1 diabetes mellitus. Seizure 2012;21(4):292–4.

[46] Keezer MR, Novy J, Sander JW. Type 1 diabetes mellitus in people with pharmacoresistant epilepsy: prevalence and clinical characteristics. Epilepsy Res 2015;115:55–7.

[47] Slingerland AS, Shields BM, Flanagan SE, Bruining GJ, Noordam K, Gach A, et al. Referral rates for diagnostic testing support an incidence of permanent neonatal diabetes in three European countries of at least 1 in 260,000 live births. Diabetologia 2009;52(8):1683–5.

[48] Gloyn AL, Pearson ER, Antcliff JF, Proks P, Bruining GJ, Slingerland AS, et al. Activating mutations in the gene encoding the ATP-sensitive potassium-channel subunit Kir6.2 and permanent neonatal diabetes. N Engl J Med 2004;350(18):1838–49.

[49] Babenko AP, Polak M, Cave H, Busiah K, Czernichow P, Scharfmann R, et al. Activating mutations in the ABCC8 gene in neonatal diabetes mellitus. N Engl J Med 2006;355(5):456–66.

[50] Hattersley AT, Ashcroft FM. Activating mutations in Kir6.2 and neonatal diabetes: new clinical syndromes, new scientific insights, and new therapy. Diabetes 2005;54(9):2503–13.

[51] Zwaveling-Soonawala N, Hagebeuk EE, Slingerland AS, Ris-Stalpers C, Vulsma T, van Trotsenburg AS. Successful transfer to sulfonylurea therapy in an infant with developmental delay, epilepsy and neonatal diabetes (DEND) syndrome and a novel ABCC8 gene mutation. Diabetologia 2011;54(2):469–71.

[52] Ashcroft FM. ATP-sensitive potassium channelopathies: focus on insulin secretion. J Clin Invest 2005;115(8):2047–58.

[53] Poulton CJ, Schot R, Kia SK, Jones M, Verheijen FW, Venselaar H, et al. Microcephaly with simplified gyration, epilepsy, and infantile diabetes linked to inappropriate apoptosis of neural progenitors. Am J Hum Genet 2011;89(2):265–76.

[54] Yiu WH, Yeung TL, Poon JW, Tsui SK, Fung KP, Waye MM. Transcriptional regulation of IER3IP1 gene by tumor necrosis factor-alpha and Sp family proteins. Cell Biochem Funct 2010;28(1):31–7.

[55] Bien CG, Scheffer IE. Autoantibodies and epilepsy. Epilepsia 2011;52(Suppl 3):18–22.

[56] Yoshimoto T, Doi M, Fukai N, Izumiyama H, Wago T, Minami I, et al. Type 1 diabetes mellitus and drug-resistant epilepsy: presence of high titer of anti-glutamic acid decarboxylase autoantibodies in serum and cerebrospinal fluid. Intern Med 2005;44(11):1174–7.

[57] Manto MU, Laute MA, Aguera M, Rogemond V, Pandolfo M, Honnorat J. Effects of anti-glutamic acid decarboxylase antibodies associated with neurological diseases. Ann Neurol 2007;61(6):544–51.

[58] Vincent A, Bien CG, Irani SR, Waters P. Autoantibodies associated with diseases of the CNS: new developments and future challenges. Lancet Neurol 2011;10(8):759–72.

[59] Liimatainen S, Peltola M, Sabater L, Fallah M, Kharazmi E, Haapala AM, et al. Clinical significance of glutamic acid decarboxylase antibodies in patients with epilepsy. Epilepsia 2010;51(5):760–7.

[60] Striano P, Errichiello L, Striano S. Autoantibodies to glutamic acid decarboxylase in patients with epilepsy: what is their clinical relevance? Epilepsy Behav 2011;20(1):145.

[61] Baekkeskov S, Aanstoot HJ, Christgau S, Reetz A, Solimena M, Cascalho M, et al. Identification of the 64K autoantigen in insulin-dependent diabetes as the GABA-synthesizing enzyme glutamic acid decarboxylase. Nature 1990;347(6289):151–6.

[62] Giometto B, Nicolao P, Macucci M, Tavolato B, Foxon R, Bottazzo GF. Temporal-lobe epilepsy associated with glutamic-acid-decarboxylase autoantibodies. Lancet 1998;352(9126):457.

[63] Northam EA, Rankins D, Cameron FJ. Therapy insight: the impact of type 1 diabetes on brain development and function. Nat Clin Pract Neurol 2006;2(2):78–86.

[64] Ho MS, Weller NJ, Ives FJ, Carne CL, Murray K, Vanden Driesen RI, et al. Prevalence of structural central nervous system abnormalities in early-onset type 1 diabetes mellitus. J Pediatr 2008;153(3):385–90.

[65] Fujioka M, Okuchi K, Hiramatsu KI, Sakaki T, Sakaguchi S, Ishii Y. Specific changes in human brain after hypoglycemic injury. Stroke 1997;28(3):584–7.

[66] Yoneda Y, Yamamoto S. Cerebral cortical laminar necrosis on diffusion-weighted MRI in hypoglycaemic encephalopathy. Diabet Med 2005;22(8):1098–100.

[67] Baviera M, Roncaglioni MC, Tettamanti M, Vannini T, Fortino I, Bortolotti A, et al. Diabetes mellitus: a risk factor for seizures in the elderly-a population-based study. Acta Diabetol 2017;54(9):863–70.

[68] Caietta E, Halbert C, Lepine A, Khammar A, Cano A, Gavaret M, et al. Association of type 1 diabetes mellitus and epilepsy in children. A cohort of 10 cases. Arch Pediatr 2012;19(1):9–16.

[69] McCorry D, Nicolson A, Smith D, Marson A, Feltbower RG, Chadwick DW. An association between type 1 diabetes and idiopathic generalized epilepsy. Ann Neurol 2006;59(1):204–6.

[70] Carter BL, Small RE, Mandel MD, Starkman MT. Phenytoin-induced hyperglycemia. Am J Hosp Pharm 1981;38(10):1508–12.

[71] Goldberg EM, Sanbar SS. Hyperglycemic, nonketotic coma following administration of dilantin (diphenylhydantoin). Diabetes 1969;18(2):101–6.

[72] Malherbe C, Burrill KC, Levin SR, Karam JH, Forsham PH. Effect of diphenylhydantoin on insulin secretion in man. N Engl J Med 1972;286(7):339–42.

[73] Kizer JS, Vargas-Gordon M, Brendel K, Bressler R. The in vitro inhibition of insulin secretion by diphenylhydantoin. J Clin Invest 1970;49(10):1942–8.

[74] Obembe A. Carbamazepine-induced diabetes mellitus. Cent Afr J Med 1991;37(3):96–8.

[75] Acikgoz M, Paksu MS, Guzel A, Alacam A, Alacam F. Severe carbamazepine intoxication in children: analysis of a 40-case series. Med Sci Monit 2016;22:4729–35.

[76] Jallon P, Picard F. Bodyweight gain and anticonvulsants: a comparative review. Drug Saf 2001; 24(13):969–78.

[77] Lima PA, Sampaio LP, Damasceno NR. Neurobiochemical mechanisms of a ketogenic diet in refractory epilepsy. Clinics (Sao Paulo) 2014;69(10):699–705.

[78] Dressler A, Reithofer E, Trimmel-Schwahofer P, Klebermasz K, Prayer D, Kasprian G, et al. Type 1 diabetes and epilepsy: efficacy and safety of the ketogenic diet. Epilepsia 2010;51(6):1086–9.

[79] Aguirre Castaneda RL, Mack KJ, Lteif A. Successful treatment of type 1 diabetes and seizures with combined ketogenic diet and insulin. Pediatrics 2012;129(2):e511–4.

[80] Aylward NM, Shah N, Sellers EA. The ketogenic diet for the treatment of myoclonic astatic epilepsy in a child with type 1 diabetes mellitus. Can J Diabetes 2014;38(4):223–4.

[81] Gribble FM, Reimann F. Sulphonylurea action revisited: the post-cloning era. Diabetologia 2003; 46(7):875–91.

[82] Shimomura K, Horster F, de Wet H, Flanagan SE, Ellard S, Hattersley AT, et al. A novel mutation causing DEND syndrome: a treatable channelopathy of pancreas and brain. Neurology 2007; 69(13):1342–9.

[83] Pearson ER, Flechtner I, Njolstad PR, Malecki MT, Flanagan SE, Larkin B, et al. Switching from insulin to oral sulfonylureas in patients with diabetes due to Kir6.2 mutations. N Engl J Med 2006;355(5):467–77.

[84] Slingerland AS, Nuboer R, Hadders-Algra M, Hattersley AT, Bruining GJ. Improved motor development and good long-term glycaemic control with sulfonylurea treatment in a patient with the syndrome of intermediate developmental delay, early-onset generalised epilepsy and neonatal diabetes associated with the V59M mutation in the KCNJ11 gene. Diabetologia 2006;49 (11):2559–63.

[85] Kanter IC, Huttner HB, Staykov D, Biermann T, Struffert T, Kerling F, et al. Cyclophosphamide for anti-GAD antibody-positive refractory status epilepticus. Epilepsia 2008;49(5):914–20.

[86] Mullur R, Liu YY, Brent GA. Thyroid hormone regulation of metabolism. Physiol Rev 2014;94(2):355–82.

[87] Pennell PB. Hormonal aspects of epilepsy. Neurol Clin 2009;27(4):941–65.

[88] Zhang YX, Shen CH, Lai QL, Fang GL, Ming WJ, Lu RY, et al. Effects of antiepileptic drug on thyroid hormones in patients with epilepsy: A meta-analysis. Seizure 2016;35:72–9.

[89] Jabbari B, Huott AD. Seizures in thyrotoxicosis. Epilepsia 1980;21(1):91–6.

[90] Song TJ, Kim SJ, Kim GS, Choi YC, Kim WJ. The prevalence of thyrotoxicosis-related seizures. Thyroid 2010;20(9):955–8.

[91] Hoffmann G, Dietzel ID. Thyroid hormone regulates excitability in central neurons from postnatal rats. Neuroscience 2004;125(2):369–79.

[92] Pekary AE, Sattin A. Regulation of TRH and TRH-related peptides in rat brain by thyroid and steroid hormones. Peptides 2001;22(7):1161–73.

[93] Obeid T, Awada A, al Rajeh S, Chaballout A. Thyroxine exacerbates absence seizures in juvenile myoclonic epilepsy. Neurology 1996;47(2):605–6.

[94] Aydin A, Cemeroglu AP, Baklan B. Thyroxine-induced hypermotor seizure. Seizure 2004;13(1):61–5.

[95] Larsen PR, Atkinson Jr. AJ, Wellman HN, Goldsmith RE. The effect of diphenylhydantoin on thyroxine metabolism in man. J Clin Invest 1970;49(6):1266–79.

[96] Rootwelt K, Ganes T, Johannessen SI. Effect of carbamazepine, phenytoin and phenobarbitone on serum levels of thyroid hormones and thyrotropin in humans. Scand J Clin Lab Invest 1978; 38(8):731–6.

[97] Caksen H, Dulger H, Cesur Y, Atas B, Tuncer O, Odabas D. Evaluation of thyroid and parathyroid functions in children receiving long-term carbamazepine therapy. Int J Neurosci 2003;113(9):1213–7.

[98] Vainionpaa LK, Mikkonen K, Rattya J, Knip M, Pakarinen AJ, Myllyla VV, et al. Thyroid function in girls with epilepsy with carbamazepine, oxcarbazepine, or valproate monotherapy and after withdrawal of medication. Epilepsia 2004;45(3):197–203.

[99] Verrotti A, Basciani F, Morresi S, Morgese G, Chiarelli F. Thyroid hormones in epileptic children receiving carbamazepine and valproic acid. Pediatr Neurol 2001;25(1):43–6.

[100] Yuksel A, Kartal A, Cenani A, Yalcin E. Serum thyroid hormones and pituitary response to thyrotropin-releasing hormone in epileptic children receiving anti-epileptic medication. Acta Paediatr Jpn 1993;35(2):108–12.

[101] Caksen H, Dulger H, Cesur Y, Odabas D, Tuncer O, Atas B. No effect of long-term valproate therapy on thyroid and parathyroid functions in children. Int J Neurosci 2002;112(11):1371–4.

[102] Shih FY, Chuang YC, Chuang MJ, Lu YT, Tsai WC, Fu TY, et al. Effects of antiepileptic drugs on thyroid hormone function in epilepsy patients. Seizure 2017;48:7–10.

[103] Simko J, Horacek J, Waberzinek G. Severe hypothyroidism as a complication of anticonvulsant treatment. Epilepsia 2004;45(3):292–3.

[104] Kose E, Guzel O, Demir K, Arslan N. Changes of thyroid hormonal status in patients receiving ketogenic diet due to intractable epilepsy. J Pediatr Endocrinol Metab 2017;30(4):411–6.

[105] Freeman ME, Kanyicska B, Lerant A, Nagy G. Prolactin: structure, function, and regulation of secretion. Physiol Rev 2000;80(4):1523–631.

[106] Ohman R, Walinder J, Balldin J, Wallin L. Prolactin response to electroconvulsive therapy. Lancet 1976;2(7992):936–7.

[107] Trimble MR. Serum prolactin in epilepsy and hysteria. Br Med J 1978;2(6153):1682.

[108] Sundararajan T, Tesar GE, Jimenez XF. Biomarkers in the diagnosis and study of psychogenic nonepileptic seizures: a systematic review. Seizure 2016;35:11–22.

[109] Parra A, Velasco M, Cervantes C, Munoz H, Cerbon MA, Velasco F. Plasma prolactin increase following electric stimulation of the amygdala in humans. Neuroendocrinology 1980;31(1):60–5.

[110] Nass RD, Sassen R, Elger CE, Surges R. The role of postictal laboratory blood analyses in the diagnosis and prognosis of seizures. Seizure 2017;47:51–65.

[111] Molaie M, Culebras A, Miller M. Nocturnal plasma prolactin and cortisol levels in epileptics with complex partial seizures and primary generalized seizures. Arch Neurol 1987;44(7):699–702.

[112] Chen DK, So YT, Fisher RS. Therapeutics, technology assessment subcommittee of the American Academy of N. Use of serum prolactin in diagnosing epileptic seizures: report of the therapeutics

and technology assessment subcommittee of the American Academy of Neurology. Neurology 2005;65(5):668–75.

[113] Verrotti A, Laus M, Coppola G, Parisi P, Mohn A, Chiarelli F. Catamenial epilepsy: hormonal aspects. Gynecol Endocrinol 2010;26(11):783–90.

[114] Scharfman HE, MacLusky NJ. The influence of gonadal hormones on neuronal excitability, seizures, and epilepsy in the female. Epilepsia 2006;47(9):1423–40.

[115] Herzog AG, Fowler KM, Sperling MR, Massaro JM, Progesterone Trial Study G. Distribution of seizures across the menstrual cycle in women with epilepsy. Epilepsia 2015;56(5):e58–62.

[116] Herzog AG, Klein P, Ransil BJ. Three patterns of catamenial epilepsy. Epilepsia 1997;38(10).1082–8.

[117] Duncan S, Read CL, Brodie MJ. How common is catamenial epilepsy? Epilepsia 1993;34(5):827–31.

[118] Herzog AG. Catamenial epilepsy: update on prevalence, pathophysiology and treatment from the findings of the NIH progesterone treatment Trial. Seizure 2015;28:18–25.

[119] Verrotti A, D'Egidio C, Agostinelli S, Verrotti C, Pavone P. Diagnosis and management of catamenial seizures: a review. Int J Womens Health 2012;4:535–41.

[120] Bangar S, Shastri A, El-Sayeh H, Cavanna AE. Women with epilepsy: clinically relevant issues. Funct Neurol 2016;31(3):127–34.

[121] Feely M, Gibson J. Intermittent clobazam for catamenial epilepsy: tolerance avoided. J Neurol Neurosurg Psychiatry 1984;47(12):1279–82.

[122] Herzog AG, Fowler KM, Smithson SD, Kalayjian LA, Heck CN, Sperling MR, et al. Progesterone vs placebo therapy for women with epilepsy: a randomized clinical trial. Neurology 2012; 78(24):1959–66.

[123] Navis A, Harden CA. Treatment approach to catamenial epilepsy. Curr Treat Options Neurol 2016;18(7):30.

Glossary

Diabetes mellitus　a spectrum of metabolic disorders that are characterized by chronic hyperglycemia resulting from impairment in insulin secretion, function, or both.

Hyperglycemic hyperosmolar state　a syndrome seen most frequently in type 2 diabetes mellitus that combines severe hyperglycemia (>33.3 mM), effective serum hyperosmolality (>320 mOsm/L), and dehydration in the absence of ketoacidosis.

Diabetic ketoacidosis　a syndrome that presents most often in type 1 diabetes mellitus as a triad of hyperglycemia (>13.9 mM), hyperketonemia, and metabolic acidosis.

Permanent neonatal diabetes mellitus　diabetes mellitus diagnosed within the first six months of life that is often associated with neurological manifestations.

Developmental delay, epilepsy, and neonatal diabetes syndrome　the most severe form of neurological manifestations associated with permanent neonatal diabetes mellitus, which comprise severe developmental delay, hypotonia, drug-resistant epilepsy, and mild dysmorphic features.

Anti-glutamic acid decarboxylase antibodies　antibodies directed against the enzyme involved in the synthesis of GABA, which may play a role in epilepsy associated with diabetes mellitus.

Thyrotoxicosis　a disorder of the thyroid gland that presents with elevated circulating thyroid hormones, suppressed thyroid-stimulating hormone, and clinical manifestations that may include epileptic seizures.

Prolactin　a polypeptide hormone synthesized and secreted by the lactotrophs of the anterior pituitary, which often shows elevated circulating levels after generalized tonic-clonic seizures and focal seizures with impaired awareness.

Catamenial epilepsy　a recurrent cyclical increase in epileptic seizure frequency during specific phases of the menstrual cycle, with phenotypes that comprise perimenstrual (C1), preovulatory (C2), and inadequate luteal (C3) phases of exacerbation.

CHAPTER 6

Epilepsy, coeliac disease and other inflammatory bowel diseases

Giuseppe Gobbi*, Paolo Mainardi[†], Pasquale Striano[‡], Alberto Preda[‡]
*IRCCS—Institute of Neurological Sciences of Bologna, Bologna, Italy
[†]Independent Researcher
[‡]Pediatric Neurology and Muscular Diseases Unit, DINOGMI-Department of Neurosciences, Rehabilitation, Ophthalmology, Genetics, Maternal and Child Health University of Genoa, "G. Gaslini" Institute, Genova, Italy

Contents

Abbreviations

AED	antiepileptic drugs
BBB	blood-brain barrier
CC	cerebral calcifications
CD	celiac disease
CEC	celiac disease, epilepsy, and cerebral calcifications
CNS	central nervous system
CrD	Crohn's disease
CSF	cerebrospinal fluid
CwG	convulsions associated with mild gastroenteritis
DGP	deamidated gliadin peptide
EMA	endomysial antibodies
ESPGHAN	European Society for Pediatric Gastroenterology, Hepatology, and Nutrition
GBA	gut-brain axis
GFD	gluten-free diet
GI	gluten intolerance

The Comorbidities of Epilepsy
https://doi.org/10.1016/B978-0-12-814877-8.00006-4

GS	gluten sensitivity
HLA	human leukocyte antigen
IBD	inflammatory bowel disease
IBS	irritable bowel syndrome
IL	interleukin
ILAE	International League Against Epilepsy
LNAA	large neutral amino acid
MGBA	microbiota gut-brain axis
NCGS	non-celiac gluten sensitivity
PCR	polymerase chain reaction
PNS	peripheral nervous system
SWS	Sturge-Weber syndrome
TG	transglutaminase
TNF	tumor necrosis factor
Trp	tryptophan
tTG	tissue-transglutaminase
UC	ulcerative colitis
WD	Whipple's disease

1. Introduction

The interactions between the gastrointestinal system and brain are a complex and complicated controversy and still a subject matter for discussion in large evolution. There are many neurologic, psychiatric, and behavioral disorders connected to pathologies of the gastrointestinal tract (GIT), liver, and pancreas. There is also a large number of theories concerning the biological basis of these interactions referring to the different organs of the gastrointestinal system.

Some inflammatory bowel diseases (IBDs), such as celiac disease (CD), ulcerative colitis (UC) and Crohn's disease (CrD) are associated with neurological symptoms, which can also forego the onset of the gastrointestinal manifestation of the disease. Particular attention was paid to CD and to gluten intolerance (GI) starting from the 1960s when the first evidence that CD could arise with extra intestinal manifestations [1], and the first comprehensive report of neurological manifestations in the context of histologically (jejunal biopsy) confirmed CD [2–4] were published [3,4]. Now, it is known that GI may present with extraintestinal signs even in absence of gastrointestinal symptoms [5–7], and, in addition, most patients present neurological manifestations of CD with no gastrointestinal symptoms [7].

Neurological manifestations can also be associated with IBDs (e.g., UC and CrD). Actually, there is a lower frequency of epilepsy in IBD conditions than in CD.

Despite the fact that for both CD and IBD there is a large amount of pathogenic hypothesis, according to the most recent acquisitions, it could be supposed that the most likely pathogenic basis of these comorbidities can be attributed to the inflammatory and autoimmune processes.

It is currently known that inflammatory responses in the brain parenchyma are associated with the etiopathogenesis of different acute and chronic neurological disorders, including epileptic seizures [8]. On the contrary, little is known about the contribution of peripheral inflammation in provoking inflammatory responses in the cerebral tissue. However, systemic inflammatory conditions have been shown to decrease seizure threshold in several experimental studies with administration of bacterial lipopolysaccharide [9], bacterial sonicates [10], different models of intestinal inflammation [11], and arthritis [12]. Moreover, it is recognized that an inflammatory bowel condition may affect the brain's physiological, behavioral, and cognitive functions (gut-brain axis (GBA)). An improving body of evidence has shown that gut microbes not only play an important role in maintaining normal healthy homeostasis but also affect the individual's mental health through stress reaction, inflammation, immune system, and particularly autoimmunity processes.

Autoimmune processes result from an aberrant immune response of the body against its own substances and tissues. The pathogenesis of autoimmune diseases has still not been determined, although factors such as the environment, drug, diet, genetics, and immune system are all deemed important provoking events. During the last decade, experimental research has demonstrated a main role of glial cells, which are activated by brain injury or proconvulsant events and release proinflammatory mediators, thus starting a cascade of inflammatory processes in brain tissue [13]. A substantial number of epilepsy cases have an autoimmune-related basis, and for these cases, additional immunotherapy was effective in slowing, halting, or even reversing the development of epilepsy and controlling seizures. Autoantibody specificities recognized in the epilepsy domain include, for example, voltage-gated potassium channel complex, N-methyl-D-aspartate receptor, and glutamic acid decarboxylase. Moreover, in epileptic patients, there are levels of proinflammatory cytokines, such as IL-6 and IFN-γ in the peripheral blood or IL-17A, both in the peripheral blood and in the cerebrospinal fluid (CSF), which are usually higher than those of control patients. It has been demonstrated that circulating cytokines (TNF-a, IL-1a, IL-6, IL1-b) may have proconvulsant action, altering neuronal excitability and promoting the generation or worsening of seizures and may contribute to neuronal cell loss, astrogliosis and blood-brain barrier (BBB) damage supporting the hypothesis that inflammation may play an active role in the pathophysiology of seizures and the associated neuropathology in human epilepsy [14–16].

Finally, a pathogenic noxa action could also be addressed, at the same time, both to brain and bowel. This is what possibly happens in Whipple's disease (WD) and in benign convulsions associated with mild gastroenteritis (CwG).

2. Epilepsy and celiac disease

2.1 Celiac disease and gluten intolerance

CD is a condition due to a permanent intolerance to gluten proteins (GI). Thanks to the latest discoveries on the immunology and genetics, the perception of CD has changed from a rather uncommon enteropathy to a common multiorgan disease with a strong genetic predisposition. Now CD is defined as an immune-mediated systemic disorder triggered by the ingestion of gluten (a heterogeneous mixture of glutenin and gliadin) and related prolamines (extrinsic trigger) in genetically susceptible individuals. It is characterized by the presence of a variable combination of gluten-dependent clinical manifestations and enteropathy with chronic inflammation in the wall of the small intestine and villous atrophy, and by CD-specific antibodies. CD-specific antibodies are against transglutaminase 2 (TG2) antibodies, endomysial antibodies (EMAs), and deamidated gliadin peptide (DGP) antibodies. Genetic susceptibility is associated with human leukocyte antigen (HLA class II) genes (genetic background): HLA-DQ2 has been found in 90% of CD patients and HLA-DQ8 in 10% of cases. Recently, nonHLA genetic factors have also been identified [17].

Clinically, CD may present with a large variety of specific and nonspecific signs and symptoms, such as chronic or intermittent diarrhea, failure to thrive, weight loss, stunted growth, delayed puberty, amenorrhea, iron-deficiency anemia, nausea or vomiting, chronic abdominal pain, cramping or distension, chronic constipation, chronic fatigue, recurrent aphthous stomatitis (mouth ulcers), dermatitis herpetiformis–like rash, fracture with inadequate traumas/osteopenia/osteoporosis, and abnormal liver biochemistry. There are also patients with a less clear clinical picture of gastroenterological involvement but with an increased risk for CD and who need, therefore, to be tested for CD. These patients may have type 1 diabetes mellitus, Down syndrome, autoimmune thyroid disease, Turner syndrome, Williams syndrome, selective immunoglobulin A (IgA) deficiency, autoimmune liver disease, otherwise unexplained neurological disorders including epilepsy, and first-degree relatives with CD [18].

In general, it has to be distinguished among the following:
- Active (typical) CD: sufficient symptoms to induce clinical suspicion of CD. Positive CD antibodies and biopsy findings.
- Silent CD: positive CD antibodies and biopsy findings, not sufficient clinical symptoms suggesting CD.
- Latent CD: positive CD antibodies, no villous atrophy. The patient had a gluten-dependent enteropathy and may or may not have symptoms.
- Potential CD: positive antibodies, but no villous atrophy. Patient may or may not have symptoms. CD may or may not develop.

Gluten sensitivity (GS) or non-celiac gluten sensitivity (NCGS) is defined as "a clinical entity induced by the ingestion of gluten leading to intestinal and/or extraintestinal symptoms that improve with GFD," once CD and wheat allergy are excluded [19,20].

Actually, NCGS is a controversial clinical condition, and some authors suggest that "non-celiac wheat sensitivity" is a more appropriate term since there is evidence that not only gliadin but also other proteins present in gluten and gluten-containing cereals (wheat, rye, barely, and their derivatives) may play a role in the development of the symptoms [20,21].

According to the European Society for Pediatric Gastroenterology, Hepatology, and Nutrition (ESPGHAN) Criteria [18], the laboratory testing for CD diagnosis includes the following: presence of IgA antitTG2 (tissue-transglutaminase type 2) antibodies, IgA EMA, and IgA and IgG DPG antibodies, positivity of HLA class II genes *(DQ2–DQ8)*, and jejunal mucosa villous atrophy, followed by resolution of villous atrophy (including clinical improvement) on a gluten-free diet (GFD), and relapse of villous atrophy (including clinical symptoms) withdrawing GFD.

In the case of children and adolescents with signs or symptoms that suggest CD and high antiTG2 titers with levels >10 times ULN, the likelihood for villous atrophy (Marsh 3) is high. In this situation it could be sufficient to perform EMA and HLA to make the diagnosis of CD without biopsy [18].

2.2 Celiac disease in epilepsy

The connection between CD and epilepsy is still now full of doubts; however, it seems possible that a cause-effect relation may exist, at least in some patients. Studies on the prevalence of CD in epileptic patients in an Italian population of children with epilepsy suggested that it is equal to the one of general population [22]. In a metaanalysis study, Lionetti et al. [23] demonstrated that the relative risk of epilepsy in individuals with CD, and of CD in individuals with epilepsy, compared to the general population, was close to zero, indicating that it was probably a chance association. Similar results have been confirmed in a southeast Serbia population of children with idiopathic epilepsy [24]. Nevertheless, a more detailed analysis of the reported cohorts of patients reveals that some conclusions could be misleading. For example, in a large multicenter series of 3969 children with CD, the prevalence of epilepsy was as high as 1%, although this falls within the range reported for the prevalence of epilepsy in the general pediatric population (0.6%–1.7%) [25]. Subgroup analysis, however, revealed that the prevalence of epilepsy increases from 0.79% of cases with typical CD diagnosed at the mean age of 5.9 years to 3.5% of those with silent CD diagnosed at the mean age of 10 years, suggesting that the later the diagnosis of the disease is made and the longer the time of exposure to gluten, the higher the risk of developing epilepsy. These results were indirectly confirmed by epidemiological studies of prevalence of CD in adult epileptic patients. In fact, Cronin et al. [26] screened for CD in a series of adult epileptic patients and found CD in 2.3% of them, and in a series of adult epileptic patients without known symptomatic etiology, Luostarinen et al. [27] showed CD in 2.5%, with 0.27% in the general population [28]. Conversely, Chapman et al. [29], studying the prevalence of epilepsy among adult CD patients, reported a prevalence of epilepsy of 5.5%. It is possible that in all these patients there was a late diagnosis of CD and, therefore, a prolonged exposure to gluten. In conclusion, these epidemiological studies seem to suggest that there may be a cause-effect interaction depending on the time of exposure to gluten in individuals genetically predisposed to GI. Consequently, in future epidemiological studies, it is mandatory to define the type of CD (i.e., typical, silent, and latent), if CD is treated or untreated, the age at diagnosis of CD, and the time of exposure to gluten before starting a GFD. In all these studies there is no mention to the type of epilepsy, while epilepsy is recognized to be a heterogeneous entity with multiple underlying etiologies. We found only three anecdotal studies. Labate et al. [30], investigating for CD by AgA and EmA antibodies 72 newly diagnosed epileptic patients with initial diagnosis of idiopathic partial epilepsy found silent CD in 9% of those with occipital epilepsy, suggesting a kind of genetic link between CD and childhood idiopathic epilepsy. Similarly, Işıkay and Kocamaz [31] studying the prevalence of CD in children with idiopathic epilepsy in southeast Turkey found that the prevalence of CD in children with idiopathic partial epilepsy with occipital paroxysms is higher than with other types of epilepsies. Peltola et al. [32], testing for CD in 48 consecutive patients with drug-resistant focal epilepsy, found that seven of them were gluten sensitive and all of these patients were affected by temporal lobe epilepsy with hippocampal sclerosis. Authors suggested that this previously unrecognized link between gluten sensitivity and temporal lobe epilepsy with hippocampal sclerosis should be added to the list of potential mechanisms leading to intractable epilepsy and hippocampal sclerosis.

2.2.1 Celiac disease, epilepsy, and cerebral calcifications syndrome

Special mention has to be reserved for celiac disease, epilepsy, and cerebral calcification (CEC) syndrome, a rare disorder, first described between 1988 and 1992 by Sammaritano et al. [33] and Gobbi et al. [34,35]. Less than 200 cases have been reported at present. This syndrome [36] is typically characterized by focal epilepsy, usually occipital in type, associated with occipital calcifications in patients affected by an unexpected silent or paucisymptomatic CD. In this condition, CD may appear at any time during a lifetime and it can evolve in silent or paucisymptomatic forms. The diagnosis is frequently made in late childhood, when specific investigations are led secondary to observation of epileptic seizures and cerebral calcifications (CCs). Epilepsy's onset is between infancy and adulthood; in most cases it occurs in early childhood. Most patients start with occipital epileptic seizures, but other varieties of focal seizures originating from temporal, rolandic, or frontal areas, and with secondary generalization, have been reported. Not better specified generalized seizures have also been reported in a few patients. CCs are bilateral, subcortical, roughly symmetrical, without contrast enhancement, and without brain atrophy. Typically located in the occipital regions, in some cases additional calcifications may be found in the frontal region, and scattered cases of unilateral occipital calcifications are reported. CCs are extremely varied in size. In a number of cases significant extension of calcifications was reported in a certain lapse, especially before GFD. In other patients calcifications appeared in new regions during evolution. Finally, some patients with an initial normal CT scan may develop bilateral parieto-occipital calcifications after the mean time of 1 year. The evolution is highly variable, with benign, drug-resistant, or epileptic encephalopathy forms. In the latter, severe intellectual deterioration and/or learning disorders have been reported. CD requires a lifetime observance of a GFD, leading to clinical and histopathological resolution of CD symptoms. Early diagnosis and good compliance of GFD greatly improve patients' outcome, can reverse the epileptic disorder, and decrease the risk of developing CCs [24,36].

Differential diagnosis of CEC includes Sturge-Weber syndrome (SWS) without nevus flammeus and other conditions, such as congenital folate malabsorption, or adverse effects of methotrexate, antifolate agents and radiotherapy of leukemic children.

Patients with CD and CCs without epilepsy are considered as having an incomplete form of CEC. Patients with epilepsy and CCs without CD are supposed to have a CEC with latent CD [36].

2.3 Pathophysiology of the interaction between epilepsy and celiac disease

Whether the association between epilepsy and CD is merely a coincidence, a genetic link, or a consequence of a cause-effect interaction is still an unresolved issue.

A genetic link with idiopathic occipital epilepsy seems to be suggested by the studies of Labate et al. and Işıkay and Kocamaz [30,31].

Concerning CEC syndrome, Tiacci et al. [37] suggested the hypothesis that CEC syndrome may be considered a separate genetically determined entity, similar to SWS phakomatosis. There has been a long discussion as to whether CEC syndrome is ethnically correlated to the Italian origin of patients. A census study of ethnic investigation [38] clearly demonstrated that this syndrome is generally found all over the world and that Argentine CEC patients and other cases reported outside of Italy do not have an Italian origin. Consequently, it may be considered that the high incidence of CEC cases in Italy is due to the high prevalence of CD in Italy and to the attention paid to this pathology in the clinical practice in Italy [39]. Finally, considering that most of the CEC patients are from the Mediterranean area (Italy and Spain) and Argentina, Martinez-Bermejo et al. [40] hypothesized that CEC syndrome could be considered a genetic, noninherited, ethnically and geographically restricted syndrome associated with environmental factors.

At present, the top-rated suggestion is that the association CD and epilepsy could depend on a cause-effect interaction on an autoimmune basis. In fact, CD is an autoimmune disease and may produce autoimmune responses even outside the GIT. In predisposed individuals, gliadin crosses the intestinal lining and accumulates under enterocytes inducing an immunological reaction against epithelial cells and damaging them. These damaged epithelial cells release the tTG, an enzyme which deamidates the native gliadin, inducing a gluten-specific D4+T lymphocytes activation. This immune response against gliadin damages the immune system and promotes a broad secretion of aggressive proinflammatory cytokines (INFg, TNFa, IL-1a, IL-1b, IL-2, IL-6) [41], which have proconvulsant action and may promote the generation of seizures. Circulating cytokines may also activate the tTG. Now we know that there are specific tTGs: TG2 is the auto-antigen in CD; TG3 is the autoantigen in dermatitis herpetiformis; and transglutaminase isoenzyme 6 (TG6) is primarily expressed in the central nervous system (CNS), and antibodies against TG6 have been detected in sera from patients with gluten ataxia [8]. Recently, high levels of immunoglobulin-A directed against TG6 were found in the serum of a patient with CEC syndrome [42].

On the one hand, these last data seem to be more and more compelling toward the supposition of a cause-effect interaction immunologically mediated between CD and epilepsy. On the other hand, the fact that there is such a strong preferential involvement of the occipital regions in the epileptogenic process remains unresolved. Considering the peculiar role of the proinflammatory and antiinflammatory cytokines in the chronic inflammation of the CNS (see further in this chapter), it could be suggested that the chronic damaged brain tissue by proinflammatory cytokines cannot be repaired by uncorrected antiinflammatory cytokines. The preferential regional brain involvement could be due to the different brain fragile areas, depending on a genetic basis.

In any case, it has to be certainly highlighted that in clinical practice it is important not to forget that most patients who have neurological manifestations of GI have no gastrointestinal symptoms and patients with CD might not have gastrointestinal symptoms either. Therefore, GI cannot just be diagnosed on a clinical basis. Several diagnostic tests are now available, and they can help to decide whether patients might have CD or GS with extraintestinal manifestations with or without enteropathy. Finally, an early diagnosis may improve the response to the GFD.

3. Epilepsy and other inflammatory bowel diseases

CrD and UC are idiopathic IBDs, and they are clearly distinct pathophysiological entities. UC, the most common form of IBD, is exclusively a colonic mucosa disease; it starts in the rectum and may extend proximally in a continuous manner throughout part or the entire colon, but usually it is less prone to complications and can be treated with colectomy. In contrast, CrD is a transmural disease of the gastrointestinal mucosa, which can affect the entire GIT from the mouth to the anus. The pathogenesis of IBD results from a complex interaction among symbiotic commensal microbiota with the host, oral tolerance, epithelial barrier function, antigen recognition, and immunoregulation by the innate and adaptive immune system. Several genes have also been identified [43,44].

The clinical presentations of CrD are widely variable, chronic diarrhea, abdominal pain, and weight loss being the most common onset symptoms. Bloody diarrhea is the characteristic symptom of UC [45]. CrD and UC should be considered systemic diseases since they are associated with clinical manifestations involving several organs outside the GIT tract (joints, skin, mouth, eyes) and coagulation system and either precede the onset of intestinal manifestations or appear and evolve in parallel with them.

Among the extraintestinal manifestations, the neurologic symptoms can involve both the peripheral nervous system (PNS) and the CNS. In general the neurological manifestations are rare but more common than previously estimated. Unfortunately, there are only a few systematic studies that have reviewed large groups of IBD patients to identify neurologic symptoms, and the available literature mainly consists of case reports and small series [46]. The major neurological complications are peripheral neuropathies, cerebrovascular disease, demyelinating disease (multiple sclerosis), restless legs syndrome, sensorineural hearing loss, optic neuritis, myasthenia gravis, whether in its ocular or generalized form [46–49].

Pathophysiologically, the neurological disorders associated with IBDs represent immune-mediated inflammatory process [50]. However, other causes, including prothrombotic and thrombotic complications [51], nutrient deficiency (vitamins, folate) due to malabsorption, and iatrogenic complications of medical and surgical management of IBDs, have also been suggested. In addition, in recent years, the use of tumor necrosis factor (TNF) inhibitors as treatment of refractory IBDs appear to predispose some patients to develop different peripheral and CNS symptoms.

The association between epilepsy and IBD is rare. On top of inflammation, seizures may be the symptoms of systemic or brain processes such as hypomagnesemia, cerebral venous thrombosis or vasculitis of the CNS [47,52], and implementation with magnesium and/or calcium in patients with seizures or tetany has also been suggested [53,54]. Coexistence of two genetically transmitted diseases, such as CrD and epilepsy, has also been suggested. Finally, according to the literature, epilepsy appears more frequently associated with CrD rather than with UC [55]. Under a semeiological point of view, the seizures may be generalized tonic-clonic, complex, simple partial, or even multifocal. However, they are clinical disorders that have to be thoroughly treated in order to prevent confusional states and epileptic encephalopathies [48]. Anecdotal status epilepticus has also been reported [56]. Very interesting is the case of a patient affected by CrD with epilepsy who reached a control of the seizures after fecal microbiota transplantation [57]. Even if this is just an anecdotal report, this finding might open a new window into disease mechanism focusing on the microbiota-GBA and inspire a new treatment for epilepsy through remodeling of gut microbiota.

In this review we have also to mention irritable bowel syndrome (IBS), which is the most commonly diagnosed gastrointestinal condition consisting of a functional bowel disorder with abdominal discomfort or pain in the absence of detectable structural and biochemical abnormalities, which generates a significant health care burden. Patients report the most distressing symptoms, such as abdominal pain, straining, myalgia, urgency, bloating, and feelings of serious illness. According to the updated Rome III criteria, IBS is a clinical diagnosis and presents as one of the three predominant subtypes: (1) IBS with constipation (IBS-C); (2) IBS with diarrhea (IBS-D); and (3) mixed IBS (IBS-M); former Rome definitions refer to IBS-M as alternating IBS (IBS-A) [58].

The risk of developing IBS increases six times after acute gastrointestinal infection. The use of antibiotics also appears to increase the risk of developing IBS. Further risk factors are young age, prolonged fever, anxiety, and depression. Psychological factors, such as depression or anxiety, have not been shown to cause or influence the onset of IBS, but may play a role in the persistence and perceived severity of symptoms. Nevertheless, they may worsen IBS symptoms and the patient quality of life. Chronic fatigue syndrome is also commonly present in these patients. A number of other comorbid conditions may occur more often than expected in subjects with IBS, including gastroesophageal reflux, genitourinary symptoms, fibromyalgia, headache, and backache.

The etiopathogenesis of IBS is still unknown. Important factors to the development of IBS include alterations of gut microbiome, intestinal permeability, gut immune function, motility, visceral sensation, brain-gut interactions, and psychosocial status. The concept of a dysregulated GBA has been adopted as a suitable model for the disorder. The gut microbiome may play an important role in the onset and exacerbation of symptoms in the disorder and has been extensively studied in this context. Research has shown that genetic defects in innate immunity and epithelial homeostasis increase the risk of developing both postinfectious and other forms of IBS [59].

The interactions between IBS and epilepsy have not been studied until some years ago. Just recently, Chen et al. [60], in a population-based cohort study, revealed that the IBS patients had greater cumulative incidence of epilepsy than the cohort without IBS (log-rank test, $P < 0.001$ and 2.54 vs 1.86 per 1000 person-years) and concluded that IBS seems to increase the risk of developing epilepsy, even if further studies are necessary to clarify whether IBS is a risk factor or an epiphenomenon for epilepsy development. More recently, Camara-Lemarroy et al. [61] compared 65 consecutive people with epilepsy with an age- and sex-healthy group control and found that IBS was significantly different between the groups (3% in controls and 16% in patients with epilepsy; $P = 0.04$). In these patients IBS did not appear to affect health-related quality of life but was associated with a greater burden of affective symptoms and insomnia.

3.1 The pathophysiological basis of the gut-brain interaction

3.1.1 Microbiota gut-brain axis

Microbiota gut-brain axis (MGBA) refers to a bidirectional information network between intestinal microbiota and brain. MGBA includes gut microbiota and their metabolic products, intestinal tract, enteric nervous system, sympathetic and parasympathetic branches within the autonomic nervous system, neural immune system, neuroendocrine system, and CNS [62] (Fig. 1).

Microbiome is the collection of all genomes of microbes in an ecosystem. Microbiota consists of the microbes that collectively inhabit a given ecosystem. A large number of different microbial species reside in the distal GIT. Surprisingly, each of us can be

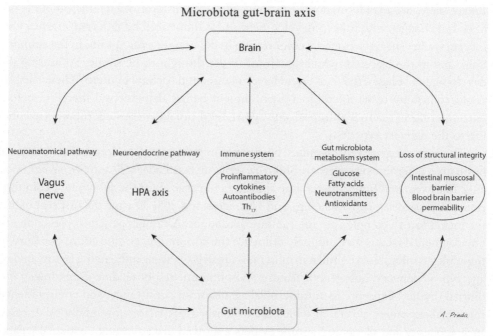

Fig. 1

identified more by the DNA of our gut microbes than by those of our cells (George Weinstock, Genoma Institute, Washington University).

In humans, the GIT represents a large microbial ecosystem, housing several trillion microbial cells. This microbiota plays a critical role in the development and continuous training of the host immune response (Th1 vs Th2 and Th17): it provides protection against pathogen overgrowth; it influences host cell proliferation and vascularization; it regulates intestinal endocrine functions, neurologic signaling and bone density; it provides a source of energetic biogenesis; it biosynthesizes vitamins, neurotransmitters, and multiple other compounds with targets yet unknown; it metabolizes bile salts; it reacts to or modifies specific drugs; and it eliminates exogenous toxins. The GIT is inhabited by trillions of microorganisms, comprising the human gut microbiota. Including roughly 9 million genes, this environment represents the human gut microbiome: a gene set 150 times larger than that of the human genome. The gut community comprises 5 phyla and 160 species in the larger intestine, weighing up to 2 kg. The dominant bacterial phyla are the *Firmicutes* (60%) and *Bacteriodetes* (20%), whereas *Actinobacteria, Proteobacteria,* and *Verrucomicrobia* are in relatively low abundance [63]. In the small intestine, there are typically high levels of acids, oxygen, and antimicrobials and a short transit time, and *Lactobacillaceae* is predominant. In contrast, in colonic conditions, the anaerobes with the ability to use complex carbohydrates, such as *Prevotellaceae, Lachnospiraceae* and

Rikenellaceae, are mainly predominant [63]. The composition of gut microbiota is not fixed but changes with human development and is influenced by different stress factors. Recent studies suggest a bacterial colonization in the nonpregnant uterus, in the amniotic fluid, and in the placenta, which previously were thought to be sterile. So, during the developmental phases, the fetus could have encountered bacteria in utero. These bacteria could contribute to its microbiota establishment before delivery and therefore before encountering all microorganisms from vaginal, fecal and cutaneous microbiotas, according to the delivery type [64].

The gut is progressively colonized by ingested environmental endotoxins and maternal facultative anaerobic or microaerophilic bacteria, such as *Lactobacilli* and *Streptococci*; soon after *Enterococci* and Enterobacteriacae appear, being crucial for the subsequent colonization of *Bifidobacteria*, *Bacteroides* spp., and *Clostridium* spp. [65]. During the first year of life, the infants form a complex gut microbiome like adults. Although genetic, epigenetic and environmental factors may uniquely influence the community composition, one third of the adult gut microbiota is similar in most individuals [66]. Some influencing factors are sex, age, type of delivery, host genetic features, host immune response, diet, drugs, infections, diurnal rhythm, exposure to antimicrobial agents, stool consistency, and environmental microbial exposures, several of which are established risk factors for childhood diseases, such as obesity and allergy [67]. Some evidence showed that stress (e.g., maternal separation) in the first few years of life could lead to changes of microbiota, and these changes may be a risk factor for stress-related disorders in adulthood [63]. Metabolome is defined as the set of metabolites (small molecules with molecular weight <1.5 kDa) produced or present in a biological system [68]. Metabolomics fits perfectly into the vision of system biology with a global approach and not guided by a priori hypothesis: it characterizes from a quantitative and qualitative point of view all metabolites present in a biological system and the interactions between them. Therefore, the "omic" science is considered the closest to phenotypic expression because it reflects both the information contained in the genetic code and the influences derived from interaction with the environment [69]. The metabolomics approach has been applied to several studies on the gut microbiota, mostly focused on the exploration of disease-related metabolites in order to obtain detailed information about the gut metabolic pathways. In other words, the way in which the gut microbiota interacts with the host metabolism and affects physiological or pathological conditions. Actually, gut microbiota dysbiosis is associated with diseases ranging from localized gastroenterologic disorders to neurologic, respiratory, metabolic, hepatic, and cardiovascular illnesses. The study of its composition helps to discriminate between unhealthy and healthy subjects. The identification of metabolites may highlight how lifestyle and dietary habits affect specific disease conditions.

In fact, the microbiota is more "medically" accessible and modifiable than the human genome, and this fact may provide a promising opportunity for preventing or treating neuropsychiatric conditions.

Over the past decade, both clinical and prenatal research showed that if the gut microbiota is damaged, there will be high-risk factors of suffering from mental illness and other CNS disorders. It has become clear that the bidirectional communication pathway between gut bacteria and the CNS, the microbiota gut-brain axis (MGBA), has a deep influence on key brain processes, such as neurotransmission, neuroinflammation, activation of the stress axes, and neurogenesis, modulating complex behaviors, such as social skills and anxiety. Gut bacteria influence these central processes through their ability to synthesize neurotransmitters (i.e., GABA, noradrenaline, and dopamine) and modulate activation of the immune system, along with their ability to produce metabolites, such as short-chain fatty acids (SCFAs), which possess neuroactive properties. Moreover, the gut microbiota and the brain are linked through neuroanatomical pathways, such as the vagus pathway, through the neuroendocrine-hypothalamic-pituitary-adrenal axis (HPA-axis), and through the modulation of key dietary amino acids, such as tryptophan (Trp). All these mechanism may also be involved in the regulation of emotions, behavior, stress response, and human brain healthy status [70] (Fig. 2).

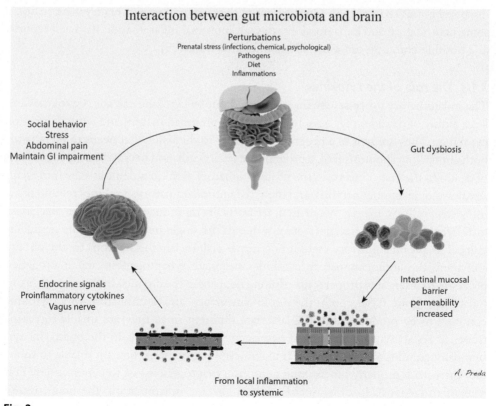

Fig. 2

3.1.2 Gut-brain axis: The role of inflammation in communicative processes between organs

It has been reported that systemic inflammation can trigger brain inflammation [71], only if BBB permeability result increased. Since BBB permeability is controlled by intestinal microbiota [72], it is clear how our microbes control all inflammation process in the brain. To better understand the underlying mechanisms, we have to refer to inflammation as a communicative process between organs, and repair is to be considered an object of communication.

Since long ago there has been evidence of the communicative ability of our organs. After 3 days, a traumatic brain injury produces the collapse of the intestinal membrane [73]. Moreover, the amount of gastric ulcers, induced by alcohol or stress, is seen to depend on the amount of epileptogenic agent (arecoline) directly injected into the brain [74]. This agent produces dose-dependent epileptic seizures; therefore, increasing the dose increases the number of seizures, and the same dose of alcohol produces more gastric ulcers. In the opposite direction, to produce an intestinal inflammation leads to a decrease in epileptogenic threshold [11]. This lowering of epileptogenic threshold is confirmed by the fact that there is an elevated risk of epilepsy in subjects affected by IBS, as previously discussed in this chapter [63]. On the basis of the common role of brain inflammation in some neurological and behavioral diseases, an intestinal inflammation has been reported as a possible common cause for all brain malfunctions [75].

3.1.3 The role of the cytokines

The inflammatory processes are mainly carried out by cytokine cascade. Cytokines are a large family of peptides that have been shared in proinflammatory and antiinflammatory cytokines. They are sent in a progressive manner to the tissue that needs to be repaired, both controlling apoptosis [76], a programmed cell death, and necrosis, an accidental type of death. In the case of necrosis, the proinflammatory cytokines demolish the more damaged tissues, increasing necrosis, and then, the antiinflammatory cytokines rebuild tissues using stem cells. Stem cells, when used, are normally reproduced. In CNS the mechanism is different, since brain functions are not due to the single neuron but to the neural circuits. The proinflammatory cytokines remove malfunctioning neurons by the circuits, and then, the antiinflammatory cytokines stimulate synaptogenesis and neurogenesis processes to insert new properly functioning neurons in the circuits. In the case of chronic inflammation in CNS, both the proinflammatory and antiinflammatory cytokines continue to be produced, but the latter are different since they are unable to rebuild tissues or restart synaptogenesis and neurogenesis processes [77]. In the brain, this type of inflammation is able to disconnect malfunctioning neurons, but it is unable to substitute them with properly functioning neurons (synaptogenesis) or to generate new neurons (neurogenesis). In other words, during chronic inflammation, the brain tissue is damaged by "corrected produced proinflammatory cytokines," but it is not repaired by "uncorrected antiinflammatory cytokines." For this reason "chronic inflammation" has been named "the mother of all diseases" [78]: it is an inflammation that is only able to damage. Interleukin-6 (IL-6) represents the turning point between proinflammatory and antiinflammatory cytokines: its cerebral high levels may be considered a marker of chronic inflammation [79] because IL-6 recalls the corrected antiinflammatory cytokines in place of those unable to work [80].

Cytokines also participate in neuronal development in brain functioning. Inappropriate activity can produce different neurological symptoms [81]. During pregnancy, the woman's intestinal microbiota undergoes deep changes, becoming similar to the one responsible for the metabolic syndrome [82], which in pregnancy are functional to the management of inflammatory processes necessary to create the tissues of the fetus. For 9 months, intestinal microbiota supports antiinflammatory processes [83]. If the woman experiences chronic inflammation during pregnancy, the tissues are created by cytokines that are unable to repair, so structural anatomical defects are generated, and, even if invisible, they are areas of future vulnerability. The impact on the offspring brain function of maternal stress during pregnancy is already known [84].

3.1.4 Gut microbiota in health and diseases
On PubMed we can find more than 4500 articles on the role of microbiota as moderator in health and diseases [67,85]. In fact, microbiota control tissue regenerative processes together with physiological functions like blood pressure, plasmatic cholesterol levels, heart and kidney functions, and neuroendocrine systems. An altered microbiota (dysbiosis) has been reported in metabolic diseases, amyotrophic lateral sclerosis, multiple sclerosis, autism, Parkinson's disease, and Alzheimer's disease. It has also been reported that different microbiota alterations can lead to different neurological diseases, such as Alzheimer's or Parkinson's disease. A different inflammatory response produces different brain damage. In detail, different types of intestinal dysbiosis, producing different inflammatory responses, may be the cause of different comorbidities between CD and other inflammatory intestinal diseases. In CD there is a low grade of chronic inflammation that is more prone to migrate and to damage other tissues than high-grade inflammations.

The interactions between intestinal microbiota and CD are complex and are not related to the topic of this paper. It is important to remember that CD patients with gastrointestinal symptoms are also known to have a different microbiota compared to patients with dermatitis herpetiformis and controls. A dysbiotic microbiota seems to be associated with persistent gastrointestinal symptoms in treated CD patients. There is an intestinal dysbiosis in CD patients, untreated and treated with a GFD, compared to healthy controls. In fact GFD itself influences gut microbiota composition, and thus constitutes an inevitable confusing factor in studies conducted in CD patients. Further studies have shown that the CD host genotype early selects colonizers of the infant's gut, which, together with environmental factors (e.g., breastfeeding, antibiotics, etc.), could influence the development of oral tolerance to gluten, and that some CD genes and/or their altered expression play a role in bacterial colonization and sensing. Conversely, intestinal dysbiosis could promote an abnormal response to gluten or other environmental CD-promoting factors (e.g., infections) in predisposed individuals [86]. Future studies on human gut microbiome, CD genetics, and possible genetic and environmental interactions, which are currently being carried out, may deeply change our knowledge on this matter.

3.1.5 Gut microbiota and epilepsy

An altered microbiota has been found in epileptic patients [87]. Gut microbiota in infants with refractory epilepsy is extremely different from that of healthy infants; epileptic patients harbored significantly enriched pathogens and decreased beneficial bacteria. In fact, the commensal bacteria in our GIT possess the ability to activate the proinflammatory Th cells in a controllable way without inducing extensive pathological inflammation; nonetheless, sometimes they may also drive our self-immune system to autoimmunity. Among these proinflammatory Th cells, Th17 cells have recently shown to be modulated by the symbiotic gut bacteria, such as *Bacteroidetes*, in a dynamic and reversible manner. Furthermore, germ-free rodents also had a decreased ability to trigger proinflammatory T-cell responses. Gut colonization with a single type of microbiota, SFB, was specifically capable of inducing Th17 cell differentiation and promoting IL-17 production either in the intestines or in other organs. Proinflammatory molecules synthesized from microbiota could act in the genesis of epilepsy, not only directly but also throughout the activation of glia. In fact, as already reported, circulating cytokines may have proconvulsant action and may play an active role in the pathophysiology of seizures [15–17].

An intestinal dysbiosis in epileptic patients, measured by urinary skatol and indican levels, a Trp metabolite, has been reported before the 1980s [88]. Oral loads of Trp-rich proteins in epileptic patients produce an increase in urinary indican levels, another Trp metabolite, and not in Trp plasmatic levels [89]. In epileptic patients it has been reported a low value of the Trp/LNAAs plasmatic ratio (LNAAs, large neutral amino acids). Since all LNAAs, Trp included, compete with the same BBB carrier, this plasmatic ratio controls Trp brain uptake rate and then the brain synthesis serotonin and melatonin. Starting from the plasmatic ratio Trp/LNAAs, a 32% reduction in brain influx rate, in epileptics respect controls, has been reported [90]. This decrease corresponds with an equal decrease in brain serotonin synthesis rate and drives our attention to the role of brain serotonin in seizure control [91].

Unfortunately, at present, despite the increased relevance of literature about this matter, there still is an evident gap between experimental and clinical evidence on the interaction between gut microbiota dysbiosis and epilepsy.

4. Epilepsy and Whipple's disease

WD is a very rare, chronic, infectious disease in which almost all organ systems of the body can be invaded by the rod-shaped bacterium *Tropheryma Whipplei* (*T. whipplei*). The disease is named after George Hoyt Whipple, who described the first case in 1907. Less than a thousand cases have been reported worldwide, and it has an annual incidence of less than one per million in Central European countries.

The circumstances facilitating this infection are unknown, however, a genetic or acquired immunological predisposition is suspected.

Clinical manifestations are protean (joint pain, fever, weight loss, abdominal pain, lymphadenopathies), and the diagnosis is often delayed. The clinical picture is variable, and the most frequent symptoms are the following: weight loss, polyarthritis, diarrhea/malabsorption, abdominal pain, fever, lymphadenopathy, cardiac valvular disease, culture-negative endocarditis, pleuritis, ocular inflammatory disease, and relapsing tenosynovitis. The different symptoms are not necessarily observed in each patient. The neurological symptoms of WD are also variable. Neurological manifestations include cognitive changes (56%–71%), of which 47% also includes psychiatric signs, abnormalities of eye movements, and involuntary movements, such as oculomasticatory myorhythmia and oculo-facial-skeletal myorhythmia (respectively 33%, 28%, and 20% of patients). These latter have been suggested as pathognomonic for CNS WD and were always accompanied by a supranuclear vertical gaze palsy [92]. Hypothalamic dysfunction, ataxia and myelopathy, cranial nerve abnormalities, sensory deficits uveitis, retinitis, optic neuritis, and papilledema have also been reported. Twenty percent of the reported cases have neurological symptoms without concurrent intestinal manifestation. Therefore, the disease may remain undiagnosed or misdiagnosed [93,94]. In fact, in the past many cases of CNS WD were not diagnosed up until postmortem [92]. Moreover, even though in the past neurological involvement has erroneously been considered a late manifestation of WD, it is frequently the initial clinical symptomatology of this disease and represents the greatest risk for long-term disability. Therefore, similar to the CD, this disease has to be studied and research has to be carried out.

Epileptic seizures are not frequent neurological manifestations of WD. However, due to the variability of the clinical manifestations of this disease, patients with epilepsy without any detectable cause associated with abdominal pain, fever, and weight loss should also be investigated for WD.

The application of a polymerase chain reaction (PCR) assay against Tropheryma whipplei has transformed the diagnosis, and nowadays, the gold standard diagnostic procedure for the diagnosis of WD is the biopsy of the duodenal mucosa through the demonstration of periodic acid–Schiff (PAS)-positive foamy macrophages. Tissue biopsy had positive results in 89% of the cases [92]. However, false positive and false negative results can arise [92]. The diagnosis of cerebral WD should be ascertained by a positive PCR for *T. whipplei* in CSF.

Possible CNS WD should be diagnosed in the setting of unexplained systemic symptoms and neurological signs (supranuclear vertical gaze palsy, rhythmic myoclonus, dementia with psychiatric symptoms, or hypothalamic manifestations). Patients with possible CNS Whipple's disease should undergo small-bowel biopsy [92]. In WD patients without neurological signs at the time of diagnosis, the CSF should be examined and evaluated for CNS WD in every patient and before antibiotic treatment [93].

CT and MR images of the CNS are normal or not specific: atrophic changes, mass lesions, focal abnormalities, and hydrocephalus.

All patients must be treated with antibiotics that cross the BBB. PCR is recognized to be a useful tool for monitoring progress, but it is sometimes difficult to reverse established neurological defects [93]. All patients should be treated and monitored as if they had CNS disease even if they are asymptomatic [93]. A long-term antibiotic treatment is required, and relapses may occur after withdrawal of antimicrobial therapy [50].

5. Benign convulsions associated with mild gastroenteritis

Benign convulsions associated with mild gastroenteritis (CwG) is a new epileptic condition that is not yet categorized by the International League Against Epilepsy (ILAE) [95]. Morooka in 1982 (reported by Verrotti et al. [96]), first described the occurrence of afebrile seizures in infants and children suffering from a mild gastroenteritis without triggering factors, such as dehydration, electrolyte imbalance, or hypoglycemia. Thereafter, this association has been extensively reported in the Far East, where it is well acknowledged as a distinct clinical entity referred to as CwG. Recently, CwG have been increasingly recognized even from nonAsian countries, demonstrating the worldwide distribution of this condition [96].

CwG occur in 3.5%–6.4% of any gastroenteritis. Age at onset ranges between 2 months and 6 years, with a peak between 12 and 24 months. The seizures show a seasonal distribution in winter and spring, which is related to the higher incidence of viral gastroenteritis during these months due to temperate climates. The interval between the onset of gastroenteritis and the onset of seizures ranges from 0 to 6 days, but the seizures may sometimes precede the onset of diarrhea by 24 h. Typically, seizures are focal seizures with secondary generalization, with an EEG focal onset originating from different cerebral regions (mostly parieto-occipital ones). The brief focal manifestations at the beginning of the seizures may be often overlooked, especially by parents, and this may lead to a misdiagnosis of generalized seizures. The seizures are isolated or in cluster lasting 24–48 h (2–20 seizures per episode). The duration of the seizures is short in most of the patients, although prolonged seizures or status epilepticus have been observed. The interictal EEG is normal in most of the cases [96,97].

The seizures may be the result of a transient alteration of neuronal excitability caused by some factors related to viral gastroenteritis. A direct viral invasion of the CNS may be supposed for rotavirus, the most common agent involved in CwG. Actually, rotaviral antigen and ribonucleic acid (RNA) have been detected in the stool, serum, and CSF in about half of the children with CwG [97]. Rotavirus RNA has also been detected in CSF whenever tested by reverse-transcriptase PCR. Other infectious agents, such as norovirus, adenovirus, sapovirus, shigella, and salmonella, have been also identified. Genetic susceptibility may be suggested by the frequent incidence of epileptic disorders in the family history of children with CwG and by family cases of CwG [96].

The clinical outcome of CwG is excellent, and children completely recover in a few days without neurological sequelae. The psychomotor development remains normal at follow-up evaluation. Given the episodic nature of CwG, their short duration, and the good prognosis, a prophylactic antiepileptic therapy and chronic antiepileptic drug (AED) administration are not necessary [96,97].

Even if this condition is not yet recognized by ILAE, probably because of the lack of high evidence that seizures are attributable to gastroenteritis, and since this association might be even random, considering the high frequency of diarrheal illness in children, the recognition of the symptoms of gastroenteritis in infants and children with a first epileptic seizure avoids intensive examinations and long-term AED treatment and gives correct prognostic information to parents.

6. Conclusion

It goes without saying that there is a link between intestinal disorders and epilepsy or epileptic manifestations.

This could come from pathogenic noxa, which acts simultaneously against both brain and bowel. This possibility has to be considered in case of children with epileptic convulsions during a gastroenteritis event and in case of the extremely rare WD.

Surely, there is also a link between epilepsy and CD, however it is under discussion which etiopathogenic basis of this comorbidity could be. Whether this association is merely a coincidence, a genetic link, or a consequence of a cause-effect interaction is still far from being demonstrated. At present, the top-rated suggestion is that CD and epilepsy association could depend on a cause-effect interaction on autoimmune basis via a proconvulsant action of proinflammatory cytokines resulting from immune response against epithelial cells induced by gliadin in predisposed individuals.

The relation between CD and intestinal microbiota is the object of many studies that can certainly improve our knowledge about the cause of this comorbidity connected with epilepsy. Whatever the cause, the presence of CD should always be considered in patients having focal epilepsy, especially if it concerns the occipital lobe. Many individuals predisposed to CD may have no gastrointestinal symptoms, apart from epilepsy or other neurological symptoms.

Epilepsy is a rare comorbidity in IBD (CrD and UC), whereas patients with IBS have greater cumulative incidence of epilepsy than the cohort without IBS. Nowadays, this link is considered to be depending on GBA, a bidirectional communication between the central and the enteric nervous system, connecting emotional and cognitive centers of the brain with peripheral intestinal functions. Both clinical evidence and recent advances in experimental research suggest that enteric microbiota has an important impact on GBA interaction, not only with intestinal cells and the enteric nervous system but also directly with CNS. In clinical practice, evidence of MGBA interactions comes from the association of dysbiosis or functional gastrointestinal disorders like the IBS with several CNS disorders. Among them epilepsy is the less frequent associated condition, but it is also true that an altered microbiota was found in epileptic patients and that gut microbiota in infants with refractory epilepsy is extremely different from that of healthy infants. Proinflammatory circulating cytokines, synthesized from microbiota in case of inflammation, may have proconvulsant action and may act in the genesis of epilepsy, not only directly but also throughout the activation of glia.

There is a need for further work to clarify the exact and complicated interactions among brain, gut, and microbiota in order to understand the etiopathogenetic events. Microbiota alterations may precede, but also may follow, the onset of the different neuropsychiatric diseases, epilepsy included, and can represent the cause but also the consequence of neurological disorders.

To conclude, due to the extremely high degree of phenotypic heterogeneity in neuropsychiatric disorders originating from the interaction between environmental risk factors and susceptible genetic loci, future studies on human gut microbiome and possible genetic and environmental interactions may deeply change our knowledge on this matter.

References

[1] Marks J, Shuster S, Watson AJ. Small bowel changes in dermatitis herpetiformis. Lancet 1966;1280–2.
[2] Cooke WT, Thomas-Smith W. Neurological disorders associated with adult coeliac disease. Brain 1966;89:683–722.
[3] Hadjivassiliou M, Mäki M, Sanders DS, Williamson CA, Grünewald RA, Woodroofe NM, Korponay-Szabó IR. Autoantibody targeting of brain and intestinal transglutaminase in gluten ataxia. Neurology 2006;66(3):373–7.
[4] Holmes GKT. Long-term health risks for unrecognized coeliac patients. In: Auricchio S, Visakorp JK, editors. Common food intolerances1: epidemiology of coeliac disease. Dynamic nutrition research Basel: Karger; 1992. p. 105–18.
[5] Maki M, Holm K, Collin P, Savilahti E. Increase in gamma deltaT cell receptor bearing lymphocytes in normal small bowel mucosa in latent coeliac disease. Gut 1991;21:1412–4.
[6] Corazza GR, Biagi F, Andfreani ML, Gasbarrini G. Clinical and biological characteristics of gluten intolerance. In: Gobbi G, Andermann F, Naccarato S, Banchini G, editors. Epilepsy and other neurological disorders in coeliac disease. London: Libbey; 1997. p. 7–12.
[7] Hadjivassiliou M, Sanders DS, Grünewald RA, Woodroofe N, Boscolo S, Aeschlimann D. Gluten sensitivity: from gut to brain. Lancet Neurol 2010;9(3):318–30.

[8] Vezzani A, French J, Bartfai T, Baram TZ. Nat Rev Neurol 2011;7(1):31–40.

[9] Sayyah M, Javad-Pour M, Ghazi-Khansari M. The bacterial endotoxin lipopolysaccharide enhances seizure susceptibility in mice: involvement of proinflammatory factors: nitric oxide and prostaglandins. Neuroscience 2003;122(4):1073–80.

[10] Balter-Seri J, Yuhas Y, Weizman A, Nofech-Mozes Y, Kaminsky E, Ashkenazi S. Role of nitric oxide in the enhancement of pentylenetetrazole-induced seizures caused by Shigella dysenteriae. Infect Immun 1999;67(12):6364–8.

[11] Riazi K, Honar H, Homayoun H, Demehri S, Bahadori M, Dehpour AR. Intestinal inflammation alters the susceptibility to pentylenetetrazole-induced seizure in mice. J Gastroenterol Hepatol 2004;19(3):270–7.

[12] Rao RS, Medhi B, Saikia UN, Arora SK, Toor JS, Khanduja KL, Pandhi P. Experimentally induced various inflammatory models and seizure: understanding the role of cytokine in rat. Eur Neuropsychopharmacol 2008;18(10):760–7.

[13] Vezzani A, Aronica E, Mazarati A, Pittman QJ. Epilepsy and brain inflammation. Exp Neurol 2013;244:11–21.

[14] Vezzani A, Moneta D, Richichi C, Aliprandi M, Burrows SJ, Ravizza T, Perego C, De Simoni MG. Functional role of inflammatory cytokines and antiinflammatory molecules in seizures and epileptogenesis. Epilepsia 2002;43(Suppl 5):30–5.

[15] Ravizza T, Gagliardi B, Noé F, Boer K, Aronica E, Vezzani A. Innate and adaptive immunity during epileptogenesis and spontaneous seizures: evidence from experimental models and human temporal lobe epilepsy. Neurobiol Dis 2008;29:142–60.

[16] Vezzani A, Balosso S, Ravizza T. The role of cytokines in the pathophysiology of epilepsy. Brain Behav Immun 2008;22:797–803.

[17] Sharma A, Liu X, Hadley D, Hagopian W, Liu E, Chen WM, Onengut-Gumuscu S, Simell V, Rewers M, Ziegler AG, Lernmark Å, Simell O, Toppari J, Krischer JP, Akolkar B, Rich SS, Agardh D, She JX, TEDDY study group. Identification of non-HLA genes associated with celiac disease and country-specific differences in a large, international pediatric cohort. PLoS One 2016;11 (3):1–20.

[18] Husby S, Koletzko S, Korponay-Szabó IR, Mearin ML, Phillips A, Shamir R, Troncone R, Giersiepen K, Branski D, Catassi C, Lelgeman M, Mäki M, Ribes-Koninckx C, Ventura A, Zimmer KP, ESPGHAN Working Group on Coeliac Disease Diagnosis, ESPGHAN Gastroenterology Committee, European Society for Pediatric Gastroenterology, Hepatology, and Nutrition. European Society for Pediatric Gastroenterology, Hepatology, and Nutrition guidelines for the diagnosis of coeliac disease. J Pediatr Gastroenterol Nutr 2012;54(1):136–60.

[19] Ludvigsson JF, Leffler DA, Bai JC, Biagi F, Fasano A, Green PH, Hadjivassiliou M, Kaukinen K, Kelly CP, Leonard JN, Lundin KE, Murray JA, Sanders DS, Walker MM, Zingone F, Ciacci C. The Oslo definitions for coeliac disease and related terms. Gut 2013;62(1):43–52.

[20] Fasano A, Sapone A, Zevallos V, Schuppan D. Non-celiac gluten sensitivity. Gastroenterology 2015;148(6):1195–204.

[21] Schuppan D, Pickert G, Ashfaq-Khan M, Zevallos V. Non-celiac wheat sensitivity: differential diagnosis, triggers and implications. Best Pract Res Clin Gastroenterol 2015;29(3):469–76.

[22] Giordano L, Valotti M, Bosetti A, Accorsi P, Caimi L, Imberti L. Celiac disease-related antibodies in Italian children with epilepsy. Pediatr Neurol 2009;41(1):34–6.

[23] Lionetti E, Francavilla R, Pavone P, Pavone L, Francavilla T, Pulvirenti A, Giugno R, Ruggieri M. The neurology of coeliac disease in childhood: what is the evidence? A systematic review and meta-analysis. Dev Med Child Neurol 2010;52(8):700–7.

[24] Djurić Z, Nagorni A, Jocić-Jakubi B, Dimić M, Novak M, Milićević R, Radenković G. Celiac disease prevalence in epileptic children from Serbia. Turk J Pediatr 2012;54(3):247–50.

[25] Vascotto M, Fois A. Epilepsy and coeliac disease. A collaborative study. In: Gobbi G, Andermann F, Naccarato S, Banchini G, editors. Epilepsy and other neurological disorders in coeliac disease. London: Libbey; 1997. p. 105–10.

[26] Cronin CC, Jackson ML, Feighery C, Shanahan F, Abuzakouk M, Rider DQ, et al. Coeliac disease and epilepsy. QJM 1998;91:303–8.

[27] Luostarinen L, Dastidar P, Collin P, Peraaho MM, Erila T, Pirttila T. Association between coeliac disease, epilepsy and brain atrophy. Eur Neurol 2001;46:187–91.

[28] Collin P, Reunala T, Rasmussen M, Kyronpalo S, Pehkonen E, Laippala P. High incidence and prevalence of adult coeliac disease: augmented diagnostic approach. Scand J Gastroenterol 1997; 30:1129–33.

[29] Chapman WR, Laidlow JM, Colin-Jones D, Eade OE, Smith CL. Increased prevalence of epilepsy in coeliac disease. Br Med J 1978;2(6132):250–1.

[30] Labate A, Gambardella A, Messina D, Tammaro S, Le Piane E, Pirritano D, et al. Silent celiac disease in patients with childhood localization-related epilepsies. Epilepsia 2001;42:1153–5.

[31] Işıkay S, Kocamaz H. Prevalence of celiac disease in children with idiopathic epilepsy in Southeast Turkey. Pediatr Neurol 2014;50(5):479–81.

[32] Peltola M, Kaukinen K, Dastidar P, Haimila K, Partanen J, Haapala AM, Mäki M, Keränen T, Peltola J. Hippocampal sclerosis in refractory temporal lobe epilepsy is associated with gluten sensitivity. J Neurol Neurosurg Psychiatry 2009;80(6):626–30.

[33] Sammaritano M, Andermann F, Melanson D, Guberman A, Tinuper P, Gastaut H. The syndrome of intractable epilepsy, bilateral occipital calcifications and folic acid deficiency. Neurology 1988;38(Suppl 1):239.

[34] Gobbi G, Sorrenti G, Santucci M, Giovanardi Rossi P, Ambrosetto P, Michelucci R, Tassinari CA. Epilepsy with bilateral occipital calcifications: a benign onset with progressive severity. Neurology 1988;38:913–20.

[35] Gobbi G, Bouquet F, Greco L, Lambertini A, Tassinari CA, Ventura A, Zaniboni MG. Coeliac disease, epilepsy and cerebral calcifications. Lancet 1992;340:439–43.

[36] Gobbi G. Coeliac disease, epilepsy and cerebral calcifications. Brain Dev 2005;27:189–200.

[37] Tiacci C, D'Alessandro P, Cantisani TA, Piccirilli M, Signorini E, Pelli MA, et al. Epilepsy with bilateral occipital calcifications: Sturge-Weber variant or a different encephalopathy? Epilepsia 1993;34:528–39.

[38] Gobbi G, Bertani G. Coeliac disease and epilepsy. In: Gobbi G, Andermann F, Naccarato S, Banchini G, editors. Epilepsy and other neurological disorders in coeliac disease. London: Libbey; 1997. p. 65–80.

[39] Greco I, Maki M, Di Donato F, VisaKorpi JK. Epidemiology of coeliac diseases in Europe and Mediterranean area. In: Auricchio S, Visakorpi JK, editors. Common food intolerances: epidemiology of coeliac disease. Basel: Karger; 1992. p. 25–44.

[40] Martinez-Bermejo A, Polanco I, Royo A, Lopez-Martin V, Arcas J, Tendero A, Fernández-Jaén A, Pascual-Castroviejo I. A study of Gobbi's syndrome in Spanish population. Rev Neurol 1999;29:105–10.

[41] Durum SK, Oppenheim JJ. Proinflammatory cytokines and immunity. In: Paul WE, editor. Fundamental immunology. 3rd ed. New York, NY: Raven Press; 1993. p. 801–36.

[42] Dale RC, Wienholt L, Hadjivassiliou M, Aeschlimann D, Lawson JA. Coeliac disease, epilepsy, and cerebral calcifications: association with TG6 autoantibodies. Dev Med Child Neurol 2013;55 (1):90–3.

[43] Baumgart DC, Carding SR. Inflammatory bowel disease: cause and immunobiology. Lancet 2007;369:1627–40.

[44] Abraham C, Cho JH. Inflammatory bowel disease. N Engl J Med 2009;361:2066–78.

[45] Ordás I, Eckmann L, Talamini M, Baumgart DC, Sandborn WJ. Ulcerative colitis. Lancet 2012;380 (9853):1606–19.

[46] Morís G. Inflammatory bowel disease: an increased risk factor for neurologic complications. World J Gastroenterol 2014;20(5):1228–37.

[47] Benavente L, Morís G. Neurologic disorders associated with inflammatory bowel disease. Eur J Neurol 2011;18(1):138–43.

[48] Zois CD, Katsanos KH, Kosmidou M, Tsianos EV. Neurologic manifestations in inflammatory bowel diseases: current knowledge and novel insights. J Crohn's Colitis 2010;4(2):115–24.

[49] Ferro JM, Oliveira SN, Correia L. Neurologic manifestations of inflammatory bowel diseases. Handb Clin Neurol 2014;120:595–605.

[50] Dietrich W, Erbguth F. Neurological complications of inflammatory intestinal diseases. Fortschr Neurol Psychiatr 2003 Aug;71(8):406–14.

[51] Akobeng AK, Miller V, Thomas AG. Epilepsy and Crohn's disease in children. J Pediatr Gastroenterol Nutr 1998;26(4):458–60.

[52] Fernández-Rodríguez E, Camarero-González E. Patient with Crohn's disease and seizures due to hypomagnesemia. Nutr Hosp 2007;22(6):720–2.

[53] Millán-Lorenzo M, Ferrero-León P, Castro-Fernández M, Ampuero-Herrojo J, Rojas-Feria M, Romero-Gómez M. Tetany and convulsions: onset symptoms in Crohn's disease. Rev Esp Enferm Dig 2014;106(8):564–6.

[54] Schluter A, Krasnianski M, Krivokuca M, Spielmann RP, Neudecker S, Hirsch W. Magnetic resonance angiography in a patient with Crohn's disease associated with cerebral vasculitis. Clin Neurol Neurosurg 2004;106:110–3.

[55] Greenstein AJ, Janowitz HD, Sachar DB. The extra-intestinal complications of Crohn's disease and ulcerative colitis: a study of 700 patients. Medicine (Baltimore) 1976;55:401–12.

[56] Akhan G, Andermann F, Gotman MJ. Ulcerative colitis, status epilepticus and intractable temporal seizures. Epileptic Disord 2002;4(2):135–7.

[57] He Z, Cui B-T, Zhang T, Li P, Long C-Y, Ji G-Z, Zhang F-M. Fecal microbiota transplantation cured epilepsy in a case with Crohn's disease: the first report. World J Gastroenterol 2017;23(19):3565–8.

[58] Saha L. Irritable bowel syndrome: pathogenesis, diagnosis, treatment, and evidence-based medicine. World J Gastroenterol 2014;20(22):6759–73.

[59] Kennedy PJ, Cryan JF, Dinan TG, Clarke G. Irritable bowel syndrome: a microbiome-gut-brain axis disorder? World J Gastroenterol 2014;20(39):14105–25.

[60] Chen CH, Lin CL, Kao CH. Irritable bowel syndrome increases the risk of epilepsy: a population-based study. Medicine (Baltimore) 2015;94(36).

[61] Camara-Lemarroy CR, Escobedo-Zúñiga N, Ortiz-Zacarias D, Peña-Avendaño J, Villarreal-Garza E, Díaz-Torres MA. Prevalence and impact of irritable bowel syndrome in people with epilepsy. Epilepsy Behav 2016;63:29–33.

[62] Wang HX, Wang YP. Gut microbiota-brain axis. Chin Med J (Engl) 2016;129(19):2373–80.

[63] Thursby E, Juge N. Introduction to the human gut microbiota. Biochem J 2017;474:1823–36.

[64] Collado MC, Rautava S, Aakko J, Isolauri E, Salminen S. Human gut colonisation may be initiated in utero by distinct microbial communities in the placenta and amniotic fluid. Sci Rep 2016;6:23129.

[65] Rodriguez JM, Murphy K, Stanton C, Ross RP, Kober OI, Juge N, Avershina E, Rudi K, Narbad A, Jenmalm MC, Marchesi JR, Collado MC. The composition of the gt microbiota throughout life, with an emphasis on early life. Microb Ecol Health Dis 2015;26:26050.

[66] Codella R, Luzi L, Terruzzi I. Exercise has the guts: how physical activity may positively modulate gut microbiota in chronic and immune-based disease. Dig Liver Dis 2018;50(4):331–41.

[67] Lynch SV, Pedersen O. The human intestinal microbiome in health and disease. N Engl J Med 2016;375:2369–79.

[68] Carraro S, Giordano G, Reniero F, et al. Metabolomics: a new frontier for research in pediatrics. J Pediatr 2009;154:638–44.

[69] Hollywood K, Brison DR, Goodacre R. Metabolomics: current technologies and future trends. Proteomics 2006;6:4716–23.

[70] Vernocchi P, Del Chierico F, Putignani L. Gut microbiota profiling: metabolomics based approach to unravel compounds affecting human health. Front Microbiol 2016;7:1144.

[71] Bañuelos-Cabrera I, Valle-Dorado MG, Aldana BI, Orozco-Suárez SA, Rocha L. Role of histaminergic system in blood-brain barrier dysfunction associated with neurological disorders. Arch Med Res 2014;45(8):677–86.

[72] Braniste V, Al-Asmakh M, Kowal C, Anuar F, Abbaspour A, Tóth M, Korecka A, Bakocevic N, Ng LG, Kundu P, Gulyás B, Halldin C, Hultenby K, Nilsson H, Hebert H, Volpe BT, Diamond B, Pettersson S. The gut microbiota influences blood-brain barrier permeability in mice. Sci Transl Med 2014;6(263):263ra158.

[73] Hang CH, Shi JX, Li JS, Wu W, Yin HX. Intestinal mucosa structure after TBI. World J Gastroenterol 2003;9(12):2776–81.

[74] Hung CR, Cheng JT, Shih CS. Gastric mucosal damage induced by arecoline seizure in rats. Life Sci 2000;66(24):2337–49.

[75] Casella G, Tontini GE, Bassotti G, Pastorelli L, Villanacci V, Spina L, Baldini V, Vecchi M. Neurological disorders and inflammatory bowel diseases. World J Gastroenterol 2014;20(27):8764–82.

[76] Hausmann M. How bacteria-induced apoptosis of intestinal epithelial cells contributes to mucosal inflammation. Int J Inflamm 2010;2010:1–9.

[77] Andreasen AS, Krabbe KS, Krogh-Madsen R, Taudorf S, Pedersen BK, Møller K. Human endotoxemia as a model of systemic inflammation. Curr Med Chem 2008;15(17):1697–705.

[78] Bengmark S. Acute and "chronic" phase reaction—a mother of disease. Clin Nutr 2004;23:1256–66.

[79] Zubarev OE, Klimenko VM. Elevation of proinflammatory cytokines level at early age as the risk factor of neurological and mental pathology development. Ross Fiziol Zh Im I M Sechenova 2011;97 (10):1048–59.

[80] Monje M, Toda H, Palmer T. Inflammatory blockade restores adult hippocampal neurogenesis. Science 2003;302:1760–5.

[81] Goines PE, Ashwood P. Cytokine dysregulation in autism spectrum disorders (ASD): possible role of the environment. Neurotoxicol Teratol 2013;36:67–81.

[82] Koren O, Goodrich JK, Cullender TC, Spor A, Laitinen K, Bäckhed HK, Gonzalez A, Werner JJ, Angenent LT, Knight R, Bäckhed F, Isolauri E, Salminen S, Ley RE. Host remodeling of the gut microbiome and metabolic changes during pregnancy. Cell 2012;150(3):470–80.

[83] Wegmann TG, Lin H, Guilbert L, Mosmann TR. Bidirectional cytokine interactions in the maternal-fetal relationship: is successful pregnancy a TH2 phenomenon? Immunol Today 1993;14:353–6.

[84] Udagawa J, Hino K. Impact of maternal stress in pregnancy on brain function of the offspring. Nihon Eiseigaku Zasshi 2016;71(3):188–94.

[85] Feng Q, Chen W-D, Wang Y-D. Gut microbiota: an integral moderator in health and disease. Front Microbiol 2018;9:151.

[86] Cenit MC, Olivares M, Codoñer-Franch P, Sanz Y. Intestinal microbiota and celiac disease: cause, consequence or co-evolution? Nutrients 2015;7(8):6900–23.

[87] Xie G, Zhou Q, Qiu CZ, Dai WK, Wang HP, Li YH, Liao JX, Lu XG, Lin SF, Ye JH, Ma ZY, Wang WJ. Ketogenic diet poses a significant effect on imbalanced gut microbiota in infants with refractory epilepsy. World J Gastroenterol 2017;23(33):6164–71.

[88] Mori A, Yasaka Y, Masamoto K, Hiramatsu M. Gas chromatography of 5-hydroxy-3-methylindole in human urine. Clin Chim Acta 1978;84(1–2):63–8.

[89] Koskiniemi ML. Deficient intestinal absorption of L-tryptophan in progressive myoclonus epilepsy without Lafora bodies. J Neurol Sci 1980;47(1):1–6.

[90] Lunardi G, Mainardi P, Rubino V, Fracassi M, Pioli F, Cultrera S, Albano C. Tryptophan and epilepsy. Adv Exp Med Biol 1996;398:101–2.

[91] Mainardi P, Leonardi A, Albano C. Potentiation of brain serotonin activity may inhibit seizures, especially in drug-resistant epilepsy. Med Hypotheses 2008;70(4):876–9.

[92] Louis ED, Lynch T, Kaufmann P, Fahn S, Odel J. Diagnostic guidelines in central nervous system Whipple's disease. Ann Neurol 1996;40(4):561–8.

[93] Vital Durand D, Gérard A, Rousset H. Neurological manifestations of Whipple disease. Rev Neurol (Paris) 2002;158:988–92.

[94] Ghezzi A, Zaffaroni M. Neurological manifestations of gastrointestinal disorders, with particular reference to the differential diagnosis of multiple sclerosis. Neurol Sci 2001;22(Suppl 2):S117–22.

[95] Berg AT, Berkovic SF, Brodie MJ, Buchhalter J, Cross JH, van Emde Boas W, Engel J, French J, Glauser TA, Mathern GW, Moshé SL, Nordli D, Plouin P, Scheffer IE. Revised terminology and concepts for organization of seizures and epilepsies: report of the ILAE commission on classification and terminology, 2005–2009. Epilepsia 2010;51:676–85.

[96] Verrotti A, Nanni G, Agostinelli S, Parisi P, Capovilla G, Beccaria F, Iannetti P, Spalice A, Coppola G, Franzoni E, Gentile V, Casellato S, Veggiotti P, Malgesini S, Crichiutti G, Balestri P, Grosso S, Zamponi N, Incorpora G, Savasta S, Costa P, Pruna D, Chiarelli F. Benign convulsions associated with mild gastroenteritis: a multicenter clinical study. Epilepsy Res 2011;93:107–14.

[97] Verrotti A, Tocco AM, Coppola GG, Altobelli E, Chiarelli F. Afebrile benign convulsions with mild gastroenteritis: a new entity? Acta Neurol Scand 2009;120:73–9.

CHAPTER 7

Epilepsy and obesity: A complex interaction

Lady Diana Ladino*, Jose Francisco Téllez-Zenteno†
*Epilepsy Program, Hospital Pablo Tobón Uribe—University of Antioquia, Neuroclínica, Medellín, Colombia
†Saskatchewan Epilepsy Program, Department of Medicine, Division of Neurology, University of Saskatchewan, Saskatoon, SK, Canada

Contents

The Comorbidities of Epilepsy
https://doi.org/10.1016/B978-0-12-814877-8.00007-6

Abbreviations

AED	antiepileptic drug
BDNF	brain-derived neurotrophic factor
BMI	body mass index
CAE	childhood absence epilepsy
CBZ	carbamazepine
CNS	central nervous system
CSF	cerebrospinal fluid
DD	developmental delay
DRE	drug-resistant epilepsy
FBM	felbamate
FS	febrile seizures
GABA	gamma-aminobutyric acid
GBP	gabapentin
HFD	high-fat diet
IL-10	interleukin-10
IL-1β	interleukin-1β
IL-6	interleukin-6
IL-8	interleukin-8
IQ	intelligence quotient
MEHMO	mental retardation, epileptic seizures, hypogenitalism, microcephaly, and obesity
NHANES	National Health and Nutrition Examination Survey
NO	nitric oxide
NPY	neuropeptide Y
OXC	oxcarbazepine
PGB	pregabaline
PTZ	pentylenetetrazol
PWE	people with epilepsy
PWS	Prader-Willi syndrome
TNFα	tumor necrosis factor alpha
TPM	topiramate
VGB	vigabatrin
VPA	valproic acid
ZM	zonisamide

1. Introduction

Nowadays obesity is one of the most serious health problems around the world. From 1999 to 2014, the Centers for Disease Control and Prevention reported an increase in obesity in adults from 30% to 38% in the United States [1]. The prevalence of obesity has also tripled in many countries of Europe since the 1980s. Based on recent estimates in European Union countries, overweight affects 30%–70% and obesity affects 10%–30% of adults [2]. The same phenomenon has been described in Latin America; currently the highest prevalence of obesity in adults is seen in Mexico (>30%) [3]. Obesity is a chronic progressive multifactorial disease. A number of hormonal, metabolic, psychological, cultural, and behavioral factors promote fat accumulation and weight gain [4]. The disease affects multiple organ systems and causes diabetes mellitus, hyperlipidemia, hypertension, heart disease, sleep apnea, and cancer, and it significantly impairs quality of life and self-esteem [5].

Neurological disorders are an important cause of disability and death worldwide. Globally, the burden of neurological diseases has increased substantially over the past 25 years because of expanding population numbers and aging. Epilepsy is not the exception, with greater rates in low-income and middle-income countries; epilepsy causes a significant burden in children and young adults [6]. Epilepsy is a disease characterized by unpredictable seizures having a profound effect on the social functioning and emotional wellbeing of patients. The disease does not have geographic, social, or racial boundaries, and it occurs in men and women and affects all ages [7]. The prevalence rates of active epilepsy in the United States and Europe varied from 3.3% in the general population in Italy to 16% in adults aged ≥18 years in Georgia, USA [8]. In Canada, 190,000 people have active epilepsy requiring medical attention [9]. Critically, the negative impact of epilepsy is disproportionate to its prevalence [10]. Persons with epilepsy (PWE) have lower quality of life, family function, and social support as compared to other chronically ill individuals [11].

Comorbidity is the simultaneous presence of two or more diseases in the same individual more frequently than the chance expectation derived from an age-matched control cohort of healthy subjects [12]. Some studies have suggested that obesity is a comorbidity of new-onset epilepsy [13, 14]. Neurologists, endocrinologists, and basic scientists have investigated the connection between the two diseases. Although the possible mechanisms of biological interaction between the endocrine system and seizures remains obscure, in this chapter we summarize the best evidence identified in the literature. See Fig. 1.

2. Association between epilepsy and obesity

Evidence about the interrelation between obesity and epilepsy is conflictive. Several investigations support the idea that obesity is more common in PWE than in the general population [15–17]. According to a Canadian population-based study, PWE have poorer health status and lower levels of health-related behaviors compared to the general population, and in some particular cases compared with other chronic conditions, such as migraine and diabetes. Overall, the prevalence of obesity is higher in those with epilepsy than in the general population [15]. A large population-based study of 8057 adults in Georgia and Tennessee showed that 170 PWE tended to be more obese than controls (34% vs. 24%) [17]. A study from Germany found similar results; 136 patients with epilepsy were compared to 145 controls in a survey. PWE tended to participate significantly less in physical activities and had a higher body mass index (BMI) [16].

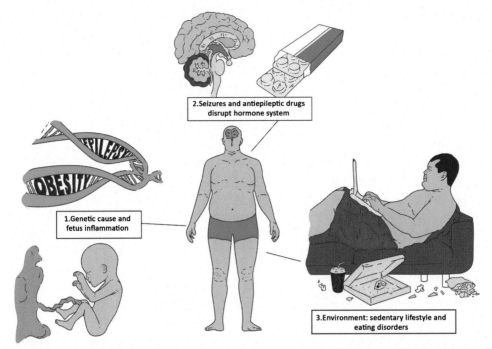

Fig. 1 Factors involved in obesity and epilepsy association. The association between epilepsy and obesity can be explained in three ways. The first factor is the genetic link between both diseases demonstrated by known genetic syndromes described in mice and humans. There is an increased prevalence of epilepsy in children with obesity, but also an increased prevalence of epilepsy in the offspring of obese mothers. The second factor is the well-known hormonal and neuronal alterations produced by seizures and antiepileptics drugs leading to overweight and obesity. The third factor is the hypothesis that environmental effects can lead to an imbalance in energy intake and expenditure. High-fat diet, fast food consumption and supersized portions, sedentary lifestyle, and lack of physical activity are elements described in people with epilepsy associated with overweight and obesity.

By contrast, a study carried out in a single epilepsy center in Bethesda, MD, USA, between 2003 and 2009 found that the frequency of overweight/obesity in PWE was high, although not higher than the general population. Unfortunately, this study did not compare PWE with an internal control group or in the same population. Nonetheless, they reported that obesity rates are higher in patients with drug-resistant epilepsy (DRE) than pharmacoresponsive epilepsy (37% vs. 25%), as well as in patients treated with polytherapy versus monotherapy (38% vs. 25%) [18].

In the same way, a longitudinal cohort study using retrospective data from the Health Improvement Network Database in the UK was conducted to examine the incidence rates of seizures across different levels of BMI in adult population. In a study period of 5 years (2000–05), 141.944 patients were included. After adjusting for age, gender, and smoking status, obesity was not associated with an increased incidence rate of seizures. By contrast, underweight patients tend to have higher epilepsy incidence rates than those with normal weight [8].

3. Epilepsy and obesity sharing a genetic etiology

There is evidence supporting the fact that overweight and obesity are more prevalent in children with newly diagnosed epilepsy than in age-matched peers, despite lower caloric and carbohydrate intake. A big epidemiological study carried out in the United States proved that children with childhood absence epilepsy (CAE) were more likely to be overweight (19% vs. 14%; $P < 0.001$) or obese (14% vs. 11%; $P < 0.001$) than National Health and Nutrition Examination Survey (NHANES) controls. The combined prevalence of overweight and obesity was 34% in the CAE cohort and 25% among controls ($P < 0.001$). Mean daily energy intake (difference 279.5 kcal/day, $P < 0.04$) and daily carbohydrate intake (difference 210.7 g/day, $P < 0.04$) were lower in the CAE group than in NHANES controls [14].

A study done at the Cincinnati Children's Hospital Medical Center also demonstrated an increased prevalence of obesity (20%) and overweight (19%) in children with newly diagnosed untreated epilepsy compared to regional healthy controls (14% and 15%, respectively). Overweight and obesity were more common in patients with idiopathic epilepsies (21%) in comparison with symptomatic epilepsies (15%) [13]. The relationship between epilepsy and obesity in the study subjects cannot be explained by drug adverse events, as these children were obese prior to starting antiepileptic drugs (AEDs).

We found a similar correlation in the Saskatchewan Epilepsy Program in Canada. In 100 adult patients with epilepsy, we demonstrated an association between obesity and generalized epilepsy (OR 2.7; CI: 1.1–6.6; $P = 0.01$), idiopathic epileptic syndrome (OR: 2.7; CI: 1.04–7.0; $P = 0.02$), and family history of epilepsy (OR: 6.1; CI: 1.5–24.2; $P = 0.002$), suggesting a potential common genetic pathway for both chronic diseases. Additionally, we found a higher prevalence of developmental delay (DD) in PWE and obesity, in comparison to PWE and normal weight (21% vs. 13%) [19].

Although causality is not well established by these studies, the association suggests that obesity may prime the brain for seizures. Consistent with this hypothesis, obese leptin receptor mutant mice and adiponectin-deficient mice on a high-fat diet (HFD) exhibit increased vulnerability of seizure-induced degeneration. Conversely, fasting can protect against seizure-induced memory impairment and neuronal degeneration. The mechanisms by which obesity endangers, while dietary energy restriction protects, neurons might involve opposite effects on adaptive cellular stress response pathways. Obesity is associated with reduced expression of brain-derived neurotrophic factor (BDNF) and elevated levels of oxidative stress and inflammatory processes in the brain. In contrast, intermittent fasting upregulates neurotrophic factors, such as BDNF, fibroblast growth factor 2, protein chaperones, and antioxidant proteins, while suppressing production of proinflammatory cytokines [20].

3.1 Research in mice

Some researchers have found a genetic role for weight gain and food intake in mutant epileptic mice. Heisler et al. demonstrated that the serotonin 5ht2c receptor null mutant in mice is associated with seizures and obesity [21]. Another group described a colony of obese mice containing a targeted deletion of the transcription factor Nescient Helix-Loop-Helix 2. These animals showed adult-onset obesity characterized by reduced spontaneous physical activity and progressive seizures [22]. Yet, the most important discovery in the area is the ob/ob mice. The obese model was a fortuitous observation in 1949 at the Jackson Laboratories in Bar Harbor. Mice homozygous for the obese spontaneous mutation, Leptin ob, exhibit obesity, hyperphagia, transient hyperglycemia, glucose intolerance, and elevated plasma insulin. Mutant mice are phenotypically indistinguishable from their unaffected littermates at birth but gain weight rapidly throughout their lives, reaching a weight three times that of unaffected mice [23]. Recently, an experimental study developed in 61 mice in the Jackson Laboratories demonstrated that ob/ob mice are more susceptible to generalized clonic and tonic-clonic seizures than wild type mice at submaximal pentylenetetrazol (PTZ) doses. These findings suggest that chronic leptin deficiency in vivo increases seizure susceptibility [24].

3.2 Research in humans

Certain epilepsy genetic syndromes in humans are related to weight gain—the best known is the Prader-Willi syndrome (PWS). PWS is a complex genetic disorder characterized by hypotonia, hypogonadism, hypomentia, obesity, and seizures. PWS affects about one in 10,000–15,000 births. It is caused by absence of expression of the paternally active genes in the PWS critical region on 15q11–q13 chromosome. In 70% of cases, the result of the deletion is related to the paternal chromosome 15. In 28%, it depends on maternal uniparental disomy of chromosome 15, and in 2%, it is attributable to a mutation or a deletion in the imprinting center or other imprinting defect. The frequency of epilepsy in PWS patients ranges from 4% to 26%. The types of seizures include generalized tonic-clonic seizures, complex partial seizures, atypical absence, myoclonic, tonic, and hemiclonic seizures [25]. It is possible that hyperphagia and obesity in PWS is correlated with high-circulating levels of ghrelin [5].

There are some case reports and case series in the literature reporting genetic associations between obesity and epilepsy in children. Vauthier et al. found a unique homozygous 80 kb deletion in the chromosomal 1p31.3 region in a 3-year-old patient with a mutation in the leptin receptor gene. The child suffered early onset severe obesity associated to hyperphagia, seizures, and DD, and had two family members affected with epilepsy [26]. Few patients with deletions of 18q12.2 have been also reported in the literature and the associated phenotype includes seizures, obesity, intellectual disability, behavioral problems, and eye manifestations, such as myopia [27]. Another research group reported a 15q24.1 BP4–BP1 microdeletion in a 10-year-old girl presenting DD, psychomotor retardation, epilepsy, overweight, and idiopathic central precocious puberty [28].

A group from the Wolfson Medical Center, Israel, reported one of the few X-linked mitochondrial syndromes cases in a child. Neurologic examination at the age of 1 year revealed an obese hypotonic baby with microcephaly, hypogenitalism and seizures. The electroencephalogram revealed a burst suppression pattern. He was treated with vigabatrin and ACTH. The syndrome is an X-linked disorder assigned to the locus Xp21.1-p22.13, called MEHMO (mental retardation, epileptic seizures, hypogenitalism, microcephaly, and pbesity) [29]. Another team reported a special mutation in CUL4B, which encodes an ubiquitin E3 ligase subunit, causing an X-linked syndrome in 39 patients from different families. The majority of patients suffered seizures, central obesity, macrocephaly, mental retardation, and hypogonadism [30]. Cornelia de Lange syndrome is another good example with several mutations in the cohesin gene complex. The syndrome is characterized by typical facial features, growth deficiency, intellectual disability, epilepsy, and major malformations. This group of patients has a clear tendency to be overweight and develop frank obesity during the first years of the disease [31].

It is possible that an unknown genetic dysfunction of neural pathways in humans could produce an increased susceptibility for seizure disorders and secondary obesity. On the other hand, obesity, mental retardation, and epilepsy could be a consequence of the same global brain dysfunction mediated by a particular genetic mutation [19].

4. Maternal obesity and epilepsy

In the United States, the prevalence of obese women aged 20–39 years old tripled between 1960 and 2000 [32]. Half of pregnant women from developed countries are either overweight or obese. Obesity during pregnancy is of major concern due to the well-characterized risk factors to both the mother and her offspring. Women who are overweight or obese early in pregnancy have an increased frequency of miscarriages, preeclampsia, gestational diabetes, infections, stillbirths, thromboembolic events, elective and emergency cesarean section, as well as postpartum hemorrhages [33].

Razaz et al. use a large population-based cohort in Sweden (1,421,551 live births included) to demonstrate an increased incidence of epilepsy in children born to obese women. The rate of childhood onset epilepsy up to age 16 years was significantly increased in the offspring of overweight and obese mothers compared to mothers with normal weight. The increase of epilepsy reached 10% in the overweight population, 20% in the population with obesity grade I, 30% in the population with obesity grade II, and

80% in the population with obesity grade III. The authors controlled for a broad range of potential confounders, including maternal characteristics, pregnancy, and neonatal complications, such as nervous system malformations (HR 46.4), hypoxic ischemic encephalopathy (HR 26.6), and neonatal convulsions (HR 33.5). Therefore, the elevated risk of epilepsy in children of obese mothers was an independent factor not explained by obesity-related pregnancy or neonatal complications [34].

Obesity has deleterious effects on the brain. It causes an inflammatory response with an elevation of interleukin-1β (IL-1β), interleukin-6 (IL-6), interleukin-8 (IL-8), tumor necrosis factor alpha (TNFα), and C-reactive protein. Fetal exposure to excessive lipid levels from the mother facilitates the activation of these cytokines. Adipocytes are altered as weight increases releasing more proinflammatory adipokines. Additionally, pregnancy leads to inflammation by triggering an increase in macrophage, neutrophil, and interleukin-10 (IL-10) levels. Therefore, obesity and pregnancy combine to result in a chronic fetal inflammatory state. This state, along with genetic factors, may create an abnormal intrauterine environment contributing to the development of epilepsy in the offspring [33, 35]. Furthermore, maternal obesity during pregnancy is associated with endothelial dysfunction and high levels of leptin that potentially could be related with direct placental dysfunction, possibly disrupting normal neurodevelopment in the children [36, 37].

This finding has already been described in mice. Maternal obesity led to increased offspring hippocampal lipid peroxidation and decreased neurogenesis due to metabolic and oxidative changes [38]. Chronic high-fat intake can lead to inflammatory changes in the brain cortex as evidenced by the presence of increased nicotinamide adenine dinucleotide phosphate oxidase-generated reactive oxygen species and accelerated prostaglandin E2 production [39]. Moroz et al. demonstrated that in mice developing obesity in response to HFD, mild neuropathological lesions were seen along with significant impairment in insulin receptor binding in the temporal lobe region [40]. HFD is associated with brain insulin resistance and compromised synaptic integrity. Mechanisms affected by obesity-induced systemic inflammation, neuroinflammation (mainly elicited by microglia in the brain), endoplasmic reticulum stress, calcium overload, and production of reactive oxygen species and proinflammatory cytokines contribute to kainic acid-induced neuronal death [41]. In summary, fetal brain development is sensitive to hormonal and inflammatory reactions, especially at the early embryonic stage.

Some studies have also reported associations between pregnancy, obesity, and other neurodevelopmental outcomes in humans, such as intellectual disability, lower cognitive performance, attention-deficit/hyperactivity disorder, cerebral palsy, and autism [42–44]. A cohort of South Carolina Medicaid-insured live births from year 2004 to 2007 found a significant association between increasing maternal BMI and cerebral palsy [45]. The same group found a significant association between prepregnancy BMI and intellectual disability in children. For every 1 unit increase in BMI, the odds of any severity of intellectual disability increased by 1.02 times (95% confidence interval = 1.01–1.02)

[46]. Interestingly, they did not observe an association between maternal obesity during pregnancy and risk of child epilepsy [45].

Lastly, according to data derived from animal models, maternal obesity has long-term consequences for offspring, predisposing or "programming" them to the development of metabolic disease in adulthood [47]. Metabolic disease is associated with a state of chronic low-grade inflammation. These metabolic changes extend to the placenta exposing the fetus to an inflammatory environment during development [48]. A child from an obese mother has a higher probability of suffering from a metabolic syndrome in the future.

5. Epilepsy as a cause of obesity

Epilepsy itself might cause weight gain through central nervous system (CNS) pathways. The regulation of food intake is a complex process involving interactions between specific brain regions. This interaction has been demonstrated through hypothalamic-mediated mechanisms in rat models with epilepsy, as well as amygdala- and hippocampus-mediated mechanisms in kindled rats [19].

Damage to specific brain nuclei results in overeating and obesity, suggesting that they play a key role in limiting food intake and body weight. These include the hypothalamic paraventricular nucleus, the ventromedial hypothalamus, the posterodorsal amygdala, the ventral noradrenergic bundle, the stria terminalis and the fibers projecting from the arcuate nucleus to the paraventricular nucleus [49].

The hypothalamus is the principal site of integration of information regulating food intake and energy expenditure. The medial hypothalamic area inhibits feeding behavior, whereas the lateral hypothalamic area activates feeding behavior. Experimental studies have shown that ventromedial lesions produced hyperphagia, lateral lesions, aphagia, and body weight loss in animals [50]. Hypothalamic neurons are modulated by neurotransmitters, neuromodulators and hormones. Gamma-aminobutyric acid (GABA) and neuropeptide Y (NPY) increase carbohydrate consumption and decrease energy expenditure. Serotonin reduces food ingestion by stimulating the medial hypothalamus. Norepinephrine can act over the medial and lateral hypothalamus depending on the situation [50].

It has been shown that epileptic seizures can change serum levels of some hormones, especially hypothalamic and pituitary hormones. These changes can be observed immediately after epileptic seizures. Repetitive seizures can also lead to chronic dysfunction in the hypothalamic-pituitary-gonadal axis, which is modulated by temporal and limbic cortices [51].

5.1 Ghrelin

Ghrelin is a hormone secreted by enterochromaffin cells lining the gastric mucosa. The hormone exerts neuroendocrine effects, such as the stimulation of appetite, satiety, fat accumulation, and control of body weight [5]. Plasma ghrelin levels increase physiologically in the early morning during the fasting state (before meals) and pathologically in patients with anorexia nervosa. Ghrelin levels decrease physiologically in the postprandial period, and pathologically due to increased calorie intake in patients with obesity. It stimulates food intake through metabolic effects, thus it ensures energy gain and storage. The increased stimulation of eating by ghrelin has been suggested to be mediated by the arcuate nucleus and with NPY and agouti-related peptide [52].

Definite relationship between ghrelin and epilepsy has been demonstrated in animals [53] and humans [51]. Ataie et al. reported that ghrelin levels decreased after PTZ-induced seizures in male Wistar rats. Ghrelin reduction might be due to release of leptin and somatostatin during seizures [53]. By contrast, Berilgen et al. found significantly increased levels of ghrelin in patients with focal and generalized epilepsy in comparison to controls [51].

5.2 Leptin

Leptin is a hormone secreted by adipocytes in direct proportion to body fat levels and activates the signal for satiety. Leptin receptors are highly expressed in the hypothalamus. The hormone inhibits food intake by acting on the arcuate nucleus (and inhibiting NPY transmission to the paraventricular nucleus) [49]. Ob/ob mice, which present mutations in the leptin gene, are obese because they fail to produce leptin. Therefore, leptin deficiency was suggested as a cause of human obesity. Interestingly, in obese individuals, leptin levels increase properly in response to body fat. Verrotti et al. demonstrated that elevation of serum leptin levels correlated well with the increase in BMI in obese patients taking valproic acid (VPA) [54]. The fact that obese patients have elevated serum leptin levels and that these high levels fail to produce changes in energy intake or expenditure that restore fat mass to normal has led to the hypothesis of leptin resistance in human obesity, possibly due to deficient hypothalamic leptin receptors [50].

Leptin receptor deficiency in humans is a congenital disorder caused by homozygous mutation of LEPR gene, on chromosome 1p31. Major symptoms include severe obesity, seizures, hyperphagia, hypogonadism, impulsivity, and impaired T-cell mediated immunity [55]. It has been established that leptin is neuroprotective, enhances neuronal survival, and is implicated in the regulation of neuronal excitability. Focal and generalized induced seizures in rats are shortened and reduced in number by administration of leptin. Leptin was found to inhibit AMPA glutamate receptor-mediated synaptic transmission in the hippocampus. The ketogenic diet, used for treatment in some types of epilepsy, increases leptin levels in serum, hinting that leptin play a role in the known beneficial effects of the ketogenic diet on suppression of seizures [55b, 56].

5.3 Adiponectin

Adiponectin, the gene product of the adipose most abundant gene transcript-1 gene, which is exclusively expressed in adipose tissue, is a 244-amino acid protein with structural homology to collagen VIII, X, and complement C1q.7. Its plasma levels negatively correlate with the degree of body fat [57]. Adiponectin regulates several metabolic processes, including glucose homeostasis and fatty acid oxidation, and has potent antiinflammatory, antidiabetic, and antiatherogenic properties [58]. Some studies suggest a role for adipokines in the genesis of seizures and neuroprotection related to seizures. Adiponectin has shown neuroprotective effects in hippocampal neurons. Adiponectin preserves the integrity of the blood-brain barrier and has neuroprotective effects after kainic acid-induced seizures. A study in 13 female patients confirmed the animal findings and demonstrated plasma adiponectin levels were increased following epileptic seizures as compared to the controls [59].

5.4 Seizure threshold

Experimental work suggests that peripheral endocrine and metabolic factors are capable of modulating seizure threshold by acting on CNS neurons to trigger intracellular signaling pathways [60]. A recent prospective cross-sectional study conducted in Egypt evaluated adipocytokine levels in children with febrile seizures (FS). The group included 100 patients with FS, and matched 100 children with febrile illness without seizures and 100 healthy controls. Serum and cerebrospinal fluid (CSF) levels of adiponectin, leptin, and IL-6 were measured. Azab et al. observed a significant association between high CSF IL-6/low CSF leptin levels and susceptibility to FS. Children with FS had significantly lower serum leptin levels in comparison to both control groups; by contrast, febrile control children had significantly elevated serum leptin levels. Fascinatingly, serum leptin levels were significantly lower in patients with complex FS compared to those with simple FS. Authors concluded that the high serum leptin levels observed in the febrile control group could be protective against seizures, whereas lower serum leptin levels were associated with seizures in susceptible children. Additionally, data revealed that children with FS had significantly higher serum IL-6 levels compared to both control groups. It seems increased brain proinflammatory cytokines decrease the threshold for individual seizures. On the other hand, elevated levels of serum adiponectin was an acute phase reactant in FS and febrile control groups that did not contribute to the development of seizures [61]. In summary, hormones may affect seizure threshold. Indeed, both leptin and ghrelin inhibit seizures in mice. The adipose hormone adiponectin also inhibits seizures and seizure-related neuropathology. Taken together, these studies suggest that seizure threshold and epilepsy may be modulated by peripheral hormones, such as leptin, ghrelin, and adiponectin, all of which are altered in obesity [20]. See Fig. 2.

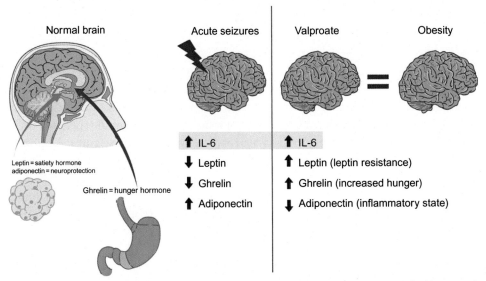

Fig. 2 Hormones interactions in epilepsy and obesity. Hunger and satiety are controlled by complex interactions between the nervous system, circadian rhythms, and hormones. Leptin and adiponectin produced by adipose tissue mediate appetite, inflammation, and fat deposition. Leptin is also known as the "satiety hormone" that regulates energy balance by inhibiting hunger; it opposes the action of ghrelin, the "hunger hormone." Adiponectin regulates several metabolic processes (including glucose homeostasis and fatty acid oxidation) and has potent antiinflammatory, antidiabetic and antiatherogenic properties. Evidence suggests that during a seizure, IL-6 is increased as an etiopathogenic factor and adiponectin is increased as an acute phase reactant. Ghrelin and leptin levels are decreased, demonstrating susceptibility in the seizure threshold of the subject. On the opposite side, ghrelin is pathologically increased in patients with obesity (increased hunger), and adiponectin is decreased as a sign of a chronic inflammatory state. Interestingly, obese patients have elevated serum leptin levels, but those high levels fail to produce changes in energy intake or expenditure, taking us to the hypothesis of leptin resistance. IL-6 is increased in obese experimental models, as well as other brain proinflammatory cytokines. The chronic inflammatory state of obesity could decrease the threshold for seizures. All the changes found in hormone levels in patients with obesity have been replicated in patients using valproic acid for epilepsy and psychiatric diseases.

6. Antiepileptic drugs producing obesity

Body weight gain is a common and undesirable effect associated with the use of AEDs. This has been observed for many years with some drugs such as VPA, gabapentin (GBP), pregabaline (PGB), and vigabatrin (VGB), and to some extent with carbamazepine (CBZ) and oxcarbazepine (OXC). Others are potentially weight neutral, such as lamotrigine, levetiracetam, and phenytoin, and a few of them are associated with weight loss, such as topiramate (TPM), zonisamide (ZM), and felbamate (FBM) [50]. According to the Columbia Comprehensive Epilepsy Center Antiepileptic Drug Database, weight gain is the most likely cosmetic side effect to result in dosage adjustment or medication discontinuation [62]. In Columbia University, weight gain was reported in 3.6% (68/1903) of PWE. Intolerability to weight gain was reported in the majority of them (92%). Patients who reported weight gain had, on average, reported an 8 kg or a 10% increase from their weight before starting an AED. Significantly more patients taking VPA (13%) and PGB (8.4%) experienced weight gain compared with the average rate of patients taking all other AEDs ($P < 0.001$) [62].

One of the difficulties when evaluating weight gain is determining whether a patient has truly gained body weight because the physician often has not weighed the patient before initiating treatment. Measurement of total body fat content is the most precise way to evaluate overweight and obesity, but this measurement is difficult and costly to be used on a routine basis. The calculation of BMI provides a quantitative way to monitor the adverse effect. BMI is calculated from the body weight in kilograms divided by the square of standing height (or supine length in small children) in meters and is reported in units of kg/m^2. Obesity is defined as BMI >25 [50].

6.1 Valproate

VPA is one of the most frequently prescribed AEDs worldwide. It has a broad spectrum of antiepileptic activity, both in partial and generalized epilepsies [63]. The rate of weight gain reported in the literature among VPA-treated patients is between 16% and 58% in children [64], and 57% and 70% in adult patients [65]. Weight gain due to VPA treatment is usually observed during the first 3 months of therapy, reaching its maximum after 6 months [66]. Patients receiving VPA increased their weight by an average of 2.0 kg in adults and 5.0 kg in children [67].

In the first place, VPA causes enhancement of GABA transmission within the hypothalamic axis, leading to deregulation of the neuroendocrine control of energy intake, consequently developing increased appetite and quenching with calorie-rich beverages [68]. Once the patients gain weight, they can develop hyperinsulinemia and insulin resistance leading to metabolic syndrome. Lowered blood glucose levels have been proposed as one basic mechanism by which VPA may lead to obesity. Low glucose levels stimulate eating through an effect on glucose-responsive neurons in the medial hypothalamus, which, in turn, reduces the efferent inhibitory output to the lateral hypothalamus [68].

In Italy, Greco et al. studied 40 patients with epilepsy treated with VPA and compared them to 40 healthy controls. At the end of follow-up (2 years), 15 PWE (37.5%) developed obesity. They showed circulating leptin ($P < 0.01$) and insulin ($P < 0.05$) levels significantly higher and ghrelin ($P < 0.01$) and adiponectin ($P < 0.001$) levels significantly lower than those patients who did not gain weight [57].

A study carried out at the outpatient clinic of the Department of Neurology, Innsbruck Medical University in Austria demonstrated that women are more prone to gain weight during VPA therapy. Serum leptin levels were higher in female than in male overweight patients with epilepsy ($P < 0.001$), possibly leading to leptin resistance and carbohydrate craving. In accordance, women revealed a higher percentage of body fat paralleled by higher plasma leptin levels compared to men [69].

A study at the department of Child Neurology, Inönü University in Turkey was carried out to investigate the effect of VPA on ghrelin and its potential effects on weight gain and growth in children. Gungor et al. found ghrelin levels were significantly increased in the prepubertal children treated with VPA. They concluded the weight gain in using VPA might be associated with the increase in ghrelin levels [52]. Increased serum levels of leptin, NPY, and galanin might also play an important role in VPA-associated weight gain in children [70]. See Fig. 3.

6.1.1 Endocrine abnormalities

Unfortunately, the problem of weight gain in VPA-treated patients is not isolated, but involves several endocrine abnormalities, such as polycystic ovary syndrome, hair loss, hyperandrogenism, amenorrhea, hyperleptinemia, leptin resistance, hyperinsulinemia, insulin resistance, dyslipidemia, elevation in the levels of uric acid, elevation in the levels of homocysteine, reduction in the levels of ghrelin and adiponectin [68], metabolic syndrome (dysglycemia, dyslipidemia, hypertension) [71], nonalcoholic fatty liver disease, and cardiovascular disorders [72].

Isojärvi et al. reported that of 29 women with epilepsy treated with VPA for a mean of 8 years, 45% had menstrual abnormalities, 43% had polycystic ovaries, and 17% had high testosterone levels. These changes were more significant when VPA was started before the 20 years of age. The authors suggested that VPA prevented the transformation of testosterone to estradiol, giving rise to hyperandrogenism [65]. El-Khayat et al. compared 66 girls with epilepsy treated with VPA for 1–5 years with a healthy age-matched control group. The VPA-treated postpubertal girls had a higher rate of obesity (37% vs. 10%, $P < 0.033$) and hyperandrogenism; 18% of those with hyperandrogenism had polycystic ovary syndrome [73]. In contrast with these findings, a prospective study carried out in Israel found that the administration of VPA in 83 girls with newly diagnosed epilepsy had no significant impact on body weight or body composition over an average follow-up of 3.2 years [74].

A study conducted in Sichuan, China evaluated the presence of metabolic syndrome among adult obese PWE on VPA. Authors found several differences between obese patients with epilepsy treated with VPA and obese patients without epilepsy. Higher fasting plasma glucose, higher insulin levels, severe insulin resistance, and higher prevalence of elevated blood pressure were detected in the patients treated with VPA. These characteristics indicate that the development of metabolic syndrome among obese patients treated with VPA is different from the general obese population [71]. Insulin is a stimulator of the vasodilator nitric oxide (NO). Insulin signaling through the PI3K pathway in insulin resistance has been proposed to be impaired, leading to decreased NO. In

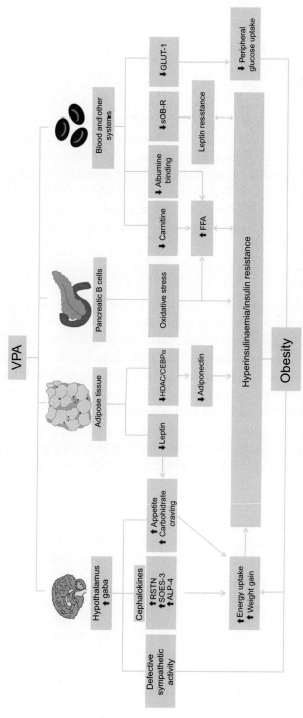

Fig. 3 Mechanisms of valproic-induced obesity. *RSTN*, resistin; *SOCS-3*, suppressor of cytokine signaling-3; *ALP-4*, angiopoietin-like protein; *HDAC*, histone deacetylase; *CEBPα*, CCAAT/enhancer binding protein-α; *FFA*, free fatty acids; *sOB-R*, soluble leptin receptor; *GLUT-1*, glucose transporter 1.

addition, hyperinsulinemia may lead to increased peripheral vascular resistance because of sympathetic overactivity and vasoconstriction from its antinatriuretic effects and increased angiotensinogen II [71].

6.2 Carbamazepine

CBZ is the drug of choice for partial onset seizures [50]. Data regarding the effect of CBZ on weight is scant and contradictory. Body weight gain during CBZ therapy has been reported in few studies: 2% in a study of 300 patients [75] 9% in a study of 480 patients [76] and 14% in a study of 300 patients [77]. Isojärvi et al. [65] reported obesity in 25% of patients taking CBZ. By the contrary, Caksen et al. proposed that CBZ treatment has no effect on body weight. They studied 19 children in Taiwan, and 2 (14%) patients complained about overeating and weight gain [78]. Similarly, a study in 56 PWE on CBZ monotherapy in Turkey showed CBZ therapy does not significantly affect BMI, leptin, and insulin plasma levels [79].

6.3 Oxcarbazepine

OXC is a new generation AED in wide use as a single-agent or combination as a treatment for focal epilepsy in patients older than 4 years. OXC metabolism is less dependent on cytochrome P-450 liver enzymes than CBZ, resulting in fewer side effects. A study conducted in Greece in 59 children with epilepsy demonstrated that similar to VPA, OXC monotherapy resulted in a significant weight gain. Eight months postOXC treatment, body weight and BMI increased significantly; the percentage of overweight/obese children climbed from 23% to 38.5% [80]. Similarly, a study of 71 children placed on OXC therapy for a minimum of 3 months demonstrated significant increases in body weight. Furthermore, this study showed that male gender, younger age, partial seizure disorder at diagnosis were risk factors for excessive weight gain with OXC [81].

6.4 Vigabatrin

VGB is an AED designed to increase the level of GABA in the brain. Studies have shown its efficacy in patients with infantile spasms and focal seizures [50]. In the Canadian Vigabatrin Study, a long-term open, add-on trial, a mean body weight gain of 3.7 ± 0.2 kg was observed by the end of the study [82].

6.5 Gabapentin

In the US Gabapentin Study carried out two decades ago, weight gain was observed in 6% of 82 patients receiving different dosages of the drug (600, 1200, and 2400 mg/day) [83]. This study did not find a clear relation between the doses and the adverse effect. By the contrary, Baulac observed that the use of GBP seems to be related to the prescribed dose. They found body weight gain in 6%, 10%, and 15% in a group of 610 adult patients with focal epilepsy who were receiving 1200 to 1600, 1600 to <2000, and 2000 mg/day, respectively, of GBP as add-on therapy [84].

6.6 Antiepileptic drugs producing loss of weight

6.6.1 Topiramate

TPM can induce emaciation and growth retardation. Different mechanisms explaining the weight loss have been published, such as decrease in body fat stores in obese patients, reduction in food intake, as well as reduction in appetite. The drug potentially can increase the insulin sensitivity and decrease the blood concentration of insulin, both of which will cause a loss of appetite and lipid metabolism. A study in China showed TPM increases the level of adiponectin to regulate metabolism in children. An increase in energy metabolism and a decrease in lipid protein cause weight to decrease [85].

6.6.2 Rufinamide

Rufinamide is a triazole derivative that can block sodium channels. It is effective as an adjunctive treatment for Lennox-Gastaut syndrome and refractory focal seizures as an add-on therapy for adults and adolescents. A study carried out in France found clinically significant weight loss in 47% of adult patients (aged 18–31 years) treated with Rufinamide as add-on therapy (800–2400 mg/day). The BMI decreased by 7.3%–18.7% [86].

6.6.3 Zonisamide

ZM is an AED chemically classified as a sulfonamide and unrelated to other AEDs. It was first used in Japan in 1972 to treat psychiatric diseases, and it has been widely used to treat epilepsy since 1990. The Food and Drug Administration approved it for use in the United States in 2000 as add-on therapy in the treatment of focal seizures in adults. Weight loss is one of the most prominent adverse effects of ZM treatment in PWE. The weight loss is not dose-related but is more prominent in overweight patients. A lower initial serum leptin level is associated with a larger weight loss. ZM can be a useful therapeutic option for overweight patients with epilepsy, and that basal serum leptin level may have a predictive role in weight loss [87]. See Table 1.

7. Physical activity limitation in people with epilepsy leading to obesity

Body weight is determined by interplay among energy intake, metabolism, and expenditure. PWE participate less frequently in sports, have poorer levels of fitness, and are more obese than those without epilepsy [16, 88]. The National Health Survey conducted in the United States in 2010 reported that PWE were less likely to follow recommendations from the American guidelines about physical activity. In fact, in the week prior to the survey only 39% of PWE had walked for at least 10 min compared to 50% of the general population [89]. A survey conducted in Ohio, USA, found that 58% of PWE

Table 1 Antiepileptic drug mechanisms of action modulating weight gain in patients [50–52, 62, 86, 87]

Drug group	Antiepileptic drug	Potential action mechanism
Antiepileptic drugs associated with weight gain	Valproic acid	• Enhance GABA transmission within the hypothalamus, causing appetite stimulation (carbohydrate craving and modified thirst), hyperinsulinemia and hyperleptinaemia • Decrease concentrations of ghrelin and adiponectin • Led to ineffective leptin action despite high leptin levels (leptin-resistance) • Defective sympathetic nervous system activity • Decrease the capacity for luxury consumption or facultative thermogenesis • Alter adipokine (adipose tissue cytokine) transmission • Direct stimulation of pancreatic beta cells • Indirect enhancement of insulin resistance by suppressing insulin-mediated peripheral glucose uptake • Elevation in fasting and postprandial insulin levels • Increase binge eating and motivation to eat • Modulation on a genetic basis for obesity • Carnitine deficiency causing impaired beta-oxidation of fatty acids
	Gabapentin	Enhancement of GABA-mediated inhibition in the medial hypothalamus
	Vigabatrine	Enhancement of GABA-mediated inhibition in the medial hypothalamus
	Carbamazepine	Induce overeating Increase fat deposition Induce water retention and edema
	Pregabalin	• Inhibit appetite-regulating effects in the CNS • Decrease energy consumption by sedation • Antidiuretic effect
	Levetiracetam	• Modify insulin secretion in response to glucose throughout its molecular target the synaptic vesicle protein 2A
Antiepileptic drugs associated with weight	Topiramate	• Reduce the food intake • Reduce energy deposition in the absence of alterations in food intake • Increase energy expenditure • Increase lipoprotein lipase activity in brown adipose tissue and muscle, which could indicate ability to enhance regulatory thermogenesis and promote substrate oxidation
	Felbamate	Reduction in food intake
	Zonisamide	Decrease leptin levels
	Rufinamide	Reduce food intake, through loss of appetite and nausea

performed physical activity in the past month as opposed to 76% of the controls. When asking whether any health professional had advised them to increase their physical activity level during the last year, the results were 47% compared to 35%, respectively [90]. In Finland, a study did not find any significant difference between PWE and controls when it came to physical activity frequency. However, it is noteworthy that 9% of PWE reported physical inactivity compared to 2% of controls. The same study found a performance below the expected level in tests of muscle strength in people with a history of seizures [88]. In California, no differences were reported between sports habits in both populations. However, this study highlighted how the topic of physical activity was not addressed during the medical consultation in the last year in the majority of appointments (56%) [91].

Wong and Wirrell determined adolescents with epilepsy were less likely to be involved in sport groups or engaged in physical activity and more likely to be overweight and obese than their siblings without the disease [92]. A population-based study in Nova Scotia, Canada, failed to show differences in the frequency of physical exercise among those affected by epilepsy and the general population but revealed that PWE were less involved in particular sports, such as hockey, weight lifting, or physical activity at home [93].

In Brazil, Arida et al. reported that 49% of patients did not perform physical activity on a regular basis. The most common explanations of this behavior included: recommendations given by relatives, friends, and physicians; fear and embarrassment of having a seizure in public; lack of time or motivation; fatigue; and absence of company [94]. Similar findings were found in a Korean study, showing that the low participation was due to different factors, including anxiety, polypharmacy, and having experienced a seizure during exercise [95]. The stigma associated with epilepsy may limit participation in activity and some PWE continue to be discouraged from exercise participation due to concerns of injury during seizures or the possibility of exercise-induced seizures [19, 94]. Finally, comorbidities of epilepsy, such as heart disease, arthritis, and depression, may also limit participation in exercise, and epilepsy in some patients is secondary to stroke or trauma, conditions that, by themselves, can result in physical or cognitive limitations to participation [15].

8. Environmental factors: eating disorder in patients with epilepsy

Physiological homeostatic mechanisms can account for only about 15% of the variance in daily food intake of freely living humans, and environmental factors account for over 85% of the variance [49]. What differentiates obese individuals from lean persons is not the chemosensory systems or the environment per se, but obese individuals' interactions with the environment, that is, their feeding responses to food-related stimuli, such as the taste, smell, texture, and sight of food, and even watching others eat. The obese individuals are much more responsive to external feeding cues than to biological control mechanisms [49]. Epilepsy is associated with several comorbid disorders, such as depression, anxiety, attention-deficit/hyperactivity disorder, low self-esteem, risk-taking behavior, and binge-eating disorder [96]. It is possible that PWE respond more to the environmental factors leading to obesity.

8.1 Adolescents

A recent cross-sectional population-based study carried out in Norway used data from a voluntary self-reported questionnaire. There were 19,995 participants aged 13–19 years, and 1.2% (247) reported a diagnosis of epilepsy. This study demonstrated that adolescents with epilepsy are at increased risk of having an eating disorder (OR 1.79, CI 1.0–3.0, $P = 0.03$). They eat less healthily (OR 1.67, 1.3–2.2, $P = 0.001$) and are less satisfied with their looks (OR 0.69, CI 0.5–0.9, $P = 0.02$). According to the research, young PWE had a significantly higher daily consumption of candy, sugar-containing soda, potato chips, and French fries than adolescents without epilepsy [97]. Interestingly, the authors did not find a significant association between eating disorders and depressive symptoms [97]. It is possible that failure to voluntarily control seizures may prompt a need in PWE to gain control over their bodies in a different way. By focusing attention on eating, PWE may feel that they are in a domain where control is possible [97].

Eating disorders among adolescents with epilepsy is a predictor of negative outcome in terms of mental health disorders, substance abuse, deliberate self-harm, impaired bone density, reduced skeletal function, impaired reproductive health in women, and overweight [97]. Referral to a nutritionist should be considered in young PWE at the time of diagnosis.

8.2 Pregnancy

Few studies in the literature have focused on eating disorders and epilepsy. Using data from the Norwegian Mother and Child Cohort Study linked to the Medical Birth Registry of Norway, Kolstad et al., studied 706 pregnancies in women with epilepsy and 106,508 pregnancies in women without epilepsy. Overall, women with epilepsy in the cohort had lower educational attainment and low income, were single parents, and had significantly higher weight and BMI than the control group. Pregnant women with epilepsy are significantly more likely to have binge-eating disorders (6.5% vs. 4.7%, $P < 0.05$). Women with epilepsy and comorbid eating disorders had significantly more preeclampsia (7.9% vs. 3.7%, $P < 0.05$), peripartum depression and/or anxiety (40.4% vs. 17.8%, $P < 0.001$), and operative delivery (38.2% vs. 23.5%, $P < 0.001$) than the reference group without epilepsy or eating disorders [98]. Rai et al. also found an increased frequency of eating disorders (OR 2.9) in PWE in a nationally representative population-based study in England [99].

8.3 Children

Pediatric epilepsy has been linked to different phenotypes, including variable degrees of intellectual disability. DD is associated with sedentary behavior and specific sedentary lifestyle patterns, such as playing digital games, using computers, and especially watching television, leading to reduced energy expenditure and increased intake of unhealthy food. Finally, the concomitant use of psychotropic medications can lead to overweight.

9. Neurological consequences of obesity in people with epilepsy

Body weight gain in children, adolescents, and adults disturbs general health, causes cosmetic adverse effects, and has serious psychological effects. Obesity is a biomarker for cardiovascular diseases that have a direct impact on cognitive function. In particular, central obesity has been associated with accelerated age-related cognitive decline from middle age onward and with an increased risk of developing dementia in old age [100, 101]. A recently published study from the UK assessed the impact of obesity on cognitive function in 81 patients with DRE. BMI was correlated with intelligence quotient (IQ) under function and slowed processing speed in these patients. The more overweight the patient, the higher the cognitive impairment in memory and verbal and visual learning [102].

9.1 Widespread neuroinflammation

When considering obesity and neuroinflammation, the focus has long been set on the hypothalamus. Neurons in the arcuate nucleus are contiguous to the third ventricle, circumventricular organs, and mediobasal eminence; thus, these cells can sense peripheral hormones, such as insulin, leptin, and ghrelin. Consequently, the arcuate nucleus can monitor the energy status of the organism, and it is responsible for weight stability [103]. Nevertheless, obesity-derived neuroinflammation affects other brain structures. It has been demonstrated in rodent models of diet-induced obesity, the presence of increased inflammatory markers, including: Toll-like receptor 4, IL-6, IL-1β, inducible nitric oxide synthase, nuclear factor-kB, TNF-a, cyclooxygenase-2, and CCL2, in the cerebral cortex, hippocampus, cerebellum, brainstem, and amygdala. Additionally, there is evidence of glial activation (gliosis and astrogliosis) and blood–brain barrier disruption [103, 104].

9.2 Structural changes secondary to obesity

It has been shown by MRI that obese subjects display increased hypothalamic gliosis. This was further confirmed using histology where individuals with a BMI of >30 presented an exacerbated microglia activation compared to individuals with a BMI of <25 [103]. Obesity measured by BMI in adults is associated with decreased ventral diencephalon and brainstem volumes [105]. Anthropometric markers have also been associated with profound architectural alterations in white and gray matters, and with microglial activation. In older adults, waist-to-hip ratio and waist circumference are associated with decreased overall brain volume [106].

9.3 Functional changes secondary to obesity

Different mechanisms of obesity have been identified as being able to alter cognitive function (learning and memory deficits), including reduced levels of BDNF, altered glutamatergic signaling, impaired insulin regulation and altered glucose transport into the CNS [107–109]. Such induced changes collectively translate into a vicious cycle of deranged metabolic control and cognitive deficits. Obesity has been clinically associated with increased occurrence of neurologic disorders, such as depression, anxiety, impaired cognitive function, reduction in executive functioning and attention, decreased global functioning, and lesser IQ [103, 104].

The hippocampus is a vital structure for cognition, processing of short- to long-term memory, learning, spatial navigation, and emotions. HFD results in increased hippocampal TNF-a expression, activated microglia, increased lipid peroxidation, proapoptotic signaling, such as increased expression of caspase-3, and gliosis in the hippocampus, particularly in the dentate gyrus. Such inflammation and cell damage lead to loss of hippocampal tissue, which could harbor accelerated cognitive impairment in late life [104]. Fascinatingly, in both hippocampus and cortex of mice, forced treadmill exercise normalized glial cell activation and rescued working memory and spatial learning [41]. Furthermore, voluntary exercise was not as efficient as mandatory physical activity for mice fed a Western diet. Voluntary running led to decreased expression of CCL2 (monocyte chemoattractant protein-1) and CXCL10 (previously known as Interferon gamma-induced protein 10) in the prefrontal cortex but had no effect on glial cell activation [110].

10. Conclusion

PWE in the general population have a twofold to fivefold risk of somatic comorbid conditions compared with people without epilepsy. There is a clear need for an integrated approach in PWE. Understanding obesity as a comorbidity of epilepsy is important from several perspectives. First, understanding obesity influences treatment, creating both therapeutic limitations and opportunities. Neurologists are often the primary care physicians for PWE, and obesity management must be a clinical priority. Identifying a problem like obesity to the attention of PWE increases the likelihood that they will initiate efforts for weight control. The use of the term overweight or elevated BMI rather than obesity may help start the discussion with patients. Body weight gain has been traditionally reported with the use of VPA, CBZ, GBP, and VGB. Patients starting these medications should be warned about possible body weight gain and should be advised to begin diet and exercise. It is also prudent to avoid combinations of VPA with CBZ, GBP, or VGB in patients who already are overweight or obese.

The study of obesity and epilepsy also provides epidemiological clues to the fundamental mechanisms of epilepsy and associated conditions. Abnormalities of brain development, feeding behavior, and energy metabolism could share some common mechanisms, offering potential for modification of gene expression with widespread benefits in the future. For instance, low serum leptin levels are associated with FS in susceptible children. The future may hold a greater promise for therapeutic success using metabolic hormones and their signaling modalities to treat seizure disorders rather than obesity. If the association between maternal obesity and offspring's epilepsy is consistent, then efforts to combat obesity on the population can have the potential to reduce the risk of epileptic syndromes and other neurodevelopmental disabilities.

Finally, patients with multiple comorbidities require a higher level of health care resources than those with one condition. Programs specifically tailored to the needs of children and adults with epilepsy and obesity are needed. The programs need to be focused on healthy living and physical activity practice, rather than management of overweight or obesity. The school and seizure clinics may be the most appropriate venues for delivering such programs. The importance of promoting healthy living styles to the students, patients, and their families is the most relevant. Interventions such as lessons on physical activity, nutrition, and healthy living in their curriculum, investing in special resources, equipment, and facilities, and investing time in upskilling staff are advised. Appropriate tools need to be developed to accurately determine physical activity, nutrition, and health behaviors in children and adults with epilepsy.

References

[1] Ogden CL, Carroll MD, Fryar CD, Flegal KM. Prevalence of obesity among adults and youth: United States, 2011–2014. NCHS Data Brief 2015;219(219):1–8.

[2] WHO European action plan for food and nutrition policy 2007–2012. Copenhagen: WHO Regional Office for Europe; 2008. Available from: http://www.euro.who.int/Document/E91153.pdf.

[3] Aschner P. Obesity in Latin America. In: Ahima RS, editor. Metabolic syndrome. Cham: Springer; 2016. p. 250.

[4] American Society for metabolic and bariatric surgery. Disease of Obesity, Available from: https://asmbs.org/patients/disease-of-obesity/2018/; 2018.

[5] Sato T, Ida T, Nakamura Y, Shiimura Y, Kangawa K, Kojima M. Physiological roles of ghrelin on obesity. Obes Res Clin Pract 2014;8(5):e405–13.

[6] GBD 2015 Neurological Disorders Collaborator Group. Global, regional, and national burden of neurological disorders during 1990–2015: a systematic analysis for the Global Burden of Disease Study 2015. Lancet Neurol 2017;16(11):877–97.

[7] Leonardi M, Ustun TB. The global burden of epilepsy. Epilepsia 2002;43(suppl 6):21–5.

[8] Gao S, Juhaeri J, Dai WS. The incidence rate of seizures in relation to BMI in UK adults. Obesity (Silver Spring) 2008;16(9):2126–32.

[9] Tellez-Zenteno JF, Pondal-Sordo M, Matijevic S, Wiebe S. National and regional prevalence of self-reported epilepsy in Canada. Epilepsia 2014;45:1623–9.

[10] Murray CJ, Lopez AD, Jamison DT. The global burden of disease in 1990: summary results, sensitivity analysis and future directions. Bull World Health Organ 1994;72:495–509.

[11] Wiebe S, Bellhouse DR, Fallahay C, Eliasziw M. Burden of epilepsy: the Ontario health survey. Can J Neurol Sci 1999;26:263–70.

[12] Jakovljevic M, Ostojic L. Comorbidity and multimorbidity in medicine today: challenges and opportunities for bringing separated branches of medicine closer to each other. Psychiatr Danub 2013;25 (suppl 1):18–28.

[13] Daniels ZS, Nick TG, Liu C, Cassedy A, Glauser TA. Obesity is a common comorbidity for pediatric patients with untreated, newly diagnosed epilepsy. Neurology 2009;73:658–64.

[14] Arya R, Gillespie CW, Cnaan A, Devarajan M, Clark P, Shinnar S, Vinks AA, Mizuno K, Glauser TA, Childhood Absence Epilepsy Study Group. Obesity and overweight as CAE comorbidities and differential drug response modifiers. Neurology 2016;86(17):1613–21.

[15] Hinnell C, Williams J, Metcalfe A, Patten SB, Parker R, Wiebe S, Jetté N. Health status and health-related behaviors in epilepsy compared to other chronic conditions–a national population-based study. Epilepsia 2010;51(5):853–61.

[16] Steinhoff BJ, Neususs K, Thegeder H, Reimers CD. Leisure time activity and physical fitness in patients with epilepsy. Epilepsia 1996;37:1221–7.

[17] Kobau R, Dilorio CA, Price PH, Thurman DJ, Martin LM, Ridings DL, Henry TR. Prevalence of epilepsy and health status of adults with epilepsy in Georgia and Tennessee: behavioral risk factor surveillance system, 2002. Epilepsy Behav 2004;5:358–66.

[18] Janousek J, Barber A, Goldman L, Klein P. Obesity in adults with epilepsy. Epilepsy Behav 2013;28 (3):391–4.

[19] Ladino LD, Hernández-Ronquillo L, Téllez-Zenteno JF. Obesity and its association with generalized epilepsy, idiopathic syndrome, and family history of epilepsy. Epileptic Disord 2014;16(3):343–53.

[20] Lee EB, Mattson MP. The neuropathology of obesity: insights from human disease. Acta Neuropathol 2014;127(1):3–28.

[21] Heisler LK, Chu HM, Tecott LH. Epilepsy and obesity in serotonin 5-HT2C receptor mutant mice. Ann N Y Acad Sci 1998;861:74–8.

[22] Pesapane R, Good DJ. Seizures in a colony of genetically obese mice. Lab Anim (NY) 2009;38 (3):81–3.

[23] Castracane VD, Henson MC. The Obese (ob/ob) mouse and the discovery of leptin. In: Castracane VD, Henson MC, editors. Leptin. Endocrine Updates, 25:Boston, MA: Springer; 2006. p. 118.

[24] Erbayat-Altay E, Yamada KA, Wong M, Thio LL. Increased severity of pentylenetetrazol induced seizures in leptin deficient Ob/Ob mice. Neurosci Lett 2008;433(2):82–6.

[25] Verrotti A, Soldani C, Laino D, d'Alonzo R, Grosso S. Epilepsy in Prader-Willi syndrome: clinical, diagnostic and treatment aspects. World J Pediatr 2014;10(2):108–13.

[26] Vauthier V, Jaillard S, Journel H, Dubourg C, Jockers R, Dam J. Homozygous deletion of an 80 kb region comprising part of DNAJC6 and LEPR genes on chromosome 1P31.3 is associated with early onset obesity, mental retardation and epilepsy. Mol Genet Metab 2012;106:345–50.

[27] Halgren C, Bache I, Bak M, Myatt MW, Anderson CM, Brøndum-Nielsen K, Tommerup N. Haploinsufficiency of CELF4 at 18q12.2 is associated with developmental and behavioral disorders, seizures, eye manifestations, and obesity. Eur J Hum Genet 2012;20(12):1315–9.

[28] Huynh MT, Lambert AS, Tosca L, Petit F, Philippe C, Parisot F, Benoît V, Linglart A, Brisset S, Tran CT, Tachdjian G, Receveur A. 15q24.1 BP4-BP1 microdeletion unmasking paternally inherited functional polymorphisms combined with distal 15q24.2q24.3 duplication in a patient with epilepsy, psychomotor delay, overweight, ventricular arrhythmia. Eur J Med Genet 2018;(17):30693–6. pii:S1769-7212.

[29] Leshinsky-Silver E, Zinger A, Bibi CN, Barash V, Sadeh M, Lev D, Sagie TL. MEHMO (mental retardation, epileptic seizures, hypogenitalism, microcephaly, obesity): a new X-linked mitochondrial disorder. Eur J Hum Genet 2002;10(4):226–30.

[30] Tarpey PS, Raymond FL, O'Meara S, Edkins S, Teague J, Butler A, Dicks E, Stevens C, Tofts C, Avis T, Barthorpe S, Buck G, Cole J, Gray K, Halliday K, Harrison R, Hills K, Jenkinson A, Jones D, Menzies A, Mironenko T, Perry J, Raine K, Richardson D, Shepherd R, Small A,

Varian J, West S, Widaa S, Mallya U, Moon J, Luo Y, Holder S, Smithson SF, Hurst JA, Clayton-Smith J, Kerr B, Boyle J, Shaw M, Vandeleur L, Rodriguez J, Slaugh R, Easton DF, Wooster R, Bobrow M, Srivastava AK, Stevenson RE, Schwartz CE, Turner G, Gecz J, Futreal PA, Stratton MR, Partington M. Mutations in CUL4B, which encodes a ubiquitin E3 ligase subunit, cause an X-linked mental retardation syndrome associated with aggressive outbursts, seizures, relative macrocephaly, central obesity, hypogonadism, pes cavus, and tremor. Am J Hum Genet 2007;80(2):345–52.

[31] Mariani M, Decimi V, Bettini LR, Maitz S, Gervasini C, Masciadri M, Ajmone P, Kullman G, Dinelli M, Panceri R, Cereda A, Selicorni A. Adolescents and adults affected by Cornelia de Lange syndrome: a report of 73 Italian patients. Am J Med Genet C Semin Med Genet 2016;172(2):206–13.

[32] Flegal KM, Carroll MD, Kit BK, Ogden CL. Prevalence of obesity and trends in the distribution of body mass index among US adults, 1999–2010. JAMA 2012;307(5):491–7.

[33] Bell WL. Maternal obesity and epilepsy. JAMA Neurol 2017;74(6):637–9.

[34] Razaz N, Tedroff K, Villamor E, Cnattingius S. Maternal body mass index in early pregnancy and risk of epilepsy in offspring. JAMA Neurol 2017;74(6):668–76.

[35] Harden CL. The plausibility of an association between maternal obesity and onset of childhood epilepsy: a well-rounded, robust argument or a thin epidemiologic association? Epilepsy Curr 2017;17(5):288–90.

[36] Ramsay JE, Ferrell WR, Crawford L, Wallace AM, Greer IA, Sattar N. Maternal obesity is associated with dysregulation of metabolic, vascular, and inflammatory pathways. J Clin Endocrinol Metab 2002;87(9):4231–7.

[37] Hauguel-de Mouzon S, Lepercq J, Catalano P. The known and unknown of leptin in pregnancy. Am J Obstet Gynecol 2006;194(6):1537–45.

[38] Tozuka Y, Wada E, Wada K. Diet-induced obesity in female miceleads to peroxidized lipid accumulations and impairment of hippocampalneurogenesis during the early life of their offspring. FASEB J 2009;23:1920–34.

[39] Zhang X, Dong F, Ren J, Driscoll MJ, Culver B. High dietary fat induces NADPH oxidase-associated oxidative stress and inflammation in rat cerebralcortex. Exp Neurol 2005;191:318–25.

[40] Moroz N, Tong M, Longato L, Xu H, de la Monte SM. Limited Alzheimer-type neurodegeneration in experimental obesity and type 2 diabetes mellitus. J Alzheimers Dis 2008;15:29–44.

[41] Kang DH, Heo RW, Yi CO, Kim H, Choi CH, Roh GS. High-fat diet-induced obesity exacerbates kainic acid-induced hippocampal cell death. BMC Neurosci 2015;16:72.

[42] Mehta SH, Kerver JM, Sokol RJ, Keating DP, Paneth N. The association between maternal obesity and neurodevelopmental outcomes of offspring. J Pediatr 2014;165(5):891–6.

[43] Pugh SJ, Richardson GA, Hutcheon JA, et al. Maternal obesity and excessive gestational weight gain are associated with components of child cognition. J Nutr 2015;145(11):2562–9.

[44] Forthun I, Wilcox AJ, Strandberg-Larsen K, Moster D, Nohr EA, Lie RT, Surén P, Tollånes MC. Maternal prepregnancy BMI and risk of cerebral palsy in offspring. Pediatrics 2016;138(4). pii:e20160874.

[45] Pan C, Deroche CB, Mann JR, McDermott S, Hardin JW. Is prepregnancy obesity associated with risk of cerebral palsy and epilepsy in children? J Child Neurol 2014;29(12):196–201.

[46] Mann JR, McDermott SW, Hardin J, Pan C, Zhang Z. Pre-pregnancy body mass index, weight change during pregnancy, and risk of intellectual disability in children. BJOG 2013;120(3):309–19.

[47] Alfaradhi MZ, Ozanne SE. Developmental programming in response to maternal overnutrition. Front Genet 2011;2:27.

[48] Segovia SA, Vickers MH, Gray C, Reynolds CM. Maternal obesity, inflammation, and developmental programming. Biomed Res Int 2014;2014:418975.

[49] King BM. The modern obesity epidemic, ancestral hunter-gatherers, and the sensory/reward control of food intake. Am Psychol 2013;68(2):88–96.

[50] Jallon P, Picard F. Bodyweight gain and anticonvulsants: a comparative review. Drug Saf 2001;24 (13):969–78.

[51] Berilgen MS, Mungen B, Ustundag B, Demir C. Serum ghrelin levels are enhanced in patients with epilepsy. Seizure 2006;15:106–11.

[52] Gungor S, Yücel G, Akinci A, Tabel Y, Ozerol IH, Yologlu S. The role of ghrelin in weight gain and growth in epileptic children using valproate. J Child Neurol 2007;22:1384–8.

[53] Ataie Z, Golzar MG, Babri S, Ebrahimi H, Mohaddes G. Does ghrelin level change after epileptic seizure in rats? Seizure 2011;20(4):347–9.

[54] Verrotti A, Basciani F, Morresi S, et al. Serum leptin changes in epileptic patients who gain weight after therapy with valproic acid. Neurology 1999;53:230–2.

[55] (a)Yakubov B, Berall G, Hwang P. Seizures in patients with leptin receptor deficiency: coincidence or close correlation? Clin Neurophysiol 2014;125:e49–52; (b)Thio LL, Erbayat-Altay E, Rensing N, Yamada KA. Leptin contributes to slower weight gain in juvenile rodents on a ketogenic diet. Pediatr Res 2006;60:413–7.

[56] Diano S, Horvath TL. Anticonvulsant effects of leptin in epilepsy. J Clin Invest 2008;118(1):26–8.

[57] Greco R, Latini G, Chiarelli F, Iannetti P, Verrotti A. Leptin, ghrelin, and adiponectin in epileptic patients treated with valproic acid. Neurology 2005;65(11):1808–9.

[58] González-Muniesa P, Mártinez-González MA, Hu FB, Després JP, Matsuzawa Y, Loos RJF, Moreno LA, Bray GA, Martinez JA. Obesity. Nat Rev Dis Primers 2017;3:.

[59] Palmio J, Vuoltenaho K, Lehtimäki K, Nieminen R, Peltola J, Moilanen E. CSF and plasma adipokines after tonic-clonic seizures. Seizure 2016;39:10–2.

[60] Xu L, Rensing N, Yang XF, Zhang HX, Thio LL, Rothman SM, Weisenfeld AE, Wong M, Yamada KA. Leptin inhibits 4-aminopyridine- and pentylenetetrazole-induced seizures and AMPAR-mediated synaptic transmission in rodents. J Clin Invest 2008;118(1):272–80.

[61] Azab SF, Abdalhady MA, Almalky MA, Amin EK, Sarhan DT, Elhindawy EM, Allah MA, Elhewala AA, Salam MM, Hashem MI, Soliman AA, Akeel NE, Abdellatif SH, Elsamad NA, Rass AA, Arafat MS. Serum and CSF adiponectin, leptin, and interleukin 6 levels as adipocytokines in Egyptian children with febrile seizures: a cross-sectional study. Ital J Pediatr 2016;42:38.

[62] Chen B, Choi H, Hirsch LJ, Moeller J, Javed A, Kato K, Legge A, Buchsbaum R, Detyniecki K. Cosmetic side effects of antiepileptic drugs in adults with epilepsy. Epilepsy Behav 2015;42:129–37.

[63] Davis R, Peters DH, McTavish D. Valproic acid. A reappraisal of its pharmacological properties and clinical efficacy in epilepsy. Drugs 1994;47:332–72.

[64] Verrotti A, la Torre R, Trotta D, Mohn A, Chiarelli F. Valproate induced insulin resistance and obesity in children. Horm Res 2009;71:125e31.

[65] Isojärvi JIT, Laatikainen TJ, Pakarinen AJ, et al. Polycystic ovaries and hyperandrogenism in women taking valproate for epilepsy. N Engl J Med 1993;329:1383–8.

[66] Dinesen H, Gram L, Andersen T, Dam M. Weight gain during treatment with valproate. Acta Neurol Scand 1984;70:65–9.

[67] Privitera M, Ficker DM. Assessment of adverse events and quality of life in epilepsy: design of a new community-based trial. Epilepsy Behav 2004;5(6):841–6.

[68] Belcastro V, D'Egidio C, Striano P, Verrotti A. Metabolic and endocrine effects of valproic acid chronic treatment. Epilepsy Res 2013;107(1–2):1–8.

[69] El-Khatib F, Rauchenzauner M, Lechleitner M, Hoppichler F, Naser A, Waldmann M, Trinka E, Unterberger I, Bauer G, Luef GJ. Valproate, weight gain and carbohydrate craving: a gender study. Seizure 2007;16(3):226–32.

[70] Cansu A, Serdaroglu A, Camurdan O, Hırfanoğlu T, Cinaz P. Serum insulin, cortisol, leptin, neuropeptide Y, galanin and ghrelin levels in epileptic children receiving valproate. Horm Res Paediatr 2011;76(1):65–71.

[71] Fang J, Chen S, Tong N, Chen L, An D, Mu J, Zhou D. Metabolic syndrome among Chinese obese patients with epilepsy on sodium valproate. Seizure 2012;21(8):578–82.

[72] Grosso S, Mostardini R, Piccini B, Balestri P. Body mass index and serum lipid changes during treatment with valproic acid in children with epilepsy. Ann Pharmacother 2009;43(1):45–50.

[73] El-Khayat HA, Abd El-Basset FZ, Tomoum HY, Tohamy SM, Zaky AA, Mohamed MS, Hakky SM, El Barbary NS, Nassef NM. Physical growth and endocrinal disorders during pubertal maturation in girls with epilepsy. Epilepsia 2004;45(9):1106–15.

[74] Goldberg-Stern H, Yaacobi E, Phillip M, de Vries L. Endocrine effects of valproic acid therapy in girls with epilepsy: a prospective study. Eur J Paediatr Neurol 2014;18(6):759–65.

[75] Richens A, Davidson DL, Cartlidge NE, Easter DJ. A multicentre comparative trial of sodium valproate and carbamazepine in adult onset epilepsy. Adult EPITEG collaborative group. J Neurol Neurosurg Psychiatry 1994;57(6):682–7.

[76] Mattson RH, Cramer JA, Collins JF. A comparison of valproate with carbamazepine for the treatment of complex partial seizures and secondarily generalized tonic-clonic seizures in adults. N Engl J Med 1992;327:765–71.

[77] Corman CL, Leung NM, Guberman AH. Weight gain in epileptic patients during treatment with valproic acid: a retrospective study. Can J Neurol Sci 1997;24(3):240–4.

[78] Caksen H, Deda G, Berberoğlu M, Içağasioğlu D, Turan EB. Serum leptin levels in children receiving long-term carbamazepine. Acta Paediatr Taiwan 2003;44(2):82–3.

[79] Uludag IF, Kulu U, Sener U, Kose S, Zorlu Y. The effect of carbamazepine treatment on serum leptin levels. Epilepsy Res 2009;86(1):48–53.

[80] Garoufi A, Vartzelis G, Tsentidis C, Attilakos A, Koemtzidou E, Kossiva L, Katsarou E, Soldatou A. Weight gain in children on oxcarbazepine monotherapy. Epilepsy Res 2016;122:110–3.

[81] Nam S, Kim Y. Weight change by oxcarbazepine monotherapy in childhood epilepsy. Epilepsia 2006;47(S3):1–272.

[82] Guberman A, Bruni J. Long-term open multicentre, add-on trial of vigabatrin in adult resistant partial epilepsy. The Canadian Vigabatrin Study Group. Seizure 2000;9(2):112–8.

[83] Beydoun A, Fischer J, Labar DR, Harden C, Cantrell D, Uthman BM, Sackellares JC, Abou-Khalil B, Ramsay RE, Hayes A, Greiner M, Garofalo E, Pierce M. Gabapentin monotherapy: II. A 26-week, double-blind, dose-controlled, multicenter study of conversion from polytherapy in outpatients with refractory complex partial or secondarily generalized seizures. The US gabapentin study group 82/83. Neurology 1997;49(3):746–52.

[84] Baulac M, Cavalcanti D, Semah F, Arzimanoglou A, Portal JJ. Gabapentin add-on therapy with adaptable dosages in 610 patients with partial epilepsy: an open, observational study. The French Gabapentin Collaborative Group. Seizure 1998;7(1):55–62.

[85] Li HF, Zou Y, Xia ZZ, Gao F, Feng JH, Yang CW. Effects of topiramate on weight and metabolism in children with epilepsy. Acta Paediatr 2009;98(9):1521–5.

[86] Mourand I, Crespel A, Gelisse P. Dramatic weight loss with rufinamide. Epilepsia 2013;54(1):e5–8.

[87] Kim DW, Yoo MW, Park KS. Low serum leptin level is associated with zonisamide-induced weight loss in overweight female epilepsy patients. Epilepsy Behav 2012;23(4):497–9.

[88] Jalava M, Sillanpää M. Physical activity, health-related fitness, and health experience in adults with childhood-onset epilepsy: a controlled study. Epilepsia 1997;38(4):424–9.

[89] Cui W, Zack MM, Kobau R, Helmers SL. Health behaviors among people with epilepsy—results from the 2010 National Health Interview Survey. Epilepsy Behav 2015;44:121–6.

[90] Elliott JO, Moore JL, Lu B. Health status and behavioral risk factors among persons with epilepsy in Ohio based on the 2006 behavioral risk factor surveillance system. Epilepsy Behav 2008;12(3):434.

[91] Elliott BJO, Lu B, Moore JL, McAuley JW, Long L. Exercise, diet, health behaviors, and risk factors among persons with epilepsy based on the California health interview survey, 2005. Epilepsy Behav 2008;13(2):307–15.

[92] Wong J, Wirrell E. Physical activity in children/teens with epilepsy compared with that in their siblings without epilepsy. Epilepsia 2006;47(3):631–9.

[93] Gordon KE, Dooley JM, Brna PM. Epilepsy and activity—a population-based study: epilepsy and activity. Epilepsia 2010;51(11):2254–9.

[94] Arida RM, Scorza FA, de Albuquerque M, Cysneiros RM, de Oliveira RJ, Cavalheiro EA. Evaluation of physical exercise habits in Brazilian patients with epilepsy. Epilepsy Behav 2003;4(5):507–10.

[95] Han K, Choi-Kwon S, Lee S-K. Leisure time physical activity in patients with epilepsy in Seoul, South Korea. Epilepsy Behav 2011;20(2):321–5.

[96] Alfstad KA, Clench-Aas J, Van Roy B, et al. Psychiatric symptoms in Norwegian children with epilepsy aged 8–13 years: effects of age and gender? Epilepsia 2011;52:1231–8.

[97] Kolstad E, Bjørk M, Gilhus NE, Alfstad K, Clench-Aas J, Lossius M. Young people with epilepsy have an increased risk of eating disorder and poor quality diet. Epilepsia Open 2017;3(1):40–5.

[98] Kolstad E, Gilhus NE, Veiby G, Reiter SF, Lossius MI, Bjørk M. Epilepsy and eating disorders during pregnancy: prevalence, complications and birth outcome. Seizure 2015;28:81–4.

[99] Rai D, Kerr MP, McManus S, Jordanova V, Lewis G, Brugha TS. Epilepsy and psychiatric comorbidity: a nationally representative population-based study. Epilepsia 2012;53(6):1095–103.

[100] Dahl A, Hassing LB, Fransson E, Berg S, Gatz M, Reynolds CA, Pedersen NL. Being overweight in midlife is associated with lower cognitive ability and steeper cognitive decline in late life. J Gerontol A Biol Sci Med Sci 2010;65(1):57–62.

[101] Birdsill AC, Carlsson CM, Willette AA, Okonkwo OC, Johnson SC, Xu G, Oh JM, Gallagher CL, Koscik RL, Jonaitis EM, Hermann BP, LaRue A, Rowley HA, Asthana S, Sager MA, Bendlin BB. Low cerebral blood flow is associated with lower memory function in metabolic syndrome. Obesity (Silver Spring) 2013;21(7):1313–20.

[102] Baxendale S, McGrath K, Donnachie E, Wintle S, Thompson P, Heaney D. The role of obesity in cognitive dysfunction in people with epilepsy. Epilepsy Behav 2015;45:187–90.

[103] Guillemot-Legris O, Muccioli GG. Obesity-induced neuroinflammation: beyond the hypothalamus. Trends Neurosci 2017;40(4):237–53.

[104] Shefer G, Marcus Y, Stern N. Is obesity a brain disease? Neurosci Biobehav Rev 2013;37(10 Pt 2): 2489–503.

[105] Marques-Iturria I. Frontal cortical thinning and subcortical volume reductions in early adulthood obesity. Psychiatry Res 2013;214:109–15.

[106] Debette S, Wolf C, Lambert JC, Crivello F, Soumaré A, Zhu YC, Schilling S, Dufouil C, Mazoyer B, Amouyel P, Tzourio C, Elbaz A. Abdominal obesity and lower gray matter volume: a Mendelian randomization study. Neurobiol Aging 2014;35(2):378–86.

[107] Miller AA, Spencer SJ. Obesity and neuroinflammation: a pathway to cognitive impairment. Brain Behav 2014;42:10–21.

[108] Kanoski SE, Davidson TL. Western diet consumption and cognitive impairment: links to hippocampal dysfunction and obesity. Physiol Behav 2011;103:59–68.

[109] Hsu TM, Kanoski SE. Blood-brain barrier disruption: mechanistic links between Western diet consumption and dementia. Front Aging Neurosci 2014;6:88.

[110] Carlin JL, Grissom N, Ying Z, Gomez-Pinilla F, Reyes TM. Voluntary exercise blocks Western diet-induced gene expression of the chemokines CXCL10 and CCL2 in the prefrontal cortex. Brain Behav Immun 2016;58:82–90.

CHAPTER 8

Epilepsy and heart diseases

Sharon Shmuely*,†, **Roland D. Thijs***,†,‡
*Stichting Epilepsie Instellingen Nederland—SEIN, Heemstede, The Netherlands
†NIHR University College London Hospitals Biomedical Research Centre, UCL Institute of Neurology, London, United Kingdom
‡Department of Neurology, LUMC Leiden University Medical Centre, Leiden, The Netherlands

Contents

1. Introduction

Well over 100 years ago, the occurrence of asystole during the course of an epileptic seizure was described: "He uttered a cry and was seen to be rubbing his hands together. His pulse was immediately examined for but was not palpable" [1]. Since then numerous associations between epilepsy and CV conditions have been identified, including this classical example of ictal asystole.

Coexisting conditions form an important part of the overall burden of epilepsy [2–5]. Several mechanisms of association between epilepsy and comorbid conditions have been described: associations can be explained by cause or effect, a shared risk factor may cause both conditions, or the mechanism of the association is unknown or spurious (i.e., coincidental) [3, 5].

This chapter serves to discuss the fascinating borderland between epileptology and cardiology and focuses on the major developments over the last 25 years and on future developments. We use the comorbidity framework [3, 5] to review all cardiac conditions known, and alleged, to be linked to epilepsy. Associations with cardiac arrhythmias are discussed first, followed by an overview of all structural cardiac conditions related to epilepsy.

The Comorbidities of Epilepsy
https://doi.org/10.1016/B978-0-12-814877-8.00008-8

2. Epilepsy and cardiac arrhythmias

Various arrhythmias have been described, occurring during (ictal) or after (postictal) seizures. Sinus tachycardia is the most common ictal pattern, seen in up to 80% of all seizures [6] and in 82% of people with epilepsy [7], but usually without symptoms. The most frequent clinically relevant arrhythmia is ictal asystole, occurring in 0.318% (95% CI 0.316%–0.320%) of people with refractory focal epilepsy admitted for video EEG [8]. Ictal asystole, bradycardia, and AV block predominantly occur in people with temporal lobe epilepsy (Table 1) [8]. Clinically, ictal asystole is characterized by sudden loss of tone during a dyscognitive seizure [11]. The circulatory pattern resembles vasovagal syncope with a transient, progressive, and self-limiting slowing of the heart rate and decrease of blood pressure [11–13]. For many years, ictal asystole was thought to be a possible mechanism underlying sudden unexpected death in epilepsy (SUDEP). This appears to be unlikely: all but one reported case so far of ictal asystole were self-limiting [8]. In this case successful resuscitation was started after 44 s of asystole and the event was classified as near-SUDEP [14]. The longest ictal asystole reported so far, however, lasted 96 s and appeared self-limiting [15]. Whether an event is classified as near-SUDEP or not will depend on interventions of medical personnel: prompt resuscitation in response to ictal asystole will likely lead to more classified as near-SUDEP cases. While there are no reports of fatal ictal asystole, it remains debatable whether ictal asystole can cause SUDEP.

The precise mechanism of ictal asystole is unknown. It may result from epileptic activity directly stimulating the central autonomic networks [6, 16]. For example, focal stimulation of parts of the limbic system (i.e., amygdala, cingulate gyrus) may provoke asystole [6, 17–19]. Alternatively, seizure-induced fear and catecholamine release [20] may evoke a vasovagal response causing cardioinhibition and vasodilation [21].

Ictal asystole is assumed to be self-limiting but may cause falls and injuries due to seizure-induced syncope [22]. Proper trials are lacking, but retrospective studies suggest that improving seizure control may prevent ictal asystole [23–25]. It also seems advisable to withdraw negative inotropic drugs and to consider the implantation of a loop recorder to monitor possible future cardioinhibitory events in individuals in whom ictal asystole has been noted. If the asystolic episodes persist, cardiac pacemaker implantation should be considered to reduce the risk of trauma [22, 23, 25, 26].

In contrast to ictal asystole, postictal asystole is less common, associated with convulsive rather than focal (temporal lobe) seizures and has a higher fatality rate; 7 of 13 reported postictal asystole cases died from SUDEP [8]. All fatal cases had a convulsive seizure with immediate postictal generalized EEG suppression and a stuttering course of transient apnea and asystole resulting in a terminal apnea followed by a terminal asystole [9].

The mechanism underlying this sequence of postictal EEG suppression, apnea, and terminal asystole has not yet been elucidated. Excessive inhibition causing brainstem depression might play a role [27]. Recent work in two animal models (mice carrying mutations in the KCNA1 gene or the SCN1A gene) demonstrated that seizures initiated

Table 1 Reported (post)ictal cardiac arrhythmias

Seizure-related arrhythmia	Reported in n cases	Associated seizure types	Reported in n cases	EEG seizure onset	Reported in n cases	SUDEP association
Ictal asystole	103	99% FDS 1% FAS	97	46% LT 31% RT 13% BT 10% Other	80	Unlikely
Postictal asystole	13	85% fbTCS 15% FDS	13	20% LT 60% RT 20% Other	10	Likely, accompanied or preceded by PGES/apnea (Ryvlin et al. [9])
Ictal bradycardia	25	100% FDS	8	52% LT 38% RT 10% Other	21	Unlikely
Ictal AV block	11	90% FDS 10% FAS	10	73% LT 18% BT 10% Other	11	Unlikely
Postictal AV block	2	100% fbTCS	2	100% RT	1	Unlikely
Atrial fibrillation	13	46% GTCS 46% fbTCS 8% FDS	13	33% LT 33% Gen 33% Non loc	3	Unlikely
(Post)ictal ventricular fibrillation	4	100% fbTCS/GTCS	4	Insufficient data	0	Probable, but in a minority of cases

FDS, focal dyscognitive seizure; *FAS*, focal autonomic seizure; *fbTCS*, focal seizure evolving to bilateral tonic–clonic seizure; *GTCS*, generalized tonic clonic seizure; *LT*, left temporal; *RT*, right temporal; *BT*, bitemporal; *Non loc*, nonlocalizing; *Gen*, generalized; *PGES*, postictal generalized EEG suppression; *in people with refractory focal epilepsy admitted for a vEEG recording. For more details see [8]. For VF/VT a recent case was added [10].

by direct cortical stimulation may evoke a spreading depression causing brain stem inhibition and cardiorespiratory collapse [28].

Another rare (post)ictal arrhythmia is ventricular tachycardia/ventricular fibrillation (VT/VF). So far four cases of postictal VT/VF leading to (near) SUDEP have been reported [8, 10]. All VT/VF occurred directly following a convulsive seizure. In three cases VT/VF was preceded by PGES/postictal apnea. No cardiac lesions were found in the case reports. There may be a publication bias, however, as cases with seizure-triggered VT/VF and cardiac lesions may not qualify as SUDEP and thus may be less likely to be reported. The mechanism of seizure-induced VT/VF is unclear. Convulsive seizures may exert proarrhythmogenic effects by triggering the sympathetic nervous system, as reflected by the peak in catecholamines and electrodermal activity [20, 29]. At the same time, convulsive seizures may increase cardiac oxygen deprivation by inducing sinus tachycardia [7] and respiratory impairment causing hypoxemia [30]. It has also been found that ECG-markers of sudden cardiac death such as QTc-lengthening and/or shortening [31, 32], and T-wave alternans are more prevalent [25] during and after convulsive seizures. The various factors might interact as seizure-related cardiac repolarization abnormalities appeared more frequent in seizures with ictal hypoxemia compared to those without [33].

Though seizure-induced VT/VF appears to be rare, a prospective community-based study of out-of-hospital cardiac arrests due to ECG-documented VT/VF showed that VT/VF risk in those with epilepsy was three times as high as the general population [34]. A further analysis of those cases with epilepsy and VT/VF showed that most were not seizure-related, but rather occurred in the context of either preexisting heart disease or as the immediate result of an acute myocardial infarction [35]. Preexisting heart disease was a stronger predictor for VT/VF in people with epilepsy than markers of epilepsy severity. In a minority of cases, however, VT/VF was unexplained and a diagnosis of (near) SUDEP was established. It thus appears that sudden cardiac arrest and SUDEP are partially overlapping disease entities.

The increased risk of nonseizure-related VF/VT episodes in people with epilepsy may be explained by high cardiovascular comorbidity [3, 36]. People with epilepsy may have a propensity for sudden cardiac death as reduced heart rate variability, a measure of cardiac sympathovagal balance that is also a risk marker of sudden cardiac death, progressively worsens over time in people with refractory epilepsy, but not in those with well-controlled epilepsy or those who become seizure-free after epilepsy surgery [37, 38]. In addition, other markers of sudden cardiac death, such as early repolarization pattern and QTc-prolongation, are more frequently found in the interictal ECGs of people with epilepsy than in those without epilepsy [39].

Another mechanism explaining the association between arrhythmias and epilepsy is a shared genetic risk factor. A rapidly increasing number of genes potentially linking epilepsy to cardiac arrhythmias has been identified. Here we discuss some relevant examples, starting with the genes predominantly known for their cardiac functions and then the "epilepsy genes."

Several genetic ion channel mutations are thought to be expressed in the brain as well as in the heart and might thus cause seizures and cardiac arrhythmias. The first reported genetic link between epilepsy and cardiac arrhythmias was the discovery of cardiac sodium channel gene *SCN5A* in the brain [40]. Subsequently, more pathogenic variants in the long QT (LQT) gene family (i.e., *KCNQ1*, *KCNH2*, and *SCN5A*) were associated with a "seizure phenotype" (e.g., self-reported diagnosis of epilepsy and AED use) [41–46]. Mice models indicated that other, nonLQT, cardiac channelopathy genes, including *RYR2* (associated with catecholaminergic polymorphic ventricular tachycardia) [47] and *HCN1-4* [48, 49], potentially predispose to epilepsy.

Several postmortem studies suggest that the LQT and nonLQT cardiac gene mutations are more common in SUDEP victims [50–55]. As ictal recordings are lacking, it remains questionable whether the fatal events were caused by arrhythmias. The same applies to the identification of "epilepsy genes" in the postmortem cohorts [50, 51]. These mutations could be markers explaining epilepsy severity or a genetically mediated liability to fatal seizures. In certain epilepsy syndromes, SUDEP risk seems particularly high. The most recognized example is the Dravet syndrome (DS), a severe epilepsy syndrome with high premature mortality, caused by *SCN1A* mutation [56]. In mutant *SCN1A* knock-out mice, postictal bradycardia, and seizure-triggered ventricular fibrillation were recorded before a death resembling SUDEP [57, 58]. In DS subjects, markers associated with the risk of sudden cardiac death (decreased HRV and increased QT-dispersion) have been found [59, 60].

Other less studied examples of "epilepsy genes" possibly mediating SUDEP risk include *KCNA1* and *SCN8A*. *KCNA1* is expressed in the vagal nerve as well as in the brain and is associated with seizures, cardiac arrhythmias, vagal hyperexcitability, and premature death in *KCNA1* null mice [61]. Mutations in this gene were found in a SUDEP case with epileptic encephalopathy and suspected cardiac arrhythmias [62].

A novel pathogenic *SCN8A* mutation was identified through whole-genome sequencing in a family affected by epileptic encephalopathy and SUDEP [63]. Before then, *SCN8A* mutations had only been linked to epilepsy in mice [64]. The *SCN8A* gene encodes a sodium channel that is expressed in hearts and brains of mice and rats and plays a role in excitation-contraction coupling, action potential propagation, and pacemaking [65, 66].

We previously discussed how seizures may cause arrhythmias. Whether the converse phenomenon exists is a subject of controversy. The major complication is the fact that syncopal events are easily mistaken for epilepsy. Misdiagnosis is a major issue in epilepsy, with reported rates of false positives of up to 71% [67]. Syncope is the most misdiagnosed condition, which is understandable as various symptoms and signs are seen in both conditions [13, 68–71]. Notably, jerking movements or signs indicative of cerebral standstill (complete flattening of the EEG), such as posturing, roving eye movements, or stertorous breathing [13, 71] are often interpreted as signs specific to epilepsy (Fig. 1).

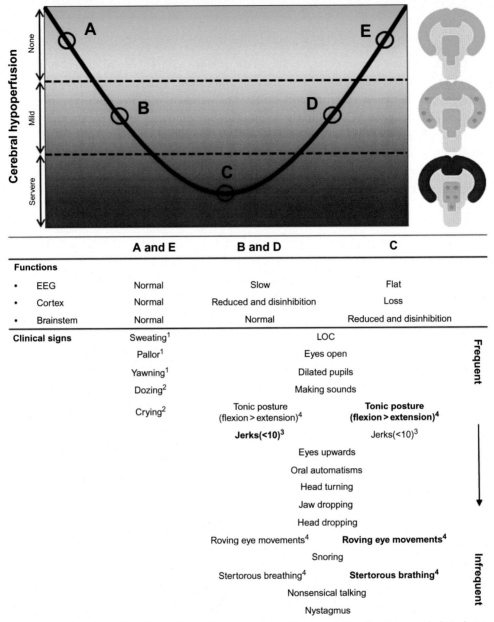

	A and E	B and D	C
Functions			
• EEG	Normal	Slow	Flat
• Cortex	Normal	Reduced and disinhibition	Loss
• Brainstem	Normal	Normal	Reduced and disinhibition
Clinical signs	Sweating[1]	LOC	
	Pallor[1]	Eyes open	
	Yawning[1]	Dilated pupils	
	Dozing[2]	Making sounds	
	Crying[2]	Tonic posture (flexion > extension)[4]	**Tonic posture (flexion > extension)[4]**
		Jerks(<10)[3]	Jerks(<10)[3]
		Eyes upwards	
		Oral automatisms	
		Head turning	
		Jaw dropping	
		Head dropping	
	Roving eye movements[4]		**Roving eye movements[4]**
		Snoring	
	Stertorous breathing[4]		**Stertorous brathing[4]**
		Nonsensical talking	
		Nystagmus	

Frequent → Infrequent

Fig. 1 Schematic illustration of the relation between cerebral hypoperfusion, functions, and clinical signs in syncope. The top graph shows a hypothetical time course of cerebral hypoperfusion (*bold line*) and the corresponding EEG phases. Three situations are distinguished in the schematic graphs of the brain: (A and E) during normal cerebral perfusion: the EEG and function of the cortex and brain stem are normal; (B and D) during mild hypoperfusion: the EEG slows and some cortical functions are impaired while cortical disinhibition also occurs, brainstem function is normal, and jerks may be observed; (C) during deeper hypoperfusion: the EEG flattens, cortical function is nearly completely lost, disinhibition occurs in the brainstem, and tonic postures may be observed. Color legend: green = normal function; yellow = reduced function with EEG slowing; blue = disinhibition; red = loss of function with flattening of the EEG. LOC: loss of consciousness[1]; more frequent prior (A) than after (E) syncope[2]; more frequent after (E) than before (A) syncope[3]; more frequent during B and D than during C[4]; more frequent during C than during B and D. (For more details, see [13, 72]). *Reproduced with permission from Neurology @Wolters Kluwer Health.*

Consequently, most seemingly overlapping presentations turn out to be an isolated phenomenon of either syncope or epilepsy, if a proper investigation is performed (e.g., ictal recording of video, heart rate, blood pressure, and EEG). Two large scale surveys of up to 2000 tilt-table tests failed to identify any adult case with syncopal-induced seizures [73, 74]. In children, however, a few cases have been reported with a cardioinhibitory reflex syncope followed by video EEG-documented clonic seizures [75–77]. The reason this phenomenon only appears to affect children is unknown. It may be that the seizure threshold is lower in children (paralleling febrile seizures that also peak in childhood). Alternatively, the depth of cerebral anoxia may be more profound in children as reflected by prolonged asystolic spells. For clinical management it is important to stress that syncope-induced seizures are extremely rare and probably only affect children. The diagnosis requires an ictal video EEG recording. While syncope may rarely trigger epilepsy, it seems that the prevalence of syncope among people with epilepsy, particularly those with refractory epilepsy, is higher than one would expect [78]. This would, however, require further studies.

Several AEDs, particularly those with sodium-blocking properties, are known to trigger conduction abnormalities or arrhythmias [79]. Atrioventricular (AV) conduction is the most frequently reported complication. ST changes, Brugada-like patterns, atrial fibrillation, and QTc prolongation have also been reported, but the association with AED treatment is less established [80–94]. Most clinically relevant arrhythmias were related to AED overdose. Carbamazepine is, however, known to cause AV conduction blocks at low levels; this is almost exclusively reported in elderly women [85, 87, 95]. Rapid administration of phenytoin may also cause sinus arrest and hypotension; elderly people and those with preexisting heart disease seem most vulnerable to these adverse effects. IV administration should, therefore, be undertaken slowly, with continuous cardiac monitoring [84, 91, 94, 96]. The above-mentioned AED effects do not seem to play a role in ictal arrhythmias. Nevertheless, it is important to take these effects into consideration in the selection of an AED and to monitor adverse effects closely, especially in elderly people and those with cardiovascular comorbidities (Table 2).

3. Epilepsy and structural cardiac conditions

Epidemiological studies have consistently shown that people with epilepsy have a higher prevalence of structural cardiac disease than those without epilepsy [4, 5, 97–100]. Cardiovascular disease seems to be a significant contributor to the increased mortality in people with epilepsy, compared with the general population [101–103].

Shared cardiovascular risk factors can account for the relationship between epilepsy and heart disease, in addition to shared genetics and etiological factors. People with a history of epilepsy are more likely to be obese, physically inactive, and current smokers [98] and have a worse cardiovascular risk profile (i.e., hypertension, hypercholesterolemia,

Table 2 Putative mechanisms of associations between epilepsy and cardiac arrhythmias

Mechanisms of association	Conditions	References
Causal	Arrhythmias → Seizures	Battaglia et al. [74], Horrocks et al. [75], Stephenson et al. [76]
Shared risk factor	Genetics → Epilepsy and arrhythmias • Important "heart genes": *KCNQ1, KCNH2, SCN5A, RYR2* • Important "epilepsy genes": *SCN1A, KCNA1, SCN8A*	Anderson et al. [41], Auerbach et al. [57], Auerbach et al. [42], Aurlien et al. [43], Heron et al. [44], Bagnall et al. [50], Benarroch [48], Delogu et al. [59], Du et al. [65], Glasscock et al. [61], Goldman et al. [96a], Hartmann et al. [39], Johnson et al. [96b], Kalume et al. [58], Keller et al. [45], Lehnart et al. [47], Leu et al. [51], Ludwig et al. [49], Noujaim et al. [96c], Papale et al. [64], Partemi et al. [46], Postma et al. [96d], Tu et al. [52], Veeramah et al. [63]
Resultant	AED → Arrhythmias • Particularly carbamazepine, phenytoin, and lacosamide	Al Aloul et al. [79], El-Menyar [81], DeGiorgio et al. [80], DeToledo et al. [95], Feldman and Gidal [82], Guldiken et al. [83], Huang et al. [96e], Ide and Kamijo [84], Kasarskis et al. [86], Kaufman et al. [87], Krause [88], Nizam et al. [89], Randazzo et al. [90], Takayanagi et al. [94], Strimel et al. [91], Swe et al. [92], Zoneraich et al. [93]
	Seizures → Arrhythmias • Ictal: tachycardia, asystole, bradycardia, and AV block. • Postictal: asystole, AV block, atrial flutter, or fibrillation and ventricular fibrillation.	Bardai et al. [34], Chaila et al. [15], Eggleston et al. [7], Lanz et al. [14], van der Lende et al. [8], Sevcencu and Struijk [6]

HRV, heart rate variability; *VT*, ventricular tachycardia; *VF*, ventricular fibrillation; *AED*, antiepileptic drug.

diabetes mellitus, stroke/TIA) than the general population [36, 98, 104, 105]. Unsurprisingly, people with epilepsy have higher rates of fatal and nonfatal cardiovascular and cerebrovascular disease than controls (mortality ratios up to 5.3 and morbidity ratio up to 7) [36, 106, 107]. The presence of cardiovascular disease (e.g., congestive heart failure and cardiac arrhythmias) was also associated with higher mortality risk in people with epilepsy [108].

Epilepsy treatment can also contribute to a poorer cardiovascular risk profile in epilepsy. Use of the enzyme-inducing AEDs, phenytoin or carbamazepine may lead to elevated serological vascular risk markers (e.g., total cholesterol, LDL, homocysteine), and, thus, result in accelerated atherosclerosis [109–112]. Certain AEDs (e.g., valproic acid, carbamazepine) are also known to cause weight gain and increase the risk of developing nonalcoholic fatty liver disease and metabolic syndrome, leading to further deterioration of the cardiovascular risk profile [110].

The cooccurrence of epilepsy and (congenital) heart disease, often accompanied by intellectual disability, may result from a multiple malformation syndrome: genetic defects may affect the development of both heart and brain, or abnormal cardiovascular function may lead to poor (intrauterine) brain growth [113].

CV disease can sometimes (indirectly) cause epilepsy through a predisposition to stroke [114, 115]. Stroke is a common risk factor for epilepsy and accounts for about a third of newly diagnosed seizures in people over the age of 60 years [115–118]. In particular, those with ischemic events with cortical involvement, cerebral hemorrhage (i.e., primary hemorrhage or hemorrhagic transformation of ischemic stroke) and early poststroke seizures have an increased risk of poststroke epilepsy [115].

Seizure activity may not only induce arrhythmias but may also lead to structural cardiac changes [79, 119–121]. Epileptic seizures have been reported to provoke cardiac ischemia via both acute and chronic effects on the heart (e.g., impaired heart rate variability, cardiac fibrosis, ST-segment depression and increased heart rate) [79, 122]. Transient myocardial ischemia, as indicated by ST-segment depression, was reported in a small-scale study in 40% of all 15 seizures [122]. Another study, however, failed to demonstrate troponin increases, suggesting that the reported ST changes do not usually cause myocardial damage [123].

Seizures are the second most frequent CNS condition known to induce the cardiomyopathy known as Takotsubo syndrome (TTS) [124]. TTS mimics myocardial infarction clinically, electrocardiographically, and chemically [125]. It is characterized by acute onset of chest pain and dyspnea, sometimes concomitant with palpitations, tiredness, edema, fever, syncope, anxiety, nausea, or vomiting [124]. TTS is most frequently triggered by tonic-clonic seizures [126, 127]. Seizures most likely cause TTS by the stress-induced release of catecholamines [128]. This abundant catecholamine release may be a contributing factor in fatal status epilepticus [129]. A relationship between TTS and SUDEP, however, does not appear likely [124] (Table 3).

Table 3 Putative mechanisms of associations between epilepsy and structural cardiac disease

Mechanisms of association	Conditions	References
Causal 	Cardiac conditions (e.g., embolism and congenital cardiac abnormalities) → Stroke	Attar et al. [113], Ferlazzo et al. [114], Gaitatzis et al. [36]
Shared risk factor 	Genetic → Malformation of cortical and cardiac development	Miller and Vogel [112]
	Shared cardiovascular risk factors → Myocardial infarction, Stroke	Centers for Disease Control and Prevention (CDC) [103], Elliott et al. [104], Gaitatzis et al. [36], Kobau et al. [97]
Resultant 	AED → Arteriosclerosis	Brodie et al. [108], Katsiki et al. [109], Lopinto-Khoury and Mintzer [110], Mintzer et al. [111]
	AED → Weight gain, nonalcoholic fatty liver disease, and metabolic syndrome	Katsiki et al. [109]
	Seizures → Transient myocardial ischemia	P-Codrea Tigaran et al. [121], Schuele [78]
	Seizures → Seizure-triggered Takotsubo syndrome (TTS)	Finsterer and Wahbi [123], Finsterer and Bersano [124], Lemke et al. [126]

4. Future concepts

Significant progress has been made since the publication of Russel's case history; the complex interrelationship between epilepsy and cardiac conditions has been explored widely, and this review aimed to capture all major discoveries made in this field. Many discoveries of coexisting conditions were made by serendipity, and underlying mechanisms are yet to be uncovered. Treatment regimens are consequently often speculative and lack a personalized approach involving all comorbid conditions. As comorbidity gains recognition, we now need to become better at noticing these symptom patterns. Today a substantial gap still remains between the specialties, but as we are now becoming aware of all overlapping syndromes, epileptologists will increasingly need to improve their cardiac skills. Pattern recognition can be fostered by incorporating validated screening instruments and guidelines, aiding the early identification and treatment of cardiovascular comorbidity in epilepsy. Concomitantly, a fundamental change in the way clinicians think of epilepsy, is crucial.

Epilepsy will soon be viewed as a collection of individual disorders that share a phenotype of an abnormal tendency for unprovoked epileptic seizures. The number of rare epilepsy syndromes with cardiac phenotypes will increase substantially. Epilepsy will be seen as a symptom-complex, and all comorbidities, even the most inconspicuous, should be considered part of the stratification and phenotyping in people with epilepsy. Cardiovascular comorbidities will provide insight into common mechanisms for epilepsy and give a window into common genetic predispositions. They may also provide important diagnostic clues. Channelopathies, for example, are increasingly identified in people with epilepsy. Genetic factors may explain both the epilepsy and the comorbid disorder(s), even in people with sporadic epilepsies [130]. Genome-wide scanning will be widely available and drive the paradigm shift in epilepsy. Certain genes might be identified as contributing to SUDEP, potentially allowing the development of individualized risk prevention strategies. Another major contributor to early identification of overlapping syndromes will be the development of new noninvasive tools to record heart function at home. The miniaturization of sensors will favor long-term home-based recordings thus aiding the early identification of cardiac arrhythmias.

Advances in seizure detection will likely take off. ECG alone will help to detect a wide variety of seizures but lacks specificity. Combining ECG with other modalities, including accelerometry and electrodermal activity, will likely improve accuracy and facilitate the widespread use of seizure-detection devices in those with refractory epilepsy [131–133].

Another unmet need relates to the treatment of epilepsy: many AEDs have proarrhythmogenic and arteriosclerogenic effects. Though nonpharmacological options exist, drug therapy is still the mainstay of epilepsy treatment, and other options are usually only explored after AEDs have failed to successfully control seizures [134]. Many new AEDs have been launched in the last two decades but have failed to improve the burden of side effects or substantially change prognosis for seizure control [135, 136]. With improved understanding of epileptogenesis, epigenetic determinants, and pharmacogenomics comes the hope for better, disease-modifying or even curative pharmacological and non-pharmacological treatment strategies. Until then, comorbidity should be considered when prescribing AEDs.

The incorporation of neurocardiology into the paroxysmal spectrum will require a critical review of the epilepsy services. We need to validate new instruments to screen for cardiovascular conditions. Modern noninvasive long-term ECG devices may help screen for cardiac conditions, and a cardiologist should review any relevant abnormalities. In cases where there is a relevant family history or abnormal ECG findings, a specialist cardiac assessment should be done. Identification and adequate treatment of cardiovascular disorders in epilepsy should, therefore, be an important part of epilepsy management.

Particular attention should be given to modifiable risk factors, such as smoking, obesity, sedentary lifestyle, high cholesterol, and hypertension. Physicians should screen for these risk factors in people with epilepsy, provide general health information, and if necessary, adjust AED treatment. Further studies are needed to improve risk profiling, thus allowing for screening in high-risk individuals (with, for example, implantable loop recorders) and targeted interventions (e.g., defibrillators).

Acknowledgments

We are grateful to M van der Lende, RJ Lamberts, and JW Sander for their contribution to a previous version of this manuscript [136].

Disclosures

SS reports no disclosures. RDT receives research support from the Dutch National Epilepsy Fund, The Netherlands Organization for Health Research and Development (ZonMW), NUTS Ohra Fund, Medtronic, and AC Thomson Foundation, and has received fees for lectures from Medtronic, UCB, and GSK.

Funding

This work was supported by the Dutch National Epilepsy Fund (project number 15-10); and Christelijke Vereniging voor de Verpleging van Lijders aan Epilepsie (The Netherlands).

References

[1] Russell AE. Cessation of the pulse during the onset of epileptic fits with remarks on the mechanism of fits. Lancet 1906;168:152–4.
[2] Forsgren L. Prevalence of epilepsy in adults in northern Sweden. Epilepsia 1992;33(3):450–8.

[3] Gaitatzis A, Sisodiya SM, Sander JW. The somatic comorbidity of epilepsy: a weighty but often unrecognized burden. Epilepsia 2012;53(8):1282–93.

[4] Kadima NKR, Zack M, Helmers S. Comorbidity in adults with epilepsy—United States. MMWR Morb Mortal Wkly Rep 2013;62(43):849–53.

[5] Keezer MR, Sisodiya SM, Sander JW. Comorbidities of epilepsy: current concepts and future perspectives. Lancet Neurol 2016;15(1):106–15.

[6] Sevcencu C, Struijk JJ. Autonomic alterations and cardiac changes in epilepsy. Epilepsia 2010; 51(5):725–37.

[7] Eggleston KS, Olin BD, Fisher RS. Ictal tachycardia: the head-heart connection. Seizure 2014;23 (7):496–505.

[8] van der Lende M, Surges R, Sander JW, Thijs RD. Cardiac arrhythmias during or after epileptic seizures. J Neurol Neurosurg Psychiatry 2016;87(1):69–74.

[9] Ryvlin P, Nashef L, Lhatoo SD, Bateman LM, Bird J, Bleasel A, et al. Incidence and mechanisms of cardiorespiratory arrests in epilepsy monitoring units (MORTEMUS): a retrospective study. Lancet Neurol 2013;12(10):966–77.

[10] Jin L, Zhang Y, Wang XL, Zhang WJ, Liu YH, Jiang Z. Postictal apnea as an important mechanism for SUDEP: a near-SUDEP with continuous EEG-ECG-EMG recording. J Clin Neurosci 2017;43:130–2.

[11] Schuele SU, Bermeo AC, Alexopoulos AV, Locatelli ER, Burgess RC, Dinner DS, et al. Video-electrographic and clinical features in patients with ictal asystole. Neurology 2007;69(5):434–41.

[12] Tinuper P, Bisulli F, Cerullo A, Carcangiu R, Marini C, Pierangeli G, et al. Ictal bradycardia in partial epileptic seizures: AUTONOMIC investigation in three cases and literature review. Brain 2001;124 (Pt 12):2361–71.

[13] van Dijk JG, Thijs RD, van Zwet E, Tannemaat MR, van Niekerk J, Benditt DG, et al. The semiology of tilt-induced reflex syncope in relation to electroencephalographic changes. Brain 2014;137 (Pt 2):576–85.

[14] Lanz M, Oehl B, Brandt A, Schulze-Bonhage A. Seizure induced cardiac asystole in epilepsy patients undergoing long term video-EEG monitoring. Seizure 2011;20(2):167–72.

[15] Chaila EBJ, Tirupathi S, Delanty N. Ictal bradycardia and asystole associated with intractable epilepsy: a case series. Br J Cardiol 2010;17:245–8.

[16] Leung H, Kwan P, Elger CE. Finding the missing link between ictal bradyarrhythmia, ictal asystole, and sudden unexpected death in epilepsy. Epilepsy Behav 2006;9(1):19–30.

[17] Altenmuller DM, Zehender M, Schulze-Bonhage A. High-grade atrioventricular block triggered by spontaneous and stimulation-induced epileptic activity in the left temporal lobe. Epilepsia 2004; 45(12):1640–4.

[18] Oppenheimer SM, Gelb A, Girvin JP, Hachinski VC. Cardiovascular effects of human insular cortex stimulation. Neurology 1992;42(9):1727–32.

[19] Pool JL, Ransohoff J. Autonomic effects on stimulating rostral portion of cingulate gyri in man. J Neurophysiol 1949;12(6):385–92.

[20] Simon RP, Aminoff MJ, Benowitz NL. Changes in plasma catecholamines after tonic-clonic seizures. Neurology 1984;34(2):255–7.

[21] Nilsson D, Sutton R, Melander O, Fedorowski A. Spontaneous vs nitroglycerin-induced vasovagal reflex on head-up tilt: are there neuroendocrine differences? Heart Rhythm 2016;13(8):1674–8.

[22] Moseley BD, Ghearing GR, Munger TM, Britton JW. The treatment of ictal asystole with cardiac pacing. Epilepsia 2011;52(4):e16–9.

[23] Bestawros M, Darbar D, Arain A, Abou-Khalil B, Plummer D, Dupont WD, et al. Ictal asystole and ictal syncope: insights into clinical management. Circ Arrhythm Electrophysiol 2015;8(1):159–64.

[24] Kohno R, Abe H, Akamatsu N, Benditt DG. Long-term follow-up of Ictal Asystole in temporal lobe epilepsy: is permanent pacemaker therapy needed? J Cardiovasc Electrophysiol 2016;27(8):930–6.

[25] Strzelczyk A, Cenusa M, Bauer S, Hamer HM, Mothersill IW, Grunwald T, et al. Management and long-term outcome in patients presenting with ictal asystole or bradycardia. Epilepsia 2011; 52(6):1160–7.

[26] Duplyakov D, Golovina G, Lyukshina N, Surkova E, Elger CE, Surges R. Syncope, seizure-induced bradycardia and asystole: two cases and review of clinical and pathophysiological features. Seizure 2014;23(7):506–11.

[27] Massey CA, Sowers LP, Dlouhy BJ, Richerson GB. Mechanisms of sudden unexpected death in epilepsy: the pathway to prevention. Nat Rev Neurol 2014;10(5):271–82.

[28] Aiba I, Noebels JL. Spreading depolarization in the brainstem mediates sudden cardiorespiratory arrest in mouse SUDEP models. Sci Transl Med 2015;7(282):282ra46.

[29] Poh MZ, Loddenkemper T, Swenson NC, Goyal S, Madsen JR, Picard RW. Continuous monitoring of electrodermal activity during epileptic seizures using a wearable sensor. Conf Proc IEEE Eng Med Biol Soc 2010;2010:4415–8.

[30] Bateman LM, Li CS, Seyal M. Ictal hypoxemia in localization-related epilepsy: analysis of incidence, severity and risk factors. Brain 2008;131(Pt 12):3239–45.

[31] Surges R, Adjei P, Kallis C, Erhuero J, Scott CA, Bell GS, et al. Pathologic cardiac repolarization in pharmacoresistant epilepsy and its potential role in sudden unexpected death in epilepsy: a case-control study. Epilepsia 2010;51(2):233–42.

[32] Surges R, Scott CA, Walker MC. Enhanced QT shortening and persistent tachycardia after generalized seizures. Neurology 2010;74(5):421–6.

[33] Seyal M, Pascual F, Lee CY, Li CS, Bateman LM. Seizure-related cardiac repolarization abnormalities are associated with ictal hypoxemia. Epilepsia 2011;52(11):2105–11.

[34] Bardai A, Lamberts RJ, Blom MT, Spanjaart AM, Berdowski J, van der Staal SR, et al. Epilepsy is a risk factor for sudden cardiac arrest in the general population. PLoS ONE 2012;7(8):e42749.

[35] Lamberts RJ, Blom MT, Wassenaar M, Bardai A, Leijten FS, de Haan GJ, et al. Sudden cardiac arrest in people with epilepsy in the community: circumstances and risk factors. Neurology 2015; 85(3):212–8.

[36] Gaitatzis A, Carroll K, Majeed A, Sander WJ. The epidemiology of the comorbidity of epilepsy in the general population. Epilepsia 2004;45(12):1613–22.

[37] Suorsa E, Korpelainen JT, Ansakorpi H, Huikuri HV, Suorsa V, Myllyla VV, et al. Heart rate dynamics in temporal lobe epilepsy-a long-term follow-up study. Epilepsy Res 2011;93(1):80–3.

[38] Hilz MJ, Platsch G, Druschky K, Pauli E, Kuwert T, Stefan H, et al. Outcome of epilepsy surgery correlates with sympathetic modulation and neuroimaging of the heart. J Neurol Sci 2003; 216(1):153–62.

[39] Lamberts RJ, Blom MT, Novy J, Belluzzo M, Seldenrijk A, Penninx BW, et al. Increased prevalence of ECG markers for sudden cardiac arrest in refractory epilepsy. J Neurol Neurosurg Psychiatry 2015;86(3):309–13.

[40] Hartmann HA, Colom LV, Sutherland ML, Noebels JL. Selective localization of cardiac SCN5A sodium channels in limbic regions of rat brain. Nat Neurosci 1999;2(7):593–5.

[41] Anderson JH, Bos JM, Cascino GD, Ackerman MJ. Prevalence and spectrum of electroencephalogram-identified epileptiform activity among patients with long QT syndrome. Heart Rhythm 2014;11(1):53–7.

[42] Auerbach DS, McNitt S, Gross RA, Zareba W, Dirksen RT, Moss AJ. Genetic biomarkers for the risk of seizures in long QT syndrome. Neurology 2016.

[43] Aurlien D, Leren TP, Tauboll E, Gjerstad L. New SCN5A mutation in a SUDEP victim with idiopathic epilepsy. Seizure 2009;18(2):158–60.

[44] Heron SE, Hernandez M, Edwards C, Edkins E, Jansen FE, Scheffer IE, et al. Neonatal seizures and long QT syndrome: a cardiocerebral channelopathy? Epilepsia 2010;51(2):293–6.

[45] Keller DI, Grenier J, Christe G, Dubouloz F, Osswald S, Brink M, et al. Characterization of novel KCNH2 mutations in type 2 long QT syndrome manifesting as seizures. Can J Cardiol 2009; 25(8):455–62.

[46] Partemi S, Cestele S, Pezzella M, Campuzano O, Paravidino R, Pascali VL, et al. Loss-of-function KCNH2 mutation in a family with long QT syndrome, epilepsy, and sudden death. Epilepsia 2013;54(8):e112–6.

[47] Lehnart SE, Mongillo M, Bellinger A, Lindegger N, Chen BX, Hsueh W, et al. Leaky Ca2+ release channel/ryanodine receptor 2 causes seizures and sudden cardiac death in mice. J Clin Invest 2008; 118(6):2230–45.

[48] Benarroch EE. HCN channels: function and clinical implications. Neurology 2013;80(3):304–10.

[49] Ludwig A, Budde T, Stieber J, Moosmang S, Wahl C, Holthoff K, et al. Absence epilepsy and sinus dysrhythmia in mice lacking the pacemaker channel HCN2. EMBO J 2003;22(2):216–24.

[50] Bagnall RD, Crompton DE, Petrovski S, Lam L, Cutmore C, Garry SI, et al. Exome-based analysis of cardiac arrhythmia, respiratory control, and epilepsy genes in sudden unexpected death in epilepsy. Ann Neurol 2016;79(4):522–34.

[51] Leu C, Balestrini S, Maher B, Hernandez-Hernandez L, Gormley P, Hamalainen E, et al. Genome-wide polygenic burden of rare deleterious variants in sudden unexpected death in epilepsy. EBioMedicine 2015;2(9):1063–70.

[52] Tu E, Waterhouse L, Duflou J, Bagnall RD, Semsarian C. Genetic analysis of hyperpolarization-activated cyclic nucleotide-gated cation channels in sudden unexpected death in epilepsy cases. Brain Pathol 2011;21(6):692–8.

[53] Hata Y, Yoshida K, Kinoshita K, Nishida N. Epilepsy-related sudden unexpected death: targeted molecular analysis of inherited heart disease genes using next-generation DNA sequencing. Brain Pathol 2017;27(3):292–304.

[54] Friedman D, Kannan K, Faustin A, Shroff S, Thomas C, Heguy A, et al. Cardiac arrhythmia and neuroexcitability gene variants in resected brain tissue from patients with sudden unexpected death in epilepsy (SUDEP). NPJ Genomic Med 2018;3:9.

[55] Coll M, Striano P, Ferrer-Costa C, Campuzano O, Mates J, Del Olmo B, et al. Targeted next-generation sequencing provides novel clues for associated epilepsy and cardiac conduction disorder/SUDEP. PLoS ONE 2017;12(12).

[56] Shmuely S, Sisodiya SM, Gunning WB, Sander JW, Thijs RD. Mortality in Dravet syndrome: a review. Epilepsy Behav 2016;64(Pt A):69–74.

[57] Auerbach DS, Jones J, Clawson BC, Offord J, Lenk GM, Ogiwara I, et al. Altered cardiac electrophysiology and SUDEP in a model of Dravet syndrome. PLoS ONE 2013;8(10).

[58] Kalume F, Westenbroek RE, Cheah CS, Yu FH, Oakley JC, Scheuer T, et al. Sudden unexpected death in a mouse model of Dravet syndrome. J Clin Invest 2013;123(4):1798–808.

[59] Delogu AB, Spinelli A, Battaglia D, Dravet C, De Nisco A, Saracino A, et al. Electrical and autonomic cardiac function in patients with Dravet syndrome. Epilepsia 2011;52(Suppl 2):55–8.

[60] Ergul Y, Ekici B, Tatli B, Nisli K, Ozmen M. QT and P wave dispersion and heart rate variability in patients with Dravet syndrome. Acta Neurol Belg 2013;113(2):161–6.

[61] Glasscock E, Yoo JW, Chen TT, Klassen TL, Noebels JL. Kv1.1 potassium channel deficiency reveals brain-driven cardiac dysfunction as a candidate mechanism for sudden unexplained death in epilepsy. J Neurosci 2010;30(15):5167–75.

[62] Klassen TL, Bomben VC, Patel A, Drabek J, Chen TT, Gu W, et al. High-resolution molecular genomic autopsy reveals complex sudden unexpected death in epilepsy risk profile. Epilepsia 2014;55(2):e6–12.

[63] Veeramah KR, O'Brien JE, Meisler MH, Cheng X, Dib-Hajj SD, Waxman SG, et al. De novo pathogenic SCN8A mutation identified by whole-genome sequencing of a family quartet affected by infantile epileptic encephalopathy and SUDEP. Am J Hum Genet 2012;90(3):502–10.

[64] Papale LA, Beyer B, Jones JM, Sharkey LM, Tufik S, Epstein M, et al. Heterozygous mutations of the voltage-gated sodium channel SCN8A are associated with spike-wave discharges and absence epilepsy in mice. Hum Mol Genet 2009;18(9):1633–41.

[65] Du Y, Huang X, Wang T, Han K, Zhang J, Xi Y, et al. Downregulation of neuronal sodium channel subunits Nav1.1 and Nav1.6 in the sinoatrial node from volume-overloaded heart failure rat. Pflugers Archiv Eur J Physiol 2007;454(3):451–9.

[66] Noujaim SF, Kaur K, Milstein M, Jones JM, Furspan P, Jiang D, et al. A null mutation of the neuronal sodium channel NaV1.6 disrupts action potential propagation and excitation-contraction coupling in the mouse heart. FASEB J 2012;26(1):63–72.

[67] Xu Y, Nguyen D, Mohamed A, Carcel C, Li Q, Kutlubaev MA, et al. Frequency of a false positive diagnosis of epilepsy: a systematic review of observational studies. Seizure 2016;41:167–74.

[68] Grubb BP, Gerard G, Roush K, Temesy-Armos P, Elliott L, Hahn H, et al. Differentiation of convulsive syncope and epilepsy with head-up tilt testing. Ann Intern Med 1991;115(11):871–6.

[69] Lempert T, Bauer M, Schmidt D. Syncope: a videometric analysis of 56 episodes of transient cerebral hypoxia. Ann Neurol 1994;36(2):233–7.

[70] Zaidi A, Clough P, Cooper P, Scheepers B, Fitzpatrick AP. Misdiagnosis of epilepsy: many seizure-like attacks have a cardiovascular cause. J Am Coll Cardiol 2000;36(1):181–4.

[71] Shmuely S, Bauer PR, van Zwet EW, van Dijk JG, Thijs RD. Differentiating motor phenomena in tilt-induced syncope and convulsive seizures. Neurology 2018;90(15):e1339–46.

[72] Blad H, Lamberts RJ, van Dijk GJ, Thijs RD. Tilt-induced vasovagal syncope and psychogenic pseudosyncope: overlapping clinical entities. Neurology 2015;85(23):2006–10.

[73] Mathias CJ, Deguchi K, Schatz I. Observations on recurrent syncope and presyncope in 641 patients. Lancet 2001;357(9253):348–53.

[74] Battaglia A, Guerrini R, Gastaut H. Epileptic seizures induced by syncopal attacks. J Epilepsy 1989;2:137–45.

[75] Horrocks IA, Nechay A, Stephenson JB, Zuberi SM. Anoxic-epileptic seizures: observational study of epileptic seizures induced by syncopes. Arch Dis Child 2005;90(12):1283–7.

[76] Stephenson J, Breningstall G, Steer C, Kirkpatrick M, Horrocks I, Nechay A, et al. Anoxic-epileptic seizures: home video recordings of epileptic seizures induced by syncopes. Epileptic Disord 2004; 6(1):15–9.

[77] Ungar A, Ceccofiglio A, Pescini F, Mussi C, Tava G, Rafanelli M, et al. Syncope and epilepsy coexist in 'possible' and 'drug-resistant' epilepsy (overlap between epilepsy and Syncope study - OESYS). BMC Neurol 2017;17(1):45.

[78] Schuele SU. Effects of seizures on cardiac function. J Clin Neurophysiol 2009;26(5):302–8.

[79] Al Aloul B, Adabag AS, Houghland MA, Tholakanahalli V. Brugada pattern electrocardiogram associated with supratherapeutic phenytoin levels and the risk of sudden death. Pacing Clin Electrophysiol 2007;30(5):713–5.

[80] DeGiorgio CM. Atrial flutter/atrial fibrillation associated with lacosamide for partial seizures. Epilepsy Behav 2010;18(3):322–4.

[81] El-Menyar A, Khan M, Al Suwaidi J, Eljerjawy E, Asaad N. Oxcarbazepine-induced resistant ventricular fibrillation in an apparently healthy young man. Am J Emerg Med 2011;29(6):693 e1–3.

[82] Feldman AE, Gidal BE. QTc prolongation by antiepileptic drugs and the risk of torsade de pointes in patients with epilepsy. Epilepsy Behav 2013;26(3):421–6.

[83] Guldiken B, Remi J, Noachtar S. Cardiovascular adverse effects of phenytoin. J Neurol 2016;263 (5):861–70.

[84] Ide A, Kamijo Y. Intermittent complete atrioventricular block after long term low-dose carbamazepine therapy with a serum concentration less than the therapeutic level. InternMed 2007; 46(9):627–9.

[85] Ishizue N, Niwano S, Saito M, Fukaya H, Nakamura H, Igarashi T, et al. Polytherapy with sodium channel-blocking antiepileptic drugs is associated with arrhythmogenic ST-T abnormality in patients with epilepsy. Seizure 2016;40:81–7.

[86] Kasarskis EJ, Kuo CS, Berger R, Nelson KR. Carbamazepine-induced cardiac dysfunction. Characterization of two distinct clinical syndromes. Arch Intern Med 1992;152(1):186–91.

[87] Kaufman KR, Velez AE, Wong S, Mani R. Low-dose lacosamide-induced atrial fibrillation: case analysis with literature review. Epilepsy Behav 2013;1:22–5.

[88] Krause LU, Brodowski KO, Kellinghaus C. Atrioventricular block following lacosamide intoxication. Epilepsy Behav 2011;20(4):725–7.

[89] Nizam A, Mylavarapu K, Thomas D, Briskin K, Wu B, Saluja D, et al. Lacosamide-induced second-degree atrioventricular block in a patient with partial epilepsy. Epilepsia 2011;52(10):e153–5.

[90] Randazzo DN, Ciccone A, Schweitzer P, Winters SL. Complete atrioventricular block with ventricular asystole following infusion of intravenous phenytoin. J Electrocardiol 1995;28(2):157–9.

[91] Strimel WJ, Woodruff A, Cheung P, Kirmani BF, Stephen Huang SK. Brugada-like electrocardiographic pattern induced by lamotrigine toxicity. Clin Neuropharmacol 2010;33(5):265–7.

[92] Swe T, Bhattarai B, Dufresne A. Type 1 Brugada pattern ECG due to supra-therapeutic phenytoin level. BMJ Case Rep 2016;2016.

[93] Zoneraich S, Zoneraich O, Siegel J. Sudden death following intravenous sodium diphenylhydantoin. Am Heart J 1976;91(3):375–7.

[94] Takayanagi K, Hisauchi I, Watanabe J, Maekawa Y, Fujito T, Sakai Y, et al. Carbamazepine-induced sinus node dysfunction and atrioventricular block in elderly women. Jpn Heart J 1998;39 (4):469–79.

[95] DeToledo JC, Lowe MR, Rabinstein A, Villaviza N. Cardiac arrest after fast intravenous infusion of phenytoin mistaken for fosphenytoin. Epilepsia 2001;42(2):288.

[96] Elliott JO, Lu B, Shneker B, Charyton C, Layne Moore J. Comorbidity, health screening, and quality of life among persons with a history of epilepsy. Epilepsy Behav 2009;14(1):125–9.

[96a] Goldman AM, Behr ER, Semsarian C, Bagnall RD, Sisodiya S, Cooper PN. Sudden unexpected death in epilepsy genetics: molecular diagnostics and prevention. Epilepsia 2016;57(Suppl. 1):17–25.

[96b] Johnson JN, Tester DJ, Bass NE, Ackerman MJ. Cardiac channel molecular autopsy for sudden unexpected death in epilepsy. J Child Neurol 2010;25(7):916–21.

[96c] Noujaim SF, Kaur K, Milstein M, Jones JM, Furspan P, Jiang D, et al. A null mutation of the neuronal sodium channel NaV1.6 disrupts action potential propagation and excitation-contraction coupling in the mouse heart. FASEB J 2012;26(1):63–72.

[96d] Postma AV, Denjoy I, Kamblock J, Alders M, Lupoglazoff JM, Vaksmann G, Dubosq-Bidot L, Sebillon P, Mannens MM, Guicheney P, Wilde AA. Catecholaminergic polymorphic ventricular tachycardia: RYR2 mutations, bradycardia, and follow up of the patients. J Med Genet 2005;42 (11):863–70.

[96e] Huang CW, Brown S, Pillay N, Campo MD, Tellez-Zenteno J, McLachlan RS. Electroencephalographic and electrocardiographic effect of intravenous Lacosamide in refractory focal epilepsy. J Clin Neurphysiol 2018;35(5):365–9.

[97] Kobau R, Zahran H, Thurman DJ, Zack MM, Henry TR, Schachter SC, et al. Epilepsy surveillance among adults—19 states, behavioral risk factor surveillance system. MMWR Surveill Summ 2008; 57(6):1–20.

[98] Strine TW, Kobau R, Chapman DP, Thurman DJ, Price P, Balluz LS. Psychological distress, comorbidities, and health behaviors among U.S. adults with seizures: results from the 2002 National Health Interview Survey. Epilepsia 2005;46(7):1133–9.

[99] Tellez-Zenteno JF, Matijevic S, Wiebe S. Somatic comorbidity of epilepsy in the general population in Canada. Epilepsia 2005;46(12):1955–62.

[100] Ding D, Wang W, Wu J, Ma G, Dai X, Yang B, et al. Premature mortality in people with epilepsy in rural China: a prospective study. Lancet Neurol 2006;5(10):823–7.

[101] Janszky I, Hallqvist J, Tomson T, Ahlbom A, Mukamal KJ, Ahnve S. Increased risk and worse prognosis of myocardial infarction in patients with prior hospitalization for epilepsy—the Stockholm heart epidemiology program. Brain 2009;132(Pt 10):2798–804.

[102] Neligan A, Bell GS, Johnson AL, Goodridge DM, Shorvon SD, Sander JW. The long-term risk of premature mortality in people with epilepsy. Brain 2011;134(Pt 2):388–95.

[103] (CDC) CfDCaP. Comorbidity in adults with epilepsy—United States, 2010. MMWR Morb Mortal Wkly Rep 2013;62(43):849–53.

[104] Elliott JO, Moore JL, Lu B. Health status and behavioral risk factors among persons with epilepsy in Ohio based on the 2006 behavioral risk factor surveillance system. Epilepsy Behav 2008;12(3):434–44.

[105] Cockerell OC, Johnson AL, Sander JW, Hart YM, Goodridge DM, Shorvon SD. Mortality from epilepsy: results from a prospective population-based study. Lancet 1994;344(8927):918–21.

[106] Nilsson L, Tomson T, Farahmand BY, Diwan V, Persson PG. Cause-specific mortality in epilepsy: a cohort study of more than 9,000 patients once hospitalized for epilepsy. Epilepsia 1997;38(10):1062–8.

[107] St Germaine-Smith C, Liu M, Quan H, Wiebe S, Jette N. Development of an epilepsy-specific risk adjustment comorbidity index. Epilepsia 2011;52(12):2161–7.

[108] Brodie MJ, Mintzer S, Pack AM, Gidal BE, Vecht CJ, Schmidt D. Enzyme induction with antiepileptic drugs: cause for concern? Epilepsia 2013;54(1):11–27.

[109] Katsiki N, Mikhailidis DP, Nair DR. The effects of antiepileptic drugs on vascular risk factors: a narrative review. Seizure 2014;23(9):677–84.

[110] Lopinto-Khoury C, Mintzer S. Antiepileptic drugs and markers of vascular risk. Curr Treat Options Neurol 2010;12(4):300–8.

[111] Mintzer S, Skidmore CT, Abidin CJ, Morales MC, Chervoneva I, Capuzzi DM, et al. Effects of antiepileptic drugs on lipids, homocysteine, and C-reactive protein. Ann Neurol 2009;65(4):448–56.

[112] Miller G, Vogel H. Structural evidence of injury or malformation in the brains of children with congenital heart disease. Semin Pediatr Neurol 1999;6(1):20–6.

[113] Attar H, Sachdeva A, Sundararajan S. Cardioembolic stroke in adults with a history of congenital heart disease. Stroke 2016;47(5):e79–81.

[114] Ferlazzo E, Gasparini S, Beghi E, Sueri C, Russo E, Leo A, et al. Epilepsy in cerebrovascular diseases: review of experimental and clinical data with meta-analysis of risk factors. Epilepsia 2016;57(8): 1205–14.

[115] Camilo O, Goldstein LB. Seizures and epilepsy after ischemic stroke. Stroke 2004;35(7):1769–75.

[116] Forsgren L, Bucht G, Eriksson S, Bergmark L. Incidence and clinical characterization of unprovoked seizures in adults: a prospective population-based study. Epilepsia 1996;37(3):224–9.

[117] Hauser WA, Annegers JF, Kurland LT. Incidence of epilepsy and unprovoked seizures in Rochester, Minnesota: 1935-1984. Epilepsia 1993;34(3):453–68.

[118] Natelson BH, Suarez RV, Terrence CF, Turizo R. Patients with epilepsy who die suddenly have cardiac disease. Arch Neurol 1998;55(6):857–60.

[119] Nei M, Sperling MR, Mintzer S, Ho RT. Long-term cardiac rhythm and repolarization abnormalities in refractory focal and generalized epilepsy. Epilepsia 2012;53(8):e137–40.

[120] Tigaran S, Molgaard H, McClelland R, Dam M, Jaffe AS. Evidence of cardiac ischemia during seizures in drug refractory epilepsy patients. Neurology 2003;60(3):492–5.

[121] P-Codrea Tigaran S, Dalager-Pedersen S, Baandrup U, Dam M, Vesterby-Charles A. Sudden unexpected death in epilepsy: is death by seizures a cardiac disease? Am J Forensic Med Pathol 2005; 26(2):99–105.

[122] Woodruff BK, Britton JW, Tigaran S, Cascino GD, Burritt MF, McConnell JP, et al. Cardiac troponin levels following monitored epileptic seizures. Neurology 2003;60(10):1690–2.

[123] Finsterer J, Wahbi K. CNS disease triggering Takotsubo stress cardiomyopathy. Int J Cardiol 2014;177(2):322–9.

[124] Finsterer J, Bersano A. Seizure-triggered Takotsubo syndrome rarely causes SUDEP. Seizure 2015;31:84–7.

[125] Le Ven F, Pennec PY, Timsit S, Blanc JJ. Takotsubo syndrome associated with seizures: an underestimated cause of sudden death in epilepsy? Int J Cardiol 2011;146(3):475–9.

[126] Lemke DM, Hussain SI, Wolfe TJ, Torbey MA, Lynch JR, Carlin A, et al. Takotsubo cardiomyopathy associated with seizures. Neurocrit Care 2008;9(1):112–7.

[127] Szardien S, Mollmann H, Willmer M, Akashi YJ, Hamm CW, Nef HM. Mechanisms of stress (takotsubo) cardiomyopathy. Heart Fail Clin 2013;9(2):197–205 [ix].

[128] Manno EM, Pfeifer EA, Cascino GD, Noe KH, Wijdicks EF. Cardiac pathology in status epilepticus. Ann Neurol 2005;58(6):954–7.

[129] Kasperaviciute D, Catarino CB, Chinthapalli K, Clayton LM, Thom M, Martinian L, et al. Uncovering genomic causes of co-morbidity in epilepsy: gene-driven phenotypic characterization of rare microdeletions. PLoS ONE 2011;6(8).

[130] Ulate-Campos A, Coughlin F, Gainza-Lein M, Fernandez IS, Pearl PL, Loddenkemper T. Automated seizure detection systems and their effectiveness for each type of seizure. Seizure 2016;40:88–101.

[131] van Andel J, Thijs RD, de Weerd A, Arends J, Leijten F. Non-EEG based ambulatory seizure detection designed for home use: what is available and how will it influence epilepsy care? Epilepsy Behav 2016;57(Pt A):82–9.

[132] Elger CE, Hoppe C. Diagnostic challenges in epilepsy: seizure under-reporting and seizure detection. Lancet Neurol 2018;17(3):279–88.

[133] Thijs RD, Surges R, O'Brien TJ, Sander JW. Epilepsy in adults. Lancet 2019;393(10172):689–701.

[134] Loscher W, Schmidt D. Modern antiepileptic drug development has failed to deliver: ways out of the current dilemma. Epilepsia 2011;52(4):657–78.

[135] Wassenaar M, van Heijl I, Leijten FS, van der Linden P, Uijl SG, Egberts AC, et al. Treatment of epilepsy in daily clinical practice: have outcomes improved over the past 10 years? J Neurol 2013;260(11):2736–43.

[136] Shmuely S, van der Lende M, Lamberts RJ, Sander JW, Thijs RD. The heart of epilepsy: current views and future concepts. Seizure 2017;44:176–83.

CHAPTER 9

Epilepsy and cancer

Ettore Beghi
Department of Neuroscience, Istituto di Ricerche Farmacologiche Mario Negri IRCCS, Milano, Italy

Contents

Abbreviations

CI	confidence interval
CNS	central nervous system
DNET	dysembryoplastic neuroepithelial tumor
IDH	isocitrate dehydrogenase
mTOR	mammalian target of rapamycin
NF1	neurofibromatosis type 1
SWS	Sturge-Weber syndrome
TSC	tuberous sclerosis complex
WHO	World Health Organization

1. Introduction

Epileptic seizures and epilepsy are common findings in people with cancer. The association between cancer and seizures/epilepsy can mostly be explained by the direct structural or functional effects of primary or metastatic tumors on the cortical areas and their connections. However, other plausible explanations can be given, including vascular complications, infection, metabolic disorders, and, not least, chemotherapy

The Comorbidities of Epilepsy
https://doi.org/10.1016/B978-0-12-814877-8.00009-X

and/or radiotherapy, and treatment of seizures. In this complex scenario, the comorbidity of epilepsy and tumors must be assessed in the light of the clinical rules that govern cause-effect mechanisms.

2. Epilepsy and cancer: Association versus causation

The association between epilepsy and cancer is not necessarily evidence of causation. Although several mechanisms can explain the association between epilepsy and a number of comorbidities, including causal relation, shared risk factors and bidirectional effects, factors clearly associated with the development of epilepsy must be identified before accepting the concept of a causal association between tumors and the occurrence of epileptic seizures [1]. Evidence of a causal relationship should be produced to exclude the possibility of a chance association even at the presence of a well-established etiological factor. This requires the satisfaction of specific criteria, including temporal sequence, strength and consistency of association, biological gradient, and plausibility.

In 1965, the English statistician Sir Austin Bradford Hill [2] proposed a set of nine criteria to provide epidemiologic evidence of a causal relationship between a presumed cause and an observed effect. The list of the criteria is given in Table 1. The present chapter is inspired by these criteria in delineating the association between epilepsy and cancer.

3. Epidemiology of epilepsy and tumors

There are only scarce data on epilepsy in patients with tumors from population-based studies. In the Rochester, Minnesota population, during the period 1935–84 the fraction of epilepsies attributable to tumors was 4% [3]. In the adult population (age 35–64 years), neoplasms were identified as antecedents with frequency equal to traumatic brain injury but were less frequent antecedents than cerebrovascular disease. Similar findings were obtained in a study on the incidence of unprovoked seizures and epilepsy in Iceland [4].

Table 1 Bradford-Hill criteria of causation

- *Strength*: The larger the association, the more likely that it is causal.
- *Consistency*: Consistent findings are observed by different persons in different places with different samples.
- *Specificity*: The more specific an association, the bigger the probability of a causal relationship.
- *Temporality*: The effect has to occur after the cause.
- *Biological gradient*: Greater exposure should generally lead to greater incidence of the effect.
- *Plausibility*: Plausible mechanism between cause and effect.
- *Coherence*: Coherence between epidemiological and laboratory findings increases the likelihood of an effect.
- *Experiment*: "Occasionally it is possible to appeal to experimental evidence."
- *Analogy*: The effect of similar factors may be considered.

Hill AB. The environment and disease: association or causation? Proc R Soc Med 1965;58(5):295–300.

The prevalence of chronic somatic conditions was investigated in people with epilepsy and compared with that in the general population using Canadian nationwide, population-based health data [5]. Epilepsy-specific and general population health data were obtained through two door-to-door health surveys, the National Population Health Survey and the Community Health Survey, which represented 98% of the Canadian population. The prevalence of epilepsy and 19 other chronic conditions, including cancer, was ascertained and compared to the prevalence of epilepsy in the general population. The prevalence ratio was 1.4 (95% CI 0.9–2.1) and 1.2 (95% CI 0.7–2.1), respectively. The prevalence ratio was 0.1 (95% CI 0.02–0.6) in men and 1.1 (95% CI 0.7–1.8) in women.

Somatic comorbidity of epilepsy was also assessed in a cross-sectional population-based study using the UK General Practice Research Database [6]. Age- and sex-standardized prevalence rates were estimated for selected conditions and groups of conditions in adults with epilepsy registered with primary care physicians. Results were compared with those in adults without epilepsy in the cohort. Somatic disorders included, among others, neoplasms and, more specifically, brain tumors and meningiomas. Brain tumors and meningiomas occurred 55 and 31 times, respectively, more often in people with epilepsy. The prevalence ratio of brain tumors was more pronounced in the younger adult epilepsy group than in the older group. The inverse picture was observed in people with meningiomas, for whom the prevalence ratio was higher in the older epilepsy group.

The inconsistency of the results of the two population-based studies may be explained by underascertainment of cases in the Canadian study. As acknowledged by the authors, cases were identified through door-to-door personal interviews, during which participants or proxies reported medical conditions diagnosed by physicians. In contrast, the generalization of the findings in the UK study was potentially limited by selection bias that possibly favored more severe cases and cases of symptomatic epilepsy that most frequently sought medical advice.

4. Factors associated with the epileptogenic potential of tumors

The epileptogenicity of tumors is related to their grade and location. Seizures are more often the presenting symptoms in low-grade tumors than in rapidly invasive tumors [7]. Seizures at disease presentation could be attributed to intrinsic glioma properties [8] and are the predominant risk factor for relapsing seizures after surgery. An association has been suggested between seizures as an opening symptom and a favorable prognosis [9].

Individuals with tumors in the temporal lobe have the highest incidence of epilepsy, followed by the frontal lobe [10]. Epilepsy is more frequent in patients with superficial and cortical tumors than those with deep and noncortical tumors. Although most seizures caused by brain tumors are focal and associated with abnormal clinical and electrophysiological changes, seizure type, neurological examination and EEG are not different in brain tumors, when compared to other causes of epilepsy, at least in children [11, 12].

Table 2 Seizure frequency by tumor type

Tumor type	Seizure frequency
Dysembryoplastic neuroepithelial tumor	100%
Ganglioglioma	80%–90%
Low-grade astrocytoma	75%
Meningioma	29%–60%
Glioblastoma multiforme	29%–49%
Metastasis	20%–35%
Leptomeningeal tumor	10%–15%
Primary CNS lymphoma	10%

van Breemen MS, Wilms EB, Vecht CJ. Epilepsy in patients with brain tumours: epidemiology, mechanisms, and management. Lancet Neurol 2007;6(5):421–30.

In clinical series, dysembryoplastic neuroepithelial tumors (DNETs) are the most epileptogenic tumors, followed by gangliogliomas and low-grade astrocytomas [13] (Table 2). Seizures are found in 20%–35% of cases with brain metastases. Primary central nervous system (CNS) lymphomas rarely cause seizures [14].

5. Mechanisms and biological plausibility

There are no straightforward explanations as to why low-grade tumors are more epileptogenic than high-grade tumors. Possible mechanisms include the site (high-grade gliomas are mostly located in subcortical white matter) and differences in survivorship (people with high-grade gliomas might survive long enough to develop epilepsy [15, 16]. Gliomas most likely associated with seizures are located in the temporal lobe, followed by the frontal lobe, the preferred sites of brain tumors [15]. The epileptogenicity of brain tumors has been extensively reviewed by Pallud and coworkers [17]. Intratumoral and peritumoral mechanisms are implicated. The infiltrated peritumoral neocortex appears to be the key structure for epileptic activity of gliomas, which depends on the interactions between the tumor and the surrounding brain. Structural reorganization and functional deafferentation with neuronal and glial losses, neurogenesis, reactive astrogliosis, and neuronal, axonal, and synaptic plasticity within the peritumoral neocortex have been described, resulting mainly in a reduction of inhibitory pathways and an increase of excitatory pathways. Glioma cells affect the surrounding environment by recruiting astrocytes, microglia, and stromal cells that facilitate tumor progression by mean of secreted factors (cytokines, growth factors, chemokines, colony-stimulating factors) and of intercellular communication. These excitatory effects are instrumental to the generation of epileptic activity in the peritumoral neocortex. The tumor itself may also affect neuronal behavior, connections, and networks through local mechanical effects. A dual pathology (gliosis, hippocampal sclerosis, cortical dysgenesis) may also play a role [18].

6. Molecular markers of epileptogenicity in brain tumors

A number of genetic factors have been implicated in the epileptogenesis of brain tumors [10]. These include, among others, a mutation of the isocitrate dehydrogenase (IDH) 1 enzyme, increased extracellular and intrasynaptic glutamate concentration, and disturbances in chloride balance secondary to changes in chloride transporters. IDH 1 mutations are frequently present in diffuse low-grade gliomas and are associated with seizures as the opening symptom. In patients with grade II astrocytoma, seizures were most common in tumors involving the temporal lobe (83%), followed by the insula (74%), the frontal lobe (73%), and the parietal lobe (59%) [19]. Multivariable analysis of three World Health Organization (WHO) grade II–IV glioma cohorts from separate institutions, including WHO grade, 1p/19q codeletion, and temporal lobe location, showed that IDH1 mutation was an independent correlate with seizures [20]. Mutant IDH1 is released by tumor cells, reduces a-ketoglutarate to 2-hydroxyglutarate (2HG) and supports the reductase rather than the oxidase activity. This results in a 100-fold raised 2HG level in gliomas with IDH1 mutation. Due to the structural similarity to glutamate, 2HG activates N-methyl-D-aspartate receptors [21], providing evidence for an epileptogenic potential of 2HG. Infiltrative glioma cells releasing this glutamate mimetic could disrupt the balance between inhibition and excitation, and potentially lead to seizures [20].

BRAF V600E mutations have been reported in glioneuronal tumors. BRAF V600E mutated protein is associated with activation of the mammalian target of rapamycin (mTOR) pathway, immunophenotype, and clinical characteristics in glioneural tumors [22].

Losses of chromosomes 1p and 19q are deemed correlated with diagnosis of oligodendroglioma. In a systematic review of the literature [23], 1p deletions and 1p19q codeletion mean rates were, respectively, 65.4% and 63.3% in oligodendrogliomas, 28.7% and 21.6% in oligoastrocytomas, 13.2% and 7.5% in astrocytomas, 11.6% and 2.9% in glioblastomas. The most favorable outcome in patients with low-grade gliomas associated with 1p/19q codeletion could explain the increased risk of seizures.

7. Primary and metastatic tumors

Primary brain tumors are, in general, more epileptogenic than metastatic tumors. In the latter, the incidence of seizures may depend on tumor pathology. In a German series of patients with primary and metastatic cancers, the incidence of seizures ranged from 16% among women with breast cancer to 67% in patients with melanoma [24]. The lower epileptogenic potential of metastases can be explained by a reduced infiltrative capability and a biochemical inability to modulate neuronal excitability [25].

8. Multiple comorbidities

The association between epilepsy and cancer can be complicated by the presence of comorbidities having epileptogenic potential. In this context, the genetic background and the interaction between genetics, epilepsy, and its comorbidities can play an important role [1]. For example, a mutation of the tuberous sclerosis complex (TSC) 1 gene in tuberous sclerosis (discussed later in this section) directly results in cortical tubers, some of which (along with surrounding cortical tissue) might result in epilepsy via a causative association.

DNETs frequently present structural abnormalities associated with cortical dysplasia, suggesting that the longstanding presence of a parenchymal lesion favors conditions that contribute to the development of seizures. DNETs are characterized by blastic changes of groups of neurons and degenerative changes of surrounding astrocytes [7].

Neurocutaneous disorders are multisystem diseases affecting brain, skin, and other organs [26]. TSC, neurofibromatosis type I (NF1) and Sturge-Weber syndrome (SWS) are the commonest clinical conditions. Epilepsy affects up to 90% of patients with TSC and SWS. The mechanisms underlying brain hyperexcitability differ between disorders, but some molecular pathways overlap. TSC is a neurocutaneous syndrome affecting the brain, skin, eyes, kidneys, heart, and lungs, with a highly variable phenotype [27]. TSC alters cellular proliferation and differentiation, resulting in hamartomas of various organs, tumor formation, and altered neuronal migration. Seizures, including infantile spasms, are present in the majority of the affected individuals. Intellectual disability and autism can be also present. TSC is inherited as an autosomal dominant trait, but spontaneous mutations are common. A mutation of either TSC1 (chromosome 9) or TSC2 (chromosome 16) leads to dysfunction of two proteins (hamartin and tuberin) that form a functional complex modulating the mTOR pathway.

SWS is a neurocutaneous syndrome identified through a facial port-wine stain involving the first division of the trigeminal nerve, ipsilateral leptomeningeal angiomata, and angioma in the ipsilateral eye [28]. Seizures are the most common neurological manifestation and typically present in the first months of life. The disease presents a variable but usually progressive course in early childhood. Stroke-like episodes, headaches, neurological and cognitive deterioration, glaucoma, and visual field defects are also present. An activating somatic mutation in the GNAQ gene has been found.

NF1 is an autosomal dominant neurocutaneous disorder caused by a mutation in the NF1 tumor suppressor gene [29]. Compared to the general population, seizures are more common in individuals with NF1 and are often focal and related to an intracranial neoplasm.

Stroke accounts for the largest fraction of burden attributable to neurological diseases [30]. Stroke is the commonest cause of seizures in the elderly and, as such, it may also occur in people with cancer. In an autopsy study of patients with cancer, 14.6% had pathologic evidence of cerebrovascular disease and 7.4% had symptoms of stroke [31]. The association between stroke and cancer is bidirectional. In a large cohort of stroke patients included in a Danish hospital discharge registry, a more than tenfold increase in brain tumors was found in the first year after a stroke [32]. The authors, however, suggested that in several occasions brain tumors could be misdiagnosed as stroke. Other authors did not confirm the association between stroke and tumors [33–35] suggesting that comorbidity may be due to misdiagnosis and/or chance. For a comprehensive review on stroke and cancer, see Grisold et al. [36].

9. Epilepsy and cancer: A bidirectional association?

While the occurrence of seizures and epilepsy as a complication of cancer cannot be contended, the role of epilepsy as a risk factor for cancer is controversial. As antiepileptic drugs have been implicated as possible risk factors for cancer in experimental animals (discussed in the following section), the role of the disease cannot be disentangled from the role of treatment.

10. Antiepileptic drugs and cancer

Most antiepileptic drugs have been found to be carcinogenic in preclinical studies. A systematic review of the Food and Drug Administration's preclinical evidence was conducted to retrieve unpublished preclinical studies on carcinogenicity of the most common marketed psychotropic drugs [37]. The anticonvulsants studied were carbamazepine, gabapentin, lamotrigine, oxcarbazepine, pregabalin, topiramate, and valproate. All compounds, except for lamotrigine, were associated with carcinogenicity. However, findings from preclinical animal studies are heterogeneous.

The potential association between antiepileptic drugs and tumors in humans has been rarely investigated. The subject has been addressed in a comprehensive review [38]. An association was found between phenobarbital and hepatocellular carcinoma, lung cancer and brain tumors. Phenytoin has been associated with lymphoma, myeloma, and neuroblastoma, the latter in the context of fetal hydantoin syndrome. However, evidence for human carcinogenicity is inconsistent, and both drugs are considered only possibly carcinogenic to humans. No carcinogenicity has been demonstrated with the newer antiepileptic drugs either during regulatory testing or in postmarketing surveillance.

The carcinogeniticy of antiepileptic drugs has been also studied in the Rochester, Minnesota population, where the observed number of subjects with cancer among people with epilepsy was compared to the number of cases expected in the local population [39]. Among 959 patients diagnosed with seizure disorders between 1935 and 1979, 65 incident cases were diagnosed with a tumor, giving a standardized morbidity ratio of 1.4. There was a 22-fold increase in the incidence of primary brain tumors, the majority of which occurring within 5 years of the occurrence of the seizure disorder. The incidence of cancer in sites other than brain was not elevated nor was there evidence of an association between cancer incidence and duration of seizures or with anticonvulsant drugs. The association between gabapentin and cancer was investigated in a US medical care program and in a UK primary care database [40]. All cancers and specific cancer types were not significantly associated with gabapentin exposure.

As the association between antiepileptic drugs and cancer in experimental animals cannot establish that these drugs can also cause cancer in humans, the possibility of chance associations cannot be excluded. However, in the absence of adequate data on humans, it is biologically plausible and prudent to regard agents for which there is sufficient evidence of carcinogenicity in experimental animals as if they presented a carcinogenic risk to humans [41].

In contrast, valproic acid has been found to exert an anticancer activity. Seizure patients with glioblastoma treated with chemotherapy experienced a moderately improved survival with the use of valproic acid, possibly due to inhibition of histone deacetylase [25, 42]. Valproic acid was found to improve survival in patients with glioblastoma [7]. In the National Health Insurance Research Database, provided by the Taiwan National Health Research Institute, patients with a diagnosis of bipolar disorder receiving valproic acid treated for less than 1 year experienced a higher than expected risk of genitourinary cancers (HR: 3.49; 95% CI: 1.04, 11.67) [43]. In the absence of plausible explanations, the possibility of a chance finding cannot be excluded.

Increased survival in patients with glioblastoma treated with temozolomide has been also found for levetiracetam [44]. The antitumor effects of the drug are mediated by the inhibition of 0–6 methylguanine DNA methyltransferase gene [45]. Brivaracetam and lacosamide showed dose-dependent antimigratory and cytotoxic effects not related to apoptosis [46]. The exposure of glioma cells to brivaracetam and lacosamide resulted in the modulation of several microRNAs. The results of these in vitro studies require confirmation in humans.

References

[1] Keezer MR, Sisodiya SM, Sander JW. Comorbidities of epilepsy: current concepts and future perspectives. Lancet Neurol 2016;15(1):106–15.

[2] Hill AB. The environment and disease: association or causation? Proc R Soc Med 1965;58(5):295–300.

[3] Hauser WA, Annegers JF, Kurland LT. Incidence of epilepsy and unprovoked seizures in Rochester, Minnesota: 1935–1984. Epilepsia 1993;34(3):453–68.

[4] Olafsson E, Ludvigsson P, Gudmundsson G, Hesdorffer D, Kjartansson O, Hauser WA. Incidence of unprovoked seizures and epilepsy in Iceland and assessment of the epilepsy syndrome classification: a prospective study. Lancet Neurol 2005;4(10):627–34.

[5] Téllez-Zenteno JF, Matijevic S, Wiebe S. Somatic comorbidity of epilepsy in the general population in Canada. Epilepsia 2005;46(12):1955–62.

[6] Gaitatzis A, Carroll K, Majeed AW, Sander J. The epidemiology of the comorbidity of epilepsy in the general population. Epilepsia 2004;45(12):1613–22.

[7] Kerkhof M, Vecht CJ. Seizure characteristics and prognostic factors of gliomas. Epilepsia 2013;54 Suppl 9:12–7.

[8] Smits A, Duffau H. Seizures and the natural history of World Health Organization grade II gliomas: a review. Neurosurgery 2011;68(5):1326–33.

[9] Rudà R, Bello L, Duffau H, Soffietti R. Seizures in low-grade gliomas: natural history, pathogenesis, and outcome after treatments. Neuro Oncol 2012;14(Suppl 4) [iv 55-64].

[10] Englot DJ, Chang EF, Vecht CJ. Epilepsy and brain tumors. Handb Clin Neurol 2016;134:267-85.

[11] Preuß M, Preiss S, Syrbe S, Nestler U, Fischer L, Merkenschlager A, Bertsche A, Christiansen H, Bernhard MK. Signs and symptoms of pediatric brain tumors and diagnostic value of preoperative EEG. Childs Nerv Syst 2015;31(11):2051-4.

[12] Fattal-Valevski A, Nissan N, Kramer U, Constantini S. Seizures as the clinical presenting symptom in children with brain tumors. J Child Neurol 2013;28(3):292-6.

[13] van Breemen MS, Wilms EB, Vecht CJ. Epilepsy in patients with brain tumours: epidemiology, mechanisms, and management. Lancet Neurol 2007;6(5):421-30.

[14] Ertürk Çetin Ö, İşler C, Uzan M, Özkara Ç. Epilepsy-related brain tumors. Seizure 2017;44:93-7.

[15] Lee JW, Wen PY, Hurwitz S, Black P, Kesari S, Drappatz J, Golby AJ, Wells 3rd WM, Warfield SK, Kikinis R, Bromfield EB. Morphological characteristics of brain tumors causing seizures. Arch Neurol 2010;67(3):336-42.

[16] Rosati A, Tomassini A, Pollo B, Ambrosi C, Schwarz A, Padovani A, Bonetti B. Epilepsy in cerebral glioma: timing of appearance and histological correlations. J Neurooncol 2009;93(3):395-400.

[17] Pallud J, Capelle L, Huberfeld G. Tumoral epileptogenicity: how does it happen? Epilepsia 2013;-54 Suppl 9:30-4.

[18] Spencer S, Huh L. Outcomes of epilepsy surgery in adults and children. Lancet Neurol 2008; 7(6):525-37.

[19] Stockhammer F, Misch M, Helms HJ, Lengler U, Prall F, von Deimling A, Hartmann C. IDH1/2 mutations in WHO grade II astrocytomas associated with localization and seizure as the initial symptom. Seizure 2012;21(3):194-7.

[20] Chen H, Judkins J, Thomas C, Wu M, Khoury L, Benjamin CG, Pacione D, Golfinos JG, Kumthekar P, Ghamsari F, Chen L, Lein P, Chetkovich DM, Snuderl M, Horbinski C. Mutant IDH1 and seizures in patients with glioma. Neurology 2017;88(19):1805-13.

[21] Kolker S, Pawlak V, Ahlemeyer B, Okun JG, Horster F, Mayatepek E, Krieglstein J, Hoffmann GF, Köhr G. NMDA receptor activation and respiratory chain complex V inhibition contribute to neurodegeneration in D-2-hydroxyglutaric aciduria. Eur J Neurosci 2002;16(1):21-8.

[22] Prabowo AS, Iyer AM, Veersema TJ, Anink JJ, Schouten-van Meeteren AY, Spliet WG, van Rijen PC, Ferrier CH, Capper D, Thom M, Aronica E. BRAF V600E mutation is associated with mTOR signaling activation in glioneuronal tumors. Brain Pathol 2014;24(1):52-66.

[23] Fontaine D, Vandenbos F, Lebrun C, Paquis V, Frenay M. Diagnostic and prognostic values of 1p and 19q deletions in adult gliomas: critical review of the literature and implications in daily clinical practice. Rev Neurol 2008;164(6-7):595-604.

[24] Oberndorfer S, Schmal T, Lahrmann H, Urbanits S, Lindner K, Grisold W. The frequency of seizures in patients with primary brain tumors or cerebral metastases. An evaluation from the Ludwig Boltzmann Institute of Neuro-Oncology and the Department of Neurology, Kaiser Franz Josef Hospital, Vienna. Wien Klin Wochenschr 2002;114(21-22):911-6.

[25] Weller M, Stupp R, Wick W. Epilepsy meets cancer: when, why, and what to do about it? Lancet Oncol 2012;13(9):e375-82.

[26] Stafstrom CE, Staedtke V, Comi AM. Epilepsy mechanisms in neurocutaneous disorders: tuberous sclerosis complex, neurofibromatosis type 1, and Sturge-Weber syndrome. Front Neurol 2017;8:87.

[27] Islam MP, Roach ES. Tuberous sclerosis complex. Handb Clin Neurol 2015;132:97-109.

[28] Sudarsanam A, Ardern-Holmes SL. Sturge-Weber syndrome: from the past to the present. Eur J Paediatr Neurol 2014;18(3):257-66.

[29] Ostendorf AP, Gutmann DH, Weisenberg JL. Epilepsy in individuals with neurofibromatosis type 1. Epilepsia 2013;54(10):1810-4.

[30] GBD 2015 Neurological Disorders Collaborator Group. Global, regional, and national burden of neurological disorders during 1990-2015: a systematic analysis for the Global Burden of Disease Study 2015. Lancet Neurol 2017;16(11):877-97.

[31] Graus F, Rogers LR, Posner JB. Cerebrovascular complications in patients with cancer. Medicine 1985;64(1):16-35.

[32] Lindvig K, Møller H, Mosbech J, Jensen OM. The pattern of cancer in a large cohort of stroke patients. Int J Epidemiol 1990;19(3):498–504.

[33] Chaturvedi S, Ansell J, Recht L. Should cerebral ischemic events in cancer patients be considered a manifestation of hypercoagulability? Stroke 1994;25(6):1215–8.

[34] Cestari DM, Weine DM, Panageas KS, Segal AZ, DeAngelis LM. Stroke in patients with cancer: incidence and etiology. Neurology 2004;62(11):2025–30.

[35] Zhang YY, Cordato D, Shen Q, Sheng AZ, Hung WT, Chan DK. Risk factor, pattern, etiology and outcome in ischemic stroke patients with cancer: a nested case-control study. Cerebrovasc Dis 2007;23 (2–3):181–7.

[36] Grisold W, Oberndorfer S, Struhal W. Stroke and cancer: a review. Acta Neurol Scand 2009;119 (1):1–16.

[37] Amerio A, Gálvez JF, Odone A, Dalley SA, Ghaemi SN. Carcinogenicity of psychotropic drugs: a systematic review of US Food and Drug Administration-required preclinical in vivo studies. Aust N Z J Psychiatry 2015;49(8):686–96.

[38] Singh G, Driever PH, Sander JW. Cancer risk in people with epilepsy: the role of antiepileptic drugs. Brain 2005;128(Pt 1):7–17.

[39] Shirts SB, Annegers JF, Hauser WA, Kurland LT. Cancer incidence in a cohort of patients with seizure disorders. J Natl Cancer Inst 1986;77(1):83–7.

[40] Irizarry MC, Webb DJ, Boudiaf N, Logie J, Habel LA, Udaltsova N, Friedman GD. Risk of cancer in patients exposed to gabapentin in two electronic medical record systems. Pharmacoepidemiol Drug Saf 2012;21(2):214–25.

[41] International Agency for Research on Cancer (IARC) and World Health Organization. IARC: IARC monographs on the evaluation of carcinogenic risks to humans. Lyon: World Health Organization; 2000.

[42] de Groot M, Reijneveld JC, Aronica E, Heimans JJ. Epilepsy in patients with a brain tumour: focal epilepsy requires focused treatment. Brain 2012;135(Pt 4):1002–16.

[43] Lin CC, Hsieh TC, Wu LS. Long-term use of valproic acid and the prevalence of cancers in bipolar disorder patients in a Taiwanese population: an association analysis using the National Health Insurance Research Database (NHIRD). J Affect Disord 2018;232:103–8.

[44] Kim YH, Kim T, Joo JD, Han JH, Kim YJ, Kim IA, Yun CH, Kim CY. Survival benefit of levetiracetam in patients treated with concomitant chemoradiotherapy and adjuvant chemotherapy with temozolomide for glioblastoma multiforme. Cancer 2015;121(17):2926–32.

[45] Bobustuc GC, Baker CH, Limaye A, Jenkins WD, Pearl G, Avgeropoulos NG, Konduri SD. Levetiracetam enhances p53-mediated MGMT inhibition and sensitizes glioblastoma cells to temozolomide. Neuro Oncol 2010;12(9):917–27.

[46] Rizzo A, Donzelli S, Girgenti V, Sacconi A, Vasco C, Salmaggi A, Blandino G, Maschio M, Ciusani E. In vitro antineoplastic effects of brivaracetam and lacosamide on human glioma cells. J Exp Clin Cancer Res 2017;36(1):76.

CHAPTER 10

Epilepsy, headache, and chronic pain

Cinzia Costa*, Paola Sarchielli*, Michele Romoli*, Stefano Caproni†, Paolo Calabresi*,‡
*Neurology Clinic, University of Perugia—S. Maria della Misericordia Hospital, Perugia, Italy
†Azienda Ospedaliera S. Maria, Terni, Italy
‡IRCCS "Santa Lucia", Rome, Italy

Contents

Abbreviations

AEDs	antiepileptic drugs
CBZ	carbamazepine
CADASIL	cerebral autosomal dominant arteriopathy with subcortical infarcts and leukoencephalopathy
CNP	clonazepam
CSD	cortical spreading depression
EEG	electroencephalogram
EPGP	epilepsy phenome/genome project
EH	epileptic headache
EA2	episodic ataxia type 2
FHM	familial hemiplegic migraine
GPT	gabapentin
GEFS+	generalized epilepsy with febrile seizures plus
LTG	lamotrigine
LEV	levetiracetam
MRI	magnetic resonance imaging
MA	migraine with aura
OCX	oxcarbazepine
PDS	paroxysmal depolarizing shift

The Comorbidities of Epilepsy
https://doi.org/10.1016/B978-0-12-814877-8.00010-6

PHT	phenytoin
PGB	pregabalin
post-IH	post-ictal
GABA	γ-aminobutyric acid
SMEI	severe myoclonic epilepsy of infancy
TTH	tension-type headache
TPM	topiramate
VPA	valproic acid
VGB	vigabatrin
ZNS	zonisamide

1. Introduction

Among the most common neurological disorders presenting with episodic attacks and affecting people at all ages worldwide, epilepsy and headaches have been recognized to co-occur decades ago. The first suggestions that both diseases shared clinical aspects have already been proposed by Gowers in 1907 [1], raising the concept of paroxysmal neurological disorders with abrupt alterations of neurological functions and return to baseline between attacks. Over the last 50 years, several authors confirmed this hypothesis, also demonstrating common pathophysiological and therapeutic features of these distinct neurological disorders [2].

Different studies have been conducted to verify the association between the two disorders, with conflicting results. This is in part due to methodological limitations, since issues emerge from small patient sample size, different setting of data collection (population or specialized centers), inconsistent design among studies (prospective or retrospective), and different classification criteria applied for both epilepsy and headache. The latter is particularly true for migraine, which, to date, seems to represent one of the most important conditions associated with epilepsy, having been the focus of intense research regarding shared mechanisms of these two disorders [2]. In this chapter we will define common pathophysiological mechanisms and treatment of pain conditions co-occurring with epilepsy.

2. Prevalence of headaches in epileptic patients

Overall, up to 50% of adults with active epilepsy have at least one comorbid medical disorder. Several large population-based studies report various conditions that are up to eight times more prevalent in people with epilepsy relative to the general population [3].

Epileptic patients frequently experience headaches, particularly migraine-type headaches, with postictal headaches occurring more frequently, with the frequency of migraine headaches being linked to the frequency of seizures and type of treatment. In patients with epilepsy, headaches are frequently overlooked, as they may be unreported to physicians in the presence of acute and dramatic seizure symptoms [4].

The majority of epidemiological research concerns the prevalence of migraine in epileptic patients, whereas limited studies investigated the prevalence of other types of primary headaches in the same patients [5].

In the general population migraine occurs in about 6% of adult patients with epilepsy <64 years old [6]. Epileptic patients with migraine usually have a longer duration of epilepsy, higher frequency of epileptic seizures, and a higher prevalence of refractory, unresponsive epilepsy than patients affected by epilepsy alone, independently from migraine severity [7]. A higher prevalence rate for migraine in epileptics compared to general population emerged from the Epilepsy Comorbidities and Health Survey conducted in United States, supported by an overall 1.32-fold increase in prevalence, higher than that detected for fibromyalgia, neuropathic pain, and chronic pain [8].

An interview-based survey, conducted on a large population sample (1.793 participants), denied a strict association between epilepsy and migraine. Nevertheless, the same study identified higher prevalence and frequency of migraine among patients with active epilepsy (45%) compared to those with epilepsy in remission or seizure-free status (14%). In addition, patients with migraine (1%), particularly those with migraine with aura (1.8%), showed a trend towards a more active epilepsy than those without migraine (0.5%), suggesting a to and fro connection between these two disorders.

The lifetime co-occurrence of epilepsy and migraine was investigated in a recent systematic review and metaanalysis involving 10 eligible studies and encompassing a total of 1,548,967 subjects [3]. An overall 52% increase in migraine prevalence was found among epileptic patients compared to those without epilepsy; on the other hand, an overall 79% increase in the prevalence of epilepsy was detected among migraineurs, strengthening the association between disorders. The lack of validated and accurate methods of epilepsy or migraine status assessment among cohorts included in the selected studies, as well as inconsistent attempts to check for potential confounders, seem to be the most relevant sources of interstudy heterogeneity in the subgroup analysis, supporting the need of additional higher quality studies overcoming these limitations.

A more recent study investigated the burden of headache in patients with epilepsy ($n = 208$) irrespective of their sex or age. Among those complaining of interictal headaches (77.9%), 39% reported tension-type headache, 31.7% migraine, 7.8% suffered from medication-overuse headache, and 16% complained of a possible persistent headache attributed to traumatic head injury. Interestingly, migraine seemed to be more common in males with epilepsy than in the general population, whereas medication-overuse headache was more common in patients with epilepsy. Headaches usually caused a moderate or severe burden as investigated by the "headache-attributed lost time questionnaire," suggesting a net clinical additional need for these patients [9].

As for other comorbid conditions that might allow for so-called prognostic anticipation, migraine can be associated with a reduced probability of early antiepileptic drug (AED) response and seizure freedom [3]. For a summary of prevalence of headache in epileptic patients in literature, see Table 1.

Table 1 Prevalence of headache in epileptic patients

Year	Method	Age	No. of patients	M/F	Prevalence	Refs.
1987	Interview	32 (mean)	100	39/61	18%	[10]
1994	Structured telephone interviews + medical records review for 60% of probands	≥18	1948	40%/60%	24%	[11]
1996	Questionnaires mailed to the subjects + medical records review	19–65 (range)	162	82/80	NA	[12]
1999	Questionnaire + interview + medical records review	38 ± 12	109	36/73	12.8%	[13]
1999	Interview with a standardized questionnaire	15–70 (range)	412	212/200	14%	[14]
2001	Interview with a standardized questionnaire	40 ± 15 (mean)	341	154/187	18.2%	[15]
2002	Questionnaire administered to patients	≥10	135	80/55	14.8%	[16]
2002	Semistandardized interview	35.2 (mean)	110	69/41	10%	[17]
2004	Structured interview with standardized questionnaire	12–81 (range)	364	163/201	8%	[18]
2007	Questionnaire + semistructured telephone interview	20–71 (range)	109	44/65	20%	[19]
2008	Interview with standardized questionnaire + seizures and headache diary over the 3-month observation period + final interview	36.0 ± 11.3 (mean)	227	98/129	6.6%	[20]
2009	Patients evaluated at the epilepsy clinic	9.5 (3–22)	72	45/17	15%	[21]
2010	Questionnaire at initial visit	≥13	597	348/249	12.4%	[22]
2011	Questionnaire administered to patients	33.4 ± 12.4	75	32/43	41%	[23]

Year	Method	Age/score	n	Ratio	%	Ref
2012	Questionnaire administered to patients	<10 49% >10 51%	400	203/197	25%	[24]
2012	Direct interview with questionnaire	≥18	492	154/338	18.3%	[25]
2013	Semistructured interview	≥18	201	106/95	11%	[26]
2013	Telephone or in-person interview + medical record abstraction	≥12	730	285/445	25.2%	[27]
2013	Patients evaluated at the epilepsy clinic	4–88 range	304	141/163	32.9%	[28]
2014	Self-administered questionnaire + standardized semistructured telephone interview	≥18	1109	607/502	12.53%	[29]
2014	Questionnaire administered to patients	37 (9–53)	150	70/80	33%	[30]
2015	Questionnaire administered to patients	37.3 (7–75)	255	128/127	73%	[31]
2016	Anonymous questionnaire	37.8±14.5 (mean)	280	108/172	83.2%	[9]
2017	Questionnaire administered to patients	30.9±13.1 (mean)	349	159/190	43.6%	[4]

3. Prevalence of epilepsy in migraineurs

Rates of prevalence of epilepsy among migraineurs range from 1% to 17% (median value: 5.9%), largely exceeding the epilepsy occurrence in population studies, which has been estimated to be of about 0.5%–1% [32, 33].

More recently, a national comorbidity face to face survey of adolescents aged from 13 to 18 years in continental United States revealed a higher rate of epilepsy in adolescents with any headaches, not only migraine (OR:2.2, CI:1.04–3.94) [34].

The prevalence rate concerning selected headache patients in clinical settings is lower, as shown by a multicenter study in Italy, reporting a co-occurrence of epilepsy and headache in only 1.6% of patients coming from headache centers against the 30.0% detected in patients attending epilepsy centers [25].

A population-based retrospective cohort study revealed a significant increase in subsequent epilepsy risk in young adults with migraine. In particular, the adjusted hazard ratio for developing epilepsy in the migraine cohort was 1.85. Moreover, this prevalence is increased for women (2.04) and in patients aged 20–44 years [35].

Focal-onset and cryptogenic epilepsies are associated with a slightly higher rate of migraine compared to generalized onset seizures (relative risk = 1.3). However, a stronger association was found for cases of epilepsy occurring after a head trauma, with overall 1.8-fold increase in risk. Such relationship can be explained by the fact that head injury is a risk for both conditions [33].

Although in the past the association was identified only between epilepsy and migraine with aura, more recent studies identified an increased prevalence of epilepsy both in adult patients with migraine with and those without aura [36, 37].

This was confirmed also in a large population of young patients (1.795), suffering from both idiopathic headaches and idiopathic epilepsy or unprovoked seizures. Children with epilepsy had a 4.5-fold increased risk of developing migraine than tension-type headache; likewise, young migraine patients had a 3.2 times higher risk of presenting epilepsy, with no differences between the two migraine subtypes. Furthermore, children with both migraine and focal epilepsy have also a threefold increased risk of presenting a cryptogenic headache than an idiopathic headache. Interestingly, epilepsy preceded migraine in 2/3 of patients with migraine. A positive family history for epilepsy (39%) and photosensitivity (12.5%) appear to be frequent in cases with comorbidity [37].

Contrary to the previously stated evidence, migraine and epilepsy infrequently co-occur in selected samples of young patients from headache and epilepsy centers [38]. In headache patients only 1.7% of children had epilepsy or unprovoked seizures, and migraine and epilepsy also co-occurred in 2.3%. A total of 11.4% of 70 patients affected by epilepsy complained of headaches but none had migraine. Furthermore, around 43% of patients with benign childhood epilepsy with centrotemporal spikes and childhood absence epilepsy had a family history of headache, which had higher prevalence in first-degree relatives of children in the former.

In a cross-sectional study estimating a prevalence of headache of 73% of patients with epilepsy, the Authors reported solely interictal headache in 49% of cases, solely seizure-related (preictal, ictal, or postictal) in 29%, and both interictal as well as seizure-related headache in 22% [31].

Moreover, in another cross-sectional study enrolling 150 epileptic patients, migraine was more common in persons with academic degrees, women, patients who were used to AEDs, and patients with high body mass index [30].

Further evidences showed that, among epileptic patients, migraine was more frequent in those who experienced more than one seizure per month and in patients receiving multitherapy compared with patients receiving monotherapy [4].

4. Genetic aspects of the migraine-epilepsy comorbidity

Common genetic and molecular substrates for migraine and epilepsy have been investigated during the last few decades, with specific focus on phenotypic-genotypic correlations for mutations in *CACNA1A, ATP1A2, SCN1A, SLC1A3, POLG,* and *C10 or F2* genes.

Migraine with and without aura is a common familial condition. Susceptibility genes have been unveiled with linkage and association studies, resulting in high genetic heterogeneity in susceptibility genes, such as *ESR1, TNF,* and *KCNK18*. Despite significant heterogeneity, familial aggregation suggests a genetic background and an oligogenic inheritance, also found in epilepsy. Nevertheless, genes involved in susceptibility to headache and migraine update and increase daily, including also new mutations reported for already known genes, such as *CACNA1H, CASR, CACNB4, GABRD, CLCN2, SLC2A1, GABRA1,* and *SLC12A5*. However, susceptibility genes identified in migraineurs are different from those of people with idiopathic generalized epilepsy. Powerful genetic studies, counting on whole genome association and exome sequencing, have not yet been performed on a large cohort of people with both migraine and epilepsy. Nevertheless, several genes associated with specific, monogenic forms of migraine have been reported to be associated with epilepsy, thus suggesting the existence of an underlying shared pathway for both disorders. Among monogenic diseases associated with both migraine and epilepsy, a broad variability in prevalence and clinical features exists with more common and widely known disorders, such as familial hemiplegic migraine (FHM) due to *CACNA1A, ATP1A2, SCN1A,* episodic ataxia type 6 (EA6) due to mutation in the *SLC1A3* gene (channelopathy), as well as more uncommon diseases, including mitochondrial disease due to MT-TL1, MT-ND5, POLG, C10orF2 mutations, or cerebral autosomal dominant arteriopathy with subcortical infarcts and leukoencephalopathy (CADASIL) due to NOTCH3 mutation.

FHM is a rare autosomal dominant subtype of migraine with aura, characterized by a fully reversible motor weakness as a specific symptom of aura. Mutations in the ion transportation genes *CACNA1A*, *ATP1A2*, and *SCN1A* are all responsible for the FHM phenotype, determining three different forms with specific prevalence of epilepsy [39], thus indicating a genetic heterogeneity for FHM. Few studies have reported on the prevalence of epilepsy among patients with FHM. Overall, about 7% of patients with FHM suffer from epilepsy, but currently no conclusive data are available regarding the possible association between hemiplegic migraine and epilepsy. A comprehensive review on FHM and epilepsy unveiled a crucial spot on the pathogenesis of both diseases. Indeed, among the FHM cases with seizure/epilepsy, mutational hot spots have been found in the transmembrane domains of CACNA1A and ATP1A2 proteins, suggesting that transmembrane domains are indeed the shared fulcrum of both diseases.

The *CACNA1A* gene encodes for the pore-forming α1 subunit of human voltage-gated Cav2.1 (P/Q type) calcium channels. Mutations in this gene were identified for the first time among patients with episodic ataxia type 2 (EA2), and then in several families suffering from FHM1. The finding of CAG repeat expansion in SCA6, the most recently reported to be associated with such gene mutation, was only recently reported, and interests the C-terminal coding region of the *CACNA1A* gene, producing altered polyglutamine sequence.

Apart from the SCA6, which is associated with a specific dynamic mutation, genotype-phenotype correlation studies have identified an association between EA2 and loss-of-function mutations. Vice versa, gain-of-function mutations have been implicated in FHM, with Cav2.1 channel activity boosted by the lower activation threshold, and consequently increased intracellular calcium concentrations, which promote and startle cortical spreading depression (CSD). On the other hand, a number of nontruncating mutations have been observed to cluster in the S5–S6 linkers and their borders even in EA2. Genotype-phenotype correlations seem to be dependent on the functional effects of the mutations as well as the positions of the modified amino acids. In particular, since no loss-of-function mutation has been linked with FHM1-epilepsy phenotype, gain-of-function is probably the mechanism implicated in moving from channel dysfunction to clinical phenotype.

Regarding shared pathogenic mechanisms, since CACNA1A variants may be responsible for repeated CSD, they might be able to trigger both FHM and epilepsy. S218L mutation promotes facilitation in activation of the calcium channel, as highlighted by the increased incidence in recurrent CSD in S218L knock-in mice. Such mutation is thus able to lead to a gain-of-function, with channels responding to even small depolarization.

Epileptic phenotypes have been associated with mutation in III and IV domains of the S4 segment, with mutations in domains I and II of the Cav2.1 channel (encoded by the *CACNA1A* gene) highly unlikely to determine epilepsy. Thus, patients with familial or sporadic forms of HM1 harboring such variants need to be closely monitored and managed [39].

The *ATP1A2* gene encodes the α2 subunit of the Na^+, K^+-ATPase, an integral membrane protein responsible for establishing and maintaining the electrochemical gradients of Na^+ and K^+ across the plasma membrane. The first identification of ATP1A2 mutation was made on an Italian family suffering from FHM2. The mutation of the *ATP1A2* gene causes an impairment of the pump, with substantial inability to clear extracellular K^+ by glial cells. Moreover, it leads to a lower turnover of the pump, which is then both unable to work and unable to be replaced by functioning transmembrane proteins. Mutations can cause heterogeneous malfunctioning, from total loss of function to simple turnover or kinetic activity reduction of the pump, but always lead to impairment in K^+ clearance. Glial and neuronal Na^+/K^+-ATPase play important roles in the clearance of extracellular K^+ to prevent depolarization of neurons during high neuronal activity. Malfunctioning of the Na^+/K^+-ATPase pump may lead to neuronal hyperexcitability and facilitate both paroxysmal depolarizing shifts, leading to both seizures and CSD/migraine. Indeed, the elevation of extracellular K^+ levels, associated with the accumulation of glutamate in the synaptic cleft, leads to a reduced threshold for activation and a longer exposure to facilitatory neurotransmitters, increasing intracellular Calcium waft. Missense mutations affecting the transmembrane domains can lead to both the perturbation of catalytic site functions and the modification of pump kinetic characteristics, and it is interesting to note that individuals carrying mutations within these domains are much more susceptible to epilepsy [39, 40].

The *SCN1A* gene encodes the $\alpha 1$ subunit of the voltage-gated Na^+ channel Nav 1.1. Mutations in this gene were first identified in people with familial epilepsy: generalized epilepsy with febrile seizures plus (GEFS +), and Dravet syndrome, also known as severe myoclonic epilepsy of infancy (SMEI). FHM has been associated with a heterozygous mutation in the *SCN1A* gene, at first identified in three European families with FHM3. Mutations can affect the protein structure in the intracellular, extracellular, and transmembrane domains. The genotype-phenotype correlation seems to depend mainly on the functional effect of the mutation rather than its position through the canal protein. Mutations leading to loss-of-function are mainly associated with SMEI whereas gain-of-function mutations are mainly associated with GEFS + or FHM3. In the case of FHM3-epilepsy comorbidity, experimental evidence suggests double functional effect of a single mutation. Indeed, the T1174S (c.3521 C > G) SCN1A mutation, which has been associated with seizures and/or FHM, can induce both a loss of function and a gain of function, a finding consistent with both epilepsy and FHM phenotypes [39].

Further genetic studies might highlight other shared pathways between epilepsy and migraine.

5. Pathophysiological aspects underlying the association between migraine and epilepsy

Migraine attacks like epileptic seizures are attributed to a state of brain hyperexcitability. This state can be induced by genetic or acquired factors (i.e., a head injury) increasing the risk of both migraine and epilepsy, and therefore potentially explaining their comorbid association.

The neurophysiological correlate linking migraine and seizures is CSD, which was first described by Leao [41] during the propagation of electrically provoked seizure discharges in the cerebral cortex. It is characterized by a slowly self-propagating wave (2–6 mm/min) of sustained strong neuronal depolarization, inducing a transient (in terms of seconds) and intense spike activity followed by a neural suppression lasting for minutes [41].

More recently CSD can be triggered in animal models by not only focal electrical stimulation but also mechanical stimulation, high extracellular K^+ or glutamate, persistent intracellular sodium influx, inhibition of the Na^+/K^+ ATPase pump in the cerebral cortex, particularly occipital regions, but also subcortical regions can be involved [42, 43].

Several pathways, including abnormalities in intrinsic neuronal activity and ionic channels, have been postulated to explain differences in the propagation of epileptic activity and SD [44, 45].

In particular some experimental evidence suggests that epileptiform activity due to an enhanced excitatory neurotransmission propagates at rates comparable to CSD whereas epileptiform activity due to reduced inhibition propagates much faster [46].

Both seizures and SD are induced by similar mechanisms, such as hypoxia, neural injury, hypoglycemia, high concentrations of K^+, and Na^+/K^+ pump inhibition [47]. Human studies have observed SD in a variety of pathological states, including epilepsy [48]. CSD has been considered the pathophysiological correlate of migraine aura [43] and perhaps of migraine without aura in which CSD seems to develop in silent brain areas [49–51]. An increase in regional cerebral blood flow is associated to the depolarization phase, whereas a reduction in regional cerebral blood flow characterizes the phase of reduced neural activity [52].

Experimental findings from Moskowitz et al. [53], Bolay et al. [54], and functional neuroimaging studies in humans [55] suggested the potential role of CSD in inducing trigeminovascular activation, which represents the common final pathway responsible for pain of migraine attacks.

Different common mechanisms have been hypothesized to potentially relate seizure and CSD onset: CSD facilitates synaptic excitability and efficacy contributing to hyperexcitability of neocortical tissues in patients suffering from migraine, supporting the efficacy of some AEDs as preventive drugs for migraine [56]. CSD can trigger epileptiform field potentials that can be prevented by gamma-Aminobutyric acid (GABA)-mediated inhibition, suggesting that SD increases neuronal excitability and facilitates synchronization of neuronal discharges in the presence a partial disinhibition of the neuronal tissues [57].

One of the potential mechanisms underlying the association between migraine and epilepsy is the inability of the Na-K pump to regulate K^+ extracellular concentration [58], and this mechanism was supported by the identification of novel mutations involving Na^+, K^+-ATPase pump gene *ATP1A2* identified in FHM and benign familial infantile convulsions and the evidence of a monogenic defect in familial occipital lobe epilepsy associated with migraine aura [59, 60].

Furthermore, calcium-sensitive current appeared to be able to promote both seizure-like discharges and CSD in experimental models [61].

An additional mechanism involved in the ionic diffusion of both epileptic depolarization and CSD onset is the "gap junctional" interactions [62, 63].

Glutamate is also believed to be a critical mediator of hyperexcitability in both focal seizures and migraine [64–67].

However, if seizure generation and propagation are mediated by excessive synaptical release of glutamate, acting on AMPA receptors and NMDA receptors, and CSD startling depends on glutamate receptors activation, then CSD and its spread do not strictly require synaptic transmission [68–70].

The difference between CSD and focal seizure activity could also be due to nonsynaptic glutamate release from glia in CSD and the synaptic glutamate release from neurons [71–73].

Several clinical findings confirm that CSD in migraine and cortical epileptic discharges can facilitate each other. Migraine occasionally triggers seizure, which often initiate postictal headache with the characteristics of migraine.

Susceptibility genes identified in migraineurs with and without aura are different from those of patients with idiopathic, generalized epilepsy. Genetic studies aimed at identifying the genetic background of multifactorial or oligogenic diseases (such as the common forms of migraine and epilepsy) are quite difficult because of the high heterogeneity and the possible influence of the environment. Larger and powerful studies on wide cohorts of patients with migraine alone, epilepsy alone, and migraine-epilepsy comorbidity are probably needed to fully elucidate the possible shared genetic substrate.

Several genes associated with specific, monogenic forms of migraine have been reported to be associated with epilepsy, thus suggesting a common pathogenetic mechanism. In fact, migraine and epilepsy are shared comorbidities in patients with some specific gene mutations involving: *CACNA1A*, *ATP1A2*, *SCN1A* in *FHM*; *SLC1A3* gene (channelopathy) in episodic ataxia type 6 (EA6); and MT-TL1, MT-ND5, POLG, C10orF2d mitochondrial diseases, and NOTCH3 in CADASIL [2, 39, 74–76].

6. Therapeutic considerations

The rational of the use of AEDs in migraine are shared pathogenic mechanisms with epilepsy such as increased excitatory glutamatergic transmission, reduced GABAergic inhibition and abnormal activation of voltage-gated channels [77, 78].

Some AEDs, such as valproic acid (VPA), topiramate (TPM), and gabapentin (GPT), are effective in the prevention of migraine, and they are overall well tolerated [77–84].

Mechanisms included modulation high-voltage-activated Ca^{2+} channels with different potencies on cortical and PAG neurons, inhibition of ligand-gated channels, in particular both ionotropic and metabotropic glutamate receptors and potentiation of GABAergic transmission [78, 85].

All the previously mentioned AEDs have been shown to inhibit CSD in a dose-dependent manner [86, 87]. Furthermore, chronic treatment with lamotrigine (LTG) has been shown to exert a marked suppressive effect on experimental CSD, which translates into a selective prophylactic effect on migraine aura [88].

TPM and VPA have been shown to be highly effective as preventive drugs for migraine, and both have been approved by the Food and Drug Administration (FDA) for migraine prophylaxis. Doses effective for migraine are general lower than those used for treating epilepsy; 880–1000 mg/day for VPA or 100 mg/day TPM. The two drugs have also been shown to be effective for chronic migraine with and without medication overuse [84, 89]. However, significant restriction of VPA use, especially among women with childbearing potential, has been imposed after the FDA and the European Medicines Agency (EMA) reports on teratogenicity.

LTG, a potent sodium channel blocker and glutamate receptor antagonist, has also been shown to be effective in patients with migraine with aura (some of them with motor aura) in open studies but not in patients with migraine without aura [90, 91]. A weaker evidence of efficacy is available for GPT and pregabalin in episodic and chronic migraine forms. Promising findings have been reported for levetiracetam and zonisamide which should be confirmed [92].

AEDs acting only via a single mechanism of action seem to be less effective in targeting migraine. Blockage of voltage-gated sodium channels alone exerted by some AEDs (i.e., carbamazepine, phenytoin, oxcarbazepine) seems to be ineffective in antagonizing migraine attacks, although their mechanism of action is relevant in preventing epileptic crises. This does not exclude that drugs targeting, but not exclusively, Na^+ currents (i.e., VPA or TPM) could exert their effectiveness in preventing migraine, including migraine with aura, also by counteracting Na^+-dependent discharges and persistent Na^+ conductance. This effect could also be for hemiplegic migraine (HM), with and without association with epilepsy [93].

Although phenytoin, oxcarbazepine, vigabatrin, and clonazepam appear to be ineffective in migraine [94], they can be useful in epileptic patients for ictal or postictal headache as demonstrated for carbamazepine, which was shown to reduce the occurrence of ictal and postictal headache [19].

In patients with epilepsy and any type of headache, in particular migraine, AEDs are the treatment of choice [95]. Conversely, tricyclic antidepressants and neuroleptic drugs should be avoided because they lower the epileptogenic threshold.

Common targets of antiepileptic treatment in the case of comorbidity are cortical hyperexcitability and CSD underlying both ictal disorders. This can also be relevant in more rare conditions, such as HM with epileptic phenotype. Despite this, for both migraine and epilepsy, 30% of patients appear unresponsive.

It should also be remembered that headache is a common side effect of some AEDs, and this may limit their use in patients with epilepsy and migraine. Gender influences drug selection, with FDA and EMA recommendations targeting valproate to be avoided in fertile women.

Among symptomatic drugs, both analgesics (from 66% to 80% of patients) and triptans have been demonstrated to be effective on postictal headache, the latter particularly for postseizure migraine-like headaches [96–99].

Among nonpharmacological approaches tried to prevent migraines in epileptic patients, vagus stimulation should be mentioned. In two studies, 3 out of 4 and 8 out of 10 patients with epilepsy and migraines, respectively, had a decrease in migraine frequency after stimulator implantation [100].

7. Clinical and instrumental assessment

Since epilepsy and migraine are often comorbid, all patients with epilepsy should be asked for the co-occurrence of migraine and the temporal relationship between seizures and presentation of migraine/headache clarified. On the other side, patients with migraine should be asked about seizure and epilepsy diagnosis.

An accurate personal history recording and clinical assessment is mandatory to provide specific diagnosis and propose diagnostic testing. Magnetic resonance imaging (MRI), including magnetic resonance angiogram, as well as laboratory or instrumental investigations might be needed in some cases for orientating the diagnosis [101].

In the case of patients with visual symptoms suggesting occipital seizures, a differential diagnosis with visual migraine aura should be considered, based on the typical traits of the two disorders [102].

MRI scans showed transient cerebral anomalies in 6% of the patients with migralepsy, which was attributed to transient alteration in blood barrier integrity eliciting edema [103]. In a series of children diagnosed with migralepsy, MRI yielded normal findings in 75%, while the remaining 25% showed brain abnormalities including neuronal migration disorder, leukoencephalopathy, periventricular gliosis, and hydrocephalus [104]. Thus, brain MRI is a mandatory diagnostic assessment to be performed.

While electroencephalogram (EEG) is crucial in epileptic patients, it is not useful to include it in the routine assessment among patients with headache. In migraine aura, however, EEG, and especially 24-h video EEG studies have shown during migraine aura, abnormalities in electrical activity not displaying typical timeline of ictal epileptiform activity, sometimes assuming an alternating pattern with its progressive increases and decreases in frequency and amplitude [105, 106].

In ictal epileptic headache the EEG pattern is not univocal. A high-voltage rhythmic activity at 11–12 Hz with alternating spikes in the right temporal-occipital region was found in some cases, but, to date, no specific pattern is consistent with the diagnosis, and one might also observe generalized slowing or discharges of spikes and continuous bilateral slow spike-waves in occipital regions, even with photoparoxysmal responses [104, 107–111]. However, it might be underlined that surface EEG is inaccurate for detecting focal epilepsy, presenting with ictal headache, originating in deep-structure like the orbitomedial frontal region or Panayiotopoulos syndrome. This supports the concept that the absence of clear epileptic activity does not exclude a diagnosis of epilepsy. In unclear cases, deep electrodes can improve the diagnostic sensitivity [15, 112, 113].

8. Conclusions

There is accumulating epidemiological evidence supporting the comorbidity of epilepsy and headache, in particular migraine, although the prevalence rate varies among studies. Future studies should be based on prospective data collection, possibly in population-based cohorts, to reduce the risk of recall bias. Moreover, misclassification of headache disorders should be minimized using available and validated screening and diagnostic methods [3].

Some research suggests that comorbid migraine negatively affects the prognosis of epilepsy [7]. Further studies to verify if the chances of achieving remission of seizures, their refractoriness to treatment, and other outcome measures really differ between epileptic patients with and without comorbid migraine would have a clear impact on patients' quality of life.

Future longitudinal studies should also be carried out to verify the causal nature of the association between epilepsy and migraine and the direction of the relation among both disorders by investigating the temporal sequence of the two disorders.

Furthermore, consensus should be achieved on the most appropriate terminology for "ictal epileptic headache" and "hemicrania epileptica," over the old term of "migralepsy." There is, therefore, the urgent need for an agreement between International Classifications of Epilepsy and Headache disorders, which requires the constructive, cooperative efforts of both the International Headache Society and the International League Against Epilepsy to overcome the old classification debate.

Common pathophysiological mechanisms understanding should be definitely pursued, focusing on brain excitability in both paroxysmal disorders and the shared genetic background besides the complex expression on the clinical phenotypes. The insight into the molecular events that underset the association between migraine and epilepsy is crucial to identify the best drug targets to improve.

There is also a need to identify the potential comorbidity of epilepsy with other painful disorders and possibly to clarify the pathophysiological basis of the association.

Final clinical efforts should focus on investigating conditions where pain is the unique manifestation of epilepsy, since this would be crucial not only for the correct diagnosis but also for setting up the most appropriate treatment.

References

[1] Gowers W. A clinical lecture on sudden cerebral lesions: their diagnosis and immediate treatment: delivered at the polyclinic. Br Med J 1907;2(2427):1–6.

[2] Bianchin MM, Londero RG, Lima JE, Bigal ME. Migraine and epilepsy: a focus on overlapping clinical, pathophysiological, molecular, and therapeutic aspects. Curr Pain Headache Rep 2010; 14(4):276–83.

[3] Keezer MR, Bauer PR, Ferrari MD, Sander JW. The comorbid relationship between migraine and epilepsy: a systematic review and meta-analysis. Eur J Neurol 2015;22(7):1038–47.

[4] Çilliler AE, Güven H, Çomoğlu SS. Epilepsy and headaches: further evidence of a link. Epilepsy Behav 2017;70(Pt A):161–5.

[5] Dalla Volta G, Di Monda V, Bariselli M, Vignolo LA. Headache and epilepsy: a case report of the unusual association of cluster headache and epilepsy. Ital J Neurol Sci 1992;13(8):699.

[6] Gaitatzis A, Carroll K, Majeed A, Sander W. The epidemiology of the comorbidity of epilepsy in the general population. Epilepsia 2004;45(12):1613–22.

[7] Velioğlu SK, Boz C, Ozmenoğlu M. The impact of migraine on epilepsy: a prospective prognosis study. Cephalalgia 2005;25(7):528–35.

[8] Ottman R, Lipton RB, Ettinger AB, Cramer JA, Reed ML, Morrison A, Wan GJ. Comorbidities of epilepsy: results from the epilepsy comorbidities and health (EPIC) survey. Epilepsia 2011; 52(2):308–15.

[9] Mameniškienė R, Karmonaitė I, Zagorskis R. The burden of headache in people with epilepsy. Seizure 2016 Oct;41:120–6.

[10] Schon F, Blau JN. Post-epileptic headache and migraine. J Neurol Neurosurg Psychiatry 1987;50:1148–52.

[11] Ottman R, Lipton RB. Comorbidity of migraine and epilepsy. Neurology 1994;44:2105–10.

[12] Ito M, Schachter SC. Frequency and characteristics of interictal headaches in patients with epilepsy. J Epilepsy 1996;9:83–6.

[13] Ito M, Nakamura F, Honma H, Takeda Y, Kobayashi R, Miyamoto T, Koyama T. A comparison of post-ictal headache between patients with occipital lobe epilepsy and temporal lobe epilepsy. Seizure 1999;8(6):343–6.

[14] Velioglu SK, Ozmenoglu M. Migraine-related seizures in an epileptic population. Cephalalgia 1999;19:797–801.

[15] Leniger T, Isbruch K, von den Driesch S, Diener HC, Hufnagel A. Seizure-associated headache in epilepsy. Epilepsia 2001;42(9):1176–9.

[16] Karaali-Savrun F, Göksan B, Yeni SN, Ertan S, Uzun N. Seizure-related headache in patients with epilepsy. Seizure 2002;11(1):67–9.

[17] Förderreuther S, Henkel A, Noachtar S, Straube A. Headache associated with epileptic seizures: epidemiology and clinical characteristics. Headache 2002;42(7):649–55.

[18] Ito M, Adachi N, Nakamura F, Koyama T, Okamura T, Kato M, Kanemoto K, Nakano T, Matsuura M, Hara S. Characteristics of postictal headache in patients with partial epilepsy. Cephalalgia 2004;24(1):23–8.

[19] Syvertsen M, Helde G, Stovner LJ, Brodtkorb E. Headaches add to the burden of epilepsy. J Headache Pain 2007;8(4):224–30.

[20] Kwan P, Man CB, Leung H, Yu E, Wong KS. Headache in patients with epilepsy: a prospective incidence study. Epilepsia 2008;49(6):1099–102.

[21] Clarke T, Baskurt Z, Strug LJ, Pal DK. Evidence of shared genetic risk factors for migraine and rolandic epilepsy. Epilepsia 2009;50(11):2428–33.

[22] HELP Study Group. Multi-center study on migraine and seizure-related headache in patients with epilepsy. Yonsei Med J 2010;51(2):219–24.

[23] Schankin CJ, Rémi J, Klaus I, Sostak P, Reinisch VM, Noachtar S, Straube A. Headache in juvenile myoclonic epilepsy. J Headache Pain 2011;12(2):227–33.

[24] Kelley SA, Hartman AL, Kossoff EH. Comorbidity of migraine in children presenting with epilepsy to a tertiary care center. Neurology 2012;79(5):468–73.

[25] Tonini MC, Giordano L, Atzeni L, Bogliun G, Perri G, Saracco MG, Tombini M, Torelli P, Turazzini M, Vernieri F, Aguggia M, Bussone G, Beghi E, EPICEF Group. Primary headache and epilepsy: a multicenter cross-sectional study. Epilepsy Behav 2012;23(3):342–7.

[26] Duchaczek B, Ghaeni L, Matzen J, Holtkamp M. Interictal and periictal headache in patients with epilepsy. Eur J Neurol 2013;20(10):1360–6.

[27] Winawer MR, Connors R, Investigators EPGP. Evidence for a shared genetic susceptibility to migraine and epilepsy. Epilepsia 2013;54:288–95.

[28] Gameleira FT, Ataíde Jr. L, Raposo MC. Relations between epileptic seizures and headaches. Seizure 2013;22:622–6.

[29] Wang XQ, Lang SY, He MW, Zhang X, Zhu F, Dai W, Shi XB, Wan M, Ma YF, Chen YN, Yu SY. High prevalence of headaches in patients with epilepsy. J Headache Pain 2014;15:70.

[30] Jabbehdari S, Hesami O, Chavoshnejad M. Prevalence of migraine headache in epileptic patients. Acta Med Iran 2015;53(6):373–5.

[31] Hofstra WA, Hageman G, de Weerd AW. Periictal and interictal headache including migraine in Dutch patients with epilepsy: a cross-sectional study. Epilepsy Behav 2015;44:155–8.

[32] Andermann F. Migraine-epilepsy relationships. Epilepsy Res 1987;1(4):213–26.

[33] Lipton RB, Ottman R, Ehrenberg BL, Hauser WA. Comorbidity of migraine: The connection between migraine and epilepsy. Neurology 1994;44(10 Suppl 7):S28–32.

[34] Lateef TM, Cui L, Nelson KB, Nakamura EF, Merikangas KR. Physical comorbidity of migraine and other headaches in US adolescents. J Pediatr 2012 Aug;161(2):308–13.

[35] Harnod T, Wang YC, Kao CH. High risk of developing subsequent epilepsy in young adults with migraine: a nationwide population-based cohort study in Taiwan. Q J Med 2015;108:449–55.

[36] Ludvigsson P, Hesdorffer D, Olafsson E, Kjartansson O, Hauser WA. Migraine with aura is a risk factor for unprovoked seizures in children. Ann Neurol 2006;59(1):210–3.

[37] Toldo I, Perissinotto E, Menegazzo F, Boniver C, Sartori S, Salviati L, Clementi M, Montagna P, Battistella PA. Comorbidity between headache and epilepsy in a pediatric headache center. J Headache Pain 2010;11(3):235–40.

[38] Papavasiliou AS, Bregianni M, Nikaina I, Kotsalis C, Paraskevoulakos E, Bazigou H. Pediatric headache and epilepsy comorbidity in the pragmatic clinical setting. Neuropediatrics 2016;47(2):107–11.

[39] Prontera P, Sarchielli P, Caproni S, Bedetti C, Cupini LM, Calabresi P, Costa C. Epilepsy in hemiplegic migraine: genetic mutations and clinical implications. Cephalalgia 2018;38(2):361–73.

[40] Costa C, Prontera P, Sarchielli P, Tonelli A, Bassi MT, Cupini LM, Caproni S, Siliquini S, Donti E, Calabresi P. A novel ATP1A2 gene mutation in familial hemiplegic migraine and epilepsy. Cephalalgia 2014 Jan;34(1):68–72.

[41] Somjen GG. Aristides Leão's discovery of cortical spreading depression. J Neurophysiol 2005; 94(1):2–4.

[42] Somjen GG. Mechanisms of spreading depression and hypoxic spreading depression-like depolarization. Physiol Rev 2001;81(3):1065–96.

[43] Richter F, Lehmenkühler A. Cortical spreading depression (CSD): a neurophysiological correlate of migraine aura. Schmerz 2008;22(5):544. -6,548-50.

[44] Barreto E, Cressman JR. Ion concentration dynamics as a mechanism for neuronal bursting. J Biol Phys 2011;37(3):361–73.

[45] Krishnan GP, Bazhenov M. Ionic dynamics mediate spontaneous termination of seizures and postictal depression state. J Neurosci 2011;3:8870–82.

[46] Trevelyan AJ, Baldeweg T, van Drongelen W, Yuste R, Whittington M. The source of after discharge activity in neocortical tonic-clonic epilepsy. J Neurosci 2007;27(49):13513–9.

[47] Dreier JP. The role of spreading depression, spreading depolarization and spreading ischemia in neurological disease. Nat Med 2011;17(4):439–47.

[48] Kramer DR, Fujii T, Ohiorhenuan I, Liu CY. Cortical spreading depolarization: pathophysiology, implications, and future directions. J Clin Neurosci 2016;24:22–7.

[49] Géraud G, Denuelle M, Fabre N, Payoux P, Chollet F. Positron emission tomographic studies of migraine. Rev Neurol 2005;161(6–7):666–70.

[50] Chalaupka FD. Reversible imaging abnormalities consistent with CSD during migraine without aura attack. Headache 2008;48(8):1229–32.

[51] Purdy RA. Migraine with and without aura share the same pathogenic mechanisms. Neurol Sci 2008;29(Suppl 1):S44–6.

[52] Tfelt-Hansen P. Intracranial vasodilation in migraine? Ann Neurol 2010;67(5):695–6.

[53] Moskowitz MA, Nozaki K, Kraig RP. Neocortical spreading depression provokes the expression of c-fos protein-like immunoreactivity within trigeminal nucleus caudalis via trigeminovascular mechanisms. J Neurosci 1993;13(3):1167–77.

[54] Bolay H, Reuter U, Dunn AK, Huang Z, Boas DA, Moskowitz MA. Intrinsic brain activity triggers trigeminal meningeal afferents in a migraine model. Nat Med 2002;8(2):136–42.

[55] Hadjikhani N, Sanchez Del Rio M, Wu O, Schwartz D, Bakker D, Fischl B, Kwong KK, Cutrer FM, Rosen BR, Tootell RB, Sorensen AG, Moskowitz MA. Mechanisms of migraine aura revealed by functional MRI in human visual cortex. Proc Natl Acad Sci U S A 2001;98(8):4687–92.

[56] Rogawski MA. Migraine and epilepsy—Shared mechanisms within the family of episodic disorders. In: Noebels JL, Avoli M, Rogawski MA, Olsen RW, Delgado-Escueta AV, editors. Jasper's basic mechanisms of the epilepsies [Internet]. 4th ed. Bethesda (MD): National Center for Biotechnology Information (US); 2012.

[57] Eickhoff M, Kovac S, Shahabi P, Ghadiri MK, Dreier JP, Stummer W, Speckmann EJ, Pape HC, Gorji A. Spreading depression triggers ictaform activity in partially disinhibited neuronal tissues. Exp Neurol 2014;253:1–15.

[58] Haglund MM, Schwartzkroin PA. Role of Na-K pump potassium regulation and IPSPs in seizures and spreading depression in immature rabbit hippocampal slices. J Neurophysiol 1990;63(2):225–39.

[59] Vanmolkot KR, Kors EE, Hottenga JJ, Terwindt GM, Haan J, Hoefnagels WA, Black DF, Sandkuijl LA, Frants RR, Ferrari MD, van den Maagdenberg AM. Novel mutations in the Na$^+$, K$^+$-ATPase pump gene ATP1A2 associated with familial hemiplegic migraine and benign familial infantile convulsions. Ann Neurol 2003;54(3):360–6.

[60] Deprez L, Peeters K, Van Paesschen W, Claeys KG, Claes LR, Suls A, Audenaert D, Van Dyck T, Goossens D, Del-Favero J, De Jonghe P. Familial occipitotemporal lobe epilepsy and migraine with visual aura: linkage to chromosome 9q. Neurology 2007;68(23):1995–2002.

[61] Somjen GG, Kager H, Wadman WJ. Calcium sensitive non-selective cation current promotes seizure-like discharges and spreading depression in a model neuron. J Comput Neurosci 2009;26 (1):139–47.

[62] Nedergaard M, Cooper AJ, Goldman SA. Gap junctions are required for the propagation of spreading depression. J Neurobiol 1995;28(4):433–44.

[63] Nilsen KE, Kelso AR, Cock HR. Antiepileptic effect of gap-junction blockers in a rat model of refractory focal cortical epilepsy. Epilepsia 2006;47(7):1169–75.

[64] Theodore WH, Fisher RS. Brain stimulation for epilepsy. Lancet Neurol 2004;3(2):111–8.

[65] Aurora SK, Ahmad BK, Welch KM, Bhardhwaj P, Ramadan NM, Aurora SK, Ahmad BK, Welch KM, Bhardhwaj P, Ramadan NM. Transcranial magnetic stimulation confirms hyperexcitability of occipital cortex in migraine. Neurology 1998;50(4):1111–4.

[66] Chronicle EP, Pearson AJ, Mulleners WM. Objective assessment of cortical excitability in migraine with and without aura. Cephalalgia 2006;26(7):801–8.

[67] Siniatchkin M, Reich AL, Shepherd AJ, van Baalen A, Siebner HR, Stephani U. Peri-ictal changes of cortical excitability in children suffering from migraine without aura. Pain 2009;147(1–3):132–40.

[68] Yamaguchi S, Donevan SD, Rogawski MA. Anticonvulsant activity of AMPA/kainate antagonists: comparison of GYKI 52466 and NBOX in maximal electroshock and chemoconvulsant seizure models. Epilepsy Res 1993;15(3):179–84.

[69] Psarropoulou C, Avoli M. CPP, an NMDA-receptor antagonist, blocks 4-aminopyridine-induced spreading depression episodes but not epileptiform activity in immature rat hippocampal slices. Neurosci Lett 1992;135(1):139–43.

[70] Peeters M, Gunthorpe MJ, Strijbos PJ, Goldsmith P, Upton N, James MF. Effects of pan- and subtype-selective N-methyl-D-aspartate receptor antagonists on cortical spreading depression in the rat: therapeutic potential for migraine. J Pharmacol Exp Ther 2007;321(2):564–72.

[71] Larrosa B, Pastor J, López-Aguado L, Herreras O. A role for glutamate and glia in the fast network oscillations preceding spreading depression. Neuroscience 2006;141(2):1057–68.

[72] Fellin T, Haydon PG. Do astrocytes contribute to excitation underlying seizures? Trends Mol Med 2005;11(12):530–3.

[73] Rogawski MA. Astrocytes get in the act in epilepsy. Nat Med 2005;11(9):919–20.

[74] Rogawski MA. Common pathophysiologic mechanisms in migraine and epilepsy. Arch Neurol 2008;65(6):709–14.

[75] Chabriat H, Joutel A, Dichgans M, Tournier-Lasserve E, Bousser MG. Cadasil. Lancet Neurol 2009; 8(7):643–53.

[76] El-Hattab AW, Adesina AM, Jones J, Scaglia F. MELAS syndrome: clinical manifestations, pathogenesis, and treatment options. Mol Genet Metab 2015;116(1–2):4–12.

[77] Welch KM. Brain hyperexcitability: the basis for antiepileptic drugs in migraine prevention. Headache 2005;45(Suppl 1):S25–32.

[78] Calabresi P, Galletti F, Rossi C, Sarchielli P, Cupini LM. Antiepileptic drugs in migraine: from clinical aspects to cellular mechanisms. Trends Pharmacol Sci 2007;28(4):188–95.

[79] Cutrer FM. Antiepileptic drugs: how they work in headache. Headache 2001;41(Suppl 1):S3–10.

[80] Rogawski MA, Löscher W. The neurobiology of antiepileptic drugs for the treatment of nonepileptic conditions. Nat Med 2004;10(7):685–92.

[81] Calabresi P, Cupini LM, Centonze D, Pisani F, Bernardi G. Antiepileptic drugs as a possible neuroprotective strategy in brain ischemia. Ann Neurol 2003;53(6):693–702.

[82] Costa C, Leone G, Saulle E, Pisani F, Bernardi G, Calabresi P. Coactivation of GABA(A) and GABA(B) receptor results in neuroprotection during in vitro ischemia. Stroke 2004;35(2):596–600.

[83] Costa C, Martella G, Picconi B, Prosperetti C, Pisani A, Di Filippo M, Pisani F, Bernardi G, Calabresi P. Multiple mechanisms underlying the neuroprotective effects of antiepileptic drugs against in vitro ischemia. Stroke 2006;37(5):1319–26.

[84] Romoli M, Costa C, Siliquini S, Corbelli I, Eusebi P, Bedetti C, Caproni S, Cupini LM, Calabresi P, Sarchielli P. Antiepileptic drugs in migraine and epilepsy: who is at increased risk of adverse events? Cephalalgia 2018;38(2):274–82.

[85] Martella G, Costa C, Pisani A, Cupini LM, Bernardi G, Calabresi P. Antiepileptic drugs on calcium currents recorded from cortical and PAG neurons: therapeutic implications for migraine. Cephalalgia 2008;28(12):1315–26.

[86] Ayata C, Jin H, Kudo C, Dalkara T, Moskowitz MA. Suppression of cortical spreading depression in migraine prophylaxis. Ann Neurol 2006;59(4):652–61.

[87] Tozzi A, de Iure A, Di Filippo M, Costa C, Caproni S, Pisani A, Bonsi P, Picconi B, Cupini LM, Materazzi S, Geppetti P, Sarchielli P, Calabresi P. Critical role of calcitonin gene-related peptide receptors in cortical spreading depression. Proc Natl Acad Sci U S A 2012;109(46):18985–90.

[88] Bogdanov VB, Multon S, Chauvel V, Bogdanova OV, Prodanov D, Makarchuk MY, Schoenen J. Migraine preventive drugs differentially affect cortical spreading depression in rat. Neurobiol Dis 2011;41(2):430–5.

[89] Sarchielli P, Messina P, Cupini LM, Tedeschi G, Di Piero V, Livrea P, Pini LA, Bernardi G, Bono G, Sandrini G, Caproni S, Corbelli I, Pisani F, Beghi E, Calabresi P, SAMOHA Study Group. Sodium valproate in migraine without aura and medication overuse headache: a randomized controlled trial. Eur Neuropsychopharmacol 2014;24(8):1289–97.

[90] D'Andrea G, Granella F, Cadaldini M, Manzoni GC. Effectiveness of lamotrigine in the prophylaxis of migraine with aura: an open pilot study. Cephalalgia 1999;19(1):64–6.

[91] Lampl C, Katsarava Z, Diener HC, Limmroth V. Lamotrigine reduces migraine aura and migraine attacks in patients with migraine with aura. J Neurol Neurosurg Psychiatry 2005;76(12):1730–2.

[92] Mohammadianinejad SE, Abbasi V, Sajedi SA, Majdinasab N, Abdollahi F, Hajmanouchehri R, Faraji A. Zonisamide versus topiramate in migraine prophylaxis: a double-blind randomized clinical trial. Clin Neuropharmacol 2011;34(4):174–7.

[93] Galletti F, Cupini LM, Corbelli I, Calabresi P, Sarchielli P. Pathophysiological basis of migraine prophylaxis. Prog Neurobiol 2009;89(2):176–92.

[94] Linde M, Mulleners WM, Chronicle EP, McCrory DC. Antiepileptics other than gabapentin, pregabalin, topiramate, and valproate for the prophylaxis of episodic migraine in adults. Cochrane Database Syst Rev 2013;6:CD010608.

[95] Vikelis M, Rapoport AM. Role of antiepileptic drugs as preventive agents for migraine. CNS Drugs 2010;24(1):21–33.

[96] Cai S, Hamiwka LD, Wirrell EC. Peri-ictal headache in children: prevalence and character. Pediatr Neurol 2008;39(2):91–6.

[97] Yankovsky AE, Andermann F, Mercho S, Dubeau F, Bernasconi A. Preictal headache in partial epilepsy. Neurology 2005;65(12):1979–81.

[98] Jacob J, Goadsby PJ, Duncan JS. Use of sumatriptan in post-ictal migraine headache. Neurology 1996;47(4):1104.

[99] Ogunyemi A, Adams D. Migraine-like symptoms triggered by occipital lobe seizures: response to sumatriptan. Can J Neurol Sci 1998;25(2):151–3.

[100] Lenaerts ME, Oommen KJ, Couch JR, Skaggs V. Can vagus nerve stimulation help migraine? Cephalalgia 2008 Apr;28(4):392–5.

[101] Caminero A, Manso-Calderón R. Links between headaches and epilepsy: current knowledge and terminology. Neurologia 2014;29(8):453–63.

[102] Panayiotopoulos CP. Visual phenomena and headache in occipital epilepsy: a review, a systematic study and differentiation from migraine. Epileptic Disord 1999;1(4):205–16.

[103] Sances G, Guaschino E, Perucca P, Allena M, Ghiotto N, Manni R. Migralepsy: a call for a revision of the definition. Epilepsia 2009;50(11):2487–96.

[104] Verrotti A, Coppola G, Di Fonzo A, Tozzi E, Spalice A, Aloisi P, Bruschi R, Iannetti P, Villa MP, Parisi P. Should "migralepsy" be considered an obsolete concept? A multicenter retrospective clinical/EEG study and review of the literature. Epilepsy Behav 2011;21(1):52–9.

[105] De Romanis F, Buzzi MG, Cerbo R, Feliciani M, Assenza S, Agnoli A. Migraine and epilepsy with infantile onset and electroencephalographic findings of occipital spike-wave complexes. Headache 1991;31(6):378–83.

[106] De Romanis F, Buzzi MG, Assenza S, Brusa L, Cerbo R. Basilar migraine with electroencephalographic findings of occipital spike-wave complexes: a long-term study in seven children. Cephalalgia 1993;13(3):192–6.

[107] Walker MC, Smith SJ, Sisodiya SM, Shorvon SD. Case of simple partial status epilepticus in occipital lobe epilepsy misdiagnosed as migraine: clinical, electrophysiological, and magnetic resonance imaging characteristics. Epilepsia 1995;36(12):1233–6.

[108] Ghofrani M, Mahvelati F, Tonekaboni H. Headache as a sole manifestation in nonconvulsive status epilepticus. J Child Neurol 2006;21(11):981–3.

[109] Parisi P, Kasteleijn-Nolst Trenité DG, Piccioli M, Pelliccia A, Luchetti A, Buttinelli C, Villa MP. A case with atypical childhood occipital epilepsy "Gastaut type": an ictal migraine manifestation with a good response to intravenous diazepam. Epilepsia 2007;48(11):2181–6.

[110] Perucca P, Terzaghi M, Manni R. Status epilepticus migrainosus: clinical, electrophysiologic, and imaging characteristics. Neurology 2010;75(4):373–4.

[111] Belcastro V, Striano P, Pierguidi L, Calabresi P, Tambasco N. Ictal epileptic headache mimicking status migrainosus: EEG and DWI-MRI findings. Headache 2011;51(1):160–2.

[112] Laplante P, Saint-Hilaire JM, Bouvier G. Headache as an epileptic manifestation. Neurology 1983;33(11):1493–5.

[113] Piccioli M, Parisi P, Tisei P, Villa MP, Buttinelli C, Kasteleijn-Nolst Trenité DG. Ictal headache and visual sensitivity. Cephalalgia 2009;29(2):194–203.

CHAPTER 11

Epilepsy, obstructive sleep apnea syndrome, and other sleep disorders

Matthew C. Walker
UCL Institute of Neurology, Queen Square, London, United Kingdom

Contents

1. Introduction

Sleep is a characteristic of almost all animals and is ubiquitous in mammals. It seems to serve critical physiological functions, and, in humans, plays an important role in cognition and mental health. Sleep in humans can be broadly divided into rapid eye movement (REM) sleep and non-REM (NREM) sleep states. These sleep states cycle over 90 min throughout the night. NREM can be subdivided into light (stages N1/N2) and deep (stage N3) sleep. As sleep progresses, deep sleep periods become shorter and are absent toward the morning, conversely, REM sleep time increases. Disruption of sleep includes not only increased arousals (decreased sleep efficiency) but also disruption to the normal sleep architecture.

Sleep disturbances are a common complaint of people with epilepsy and are about twice as common in focal epilepsy as in the general population [1, 2]. Approximately 30%–40% of people with focal epilepsy describe a disturbance of sleep in the past 6 months [1]. People with epilepsy with a sleep disturbance have significantly impaired quality of life compared to those without [1, 2]; indeed anxiety, depression, and sleep disturbance together have a greater effect than seizure control on quality of life in people with epilepsy [3]. Importantly, many of the sleep complaints are not appreciated by physicians. As with many comorbidities, physicians do not screen or even ask about sleep

The Comorbidities of Epilepsy
https://doi.org/10.1016/B978-0-12-814877-8.00011-8

Table 1 Epworth sleepiness scale

How likely are you to doze off or fall asleep in the following situations?

0 = Would never doze
1 = Slight chance of dozing
2 = Moderate chance of dozing
3 = High chance of dozing

(i) Sitting and reading
(ii) Watching TV
(iii) Sitting inactive in a public place
(iv) As a passenger in car for an hour without a break
(v) Lying down to rest in the afternoon when circumstances permit
(vi) Sitting and talking to someone
(vii) Sitting quietly after lunch without alcohol
(viii) In a car, while stopped for a few minutes in traffic

Score
    0–10 Normal daytime sleepiness
    11–12 Mild excessive daytime sleepiness
    13–15 Moderate excessive daytime sleepiness
    16–24 Severe excessive daytime sleepiness

complaints, focusing instead on seizures and seizure frequency. Interestingly, it is my experience that patients will often not volunteer sleep complaints without prompting. Given that most of the sleep complaints are treatable and that treatment will likely lead to an improvement in quality of life and also possibly even seizure control (discussed in this chapter), at the very least, a brief inquiry for sleep complaints/problems should be part of every consultation. There are numerous sleep screening tools and scales available [4]; however, it is often much easier and more appropriate just to ask if people have problems falling asleep or remaining asleep, do anything unusual during sleep and/or are sleepy during the day. If people complain of daytime somnolence, then the Epworth sleepiness scale should be carried out (see Table 1) [5]. Any assessment of sleepiness should also include an assessment for psychiatric illness.

The commonest complaints in people with epilepsy are excessive daytime sleepiness and psychiatric sleep disorders (i.e., having stress, anxiety, depression, gloomy thoughts, etc. at night) [1]. Indeed, the latter emphasizes the close links between sleep, psychiatric illness, and epilepsy. Both sleep disturbances and epilepsy are associated with psychiatric disease; psychiatric disease can worsen sleep complaints, and, conversely, sleep disturbance can worsen psychiatric disease [6]. This relationship is not, however, the whole story as, in one study, the frequency of psychiatric disturbances could not account for the high prevalence of sleep disturbances in people with focal epilepsy [1], and it is likely that seizures, epilepsy, and antiepileptic drugs also play an important part in disrupting and disturbing sleep. Indeed, unrecognized seizures at night can present as daytime somnolence and

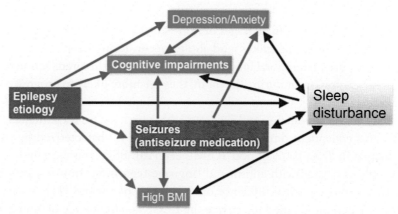

Fig. 1 Complex interaction between sleep epilepsy, seizures, and other comorbidities. Sleep often has a bidirectional association.

insomnia [7]. This complex interaction of epilepsy, sleep, and other comorbidities is important to bear in mind when developing treatment strategies (see Fig. 1).

Importantly, unrecognized sleep disorders, such as periodic limb movements and obstructive sleep apnea (OSA), are common causes of sleep disturbances in people with epilepsy [8]. This and the value of polysomnography in diagnosing these conditions suggest that there should be a lower threshold for polysomnography in people with epilepsy; however, it is my experience that investigations of sleep disorders in people with epilepsy remain underutilized.

This chapter will first discuss the impact of sleep on epilepsy and the impact of seizures and interictal abnormalities on sleep and sleep physiology. A discussion of some of the commoner associated sleep disorders will follow.

2. Seizures, interictal discharges, and sleep

People with epilepsy report sleep deprivation as one of the main factors that exacerbate their seizures [9], and there is good evidence in generalized epilepsies that sleep deprivation can precipitate seizures. Seizures also tend to occur more commonly at different points during the circadian cycle; the seizures in genetic generalized epilepsies tend to occur more commonly in the morning, shortly after waking, and, in certain epilepsies, seizures can occur exclusively during sleep. Approximately 20% of patients with epilepsy have predominantly and 6% have exclusively nocturnal seizures [10, 11]. Those with only nocturnal seizures have approximately a 2% risk of daytime seizures per year, and this risk is increased with more frequent seizures and antiepileptic drug withdrawal [12].

The predominant occurrence of seizures during sleep is a characteristic of specific epilepsy syndromes/types. Notably, clusters of nocturnal seizures are a typical feature of frontal lobe epilepsy [13]. When seizures occur at night, they tend to occur in non-REM rather than REM sleep, and in all stages of non-REM sleep [14]. Seizures in childhood epilepsy with centrotemporal spikes tend also to occur during sleep or drowsiness [15]. Although the seizures in temporal lobe epilepsy do not show this predilection for sleep, if temporal lobe seizures occur during the night, they are more likely to progress to bilateral tonic-clonic seizures [14]. Certain epileptic encephalopathies also show marked diurnal variation in seizure manifestation and electrographic activity. This is a particular feature of electrical status epilepticus during sleep (ESES), which is characterized by spike-and-wave discharges in 85%–100% of non-REM sleep [16]. ESES is important to recognize as it is strongly associated with autism and language regression. In many patients, there may also be a strong circadian influence on the timing of seizures [17]. Sleep and sleep deprivation are commonly used to activate the EEG. The frequency of interictal epileptiform discharges (IEDs) and pathological high-frequency oscillations increase with depth of non-REM sleep [18, 19].

Does the relationship hold in the other direction, that is, do seizures and interictal abnormalities have a direct impact on sleep and sleep phenomena? Patients with more frequents seizures are more likely to report sleep disturbance than control subjects or patients with less frequent seizures, regardless of epilepsy syndrome [20]. Patients with epilepsy have an increased number of awakenings during the night and a reduction or fragmentation of REM sleep [21]. Seizures and frequent interictal epileptiform activity can also change sleep architecture, causing more unstable sleep periods as measured with cyclic alternating patterns (a measure of the ultrastructure of sleep) in both partial and generalized epilepsies [22]. Moreover, polysomnography following complex partial seizures has revealed reduced amounts of REM sleep after seizures [21]. The effect was most pronounced after nocturnal seizures but was also significant after seizures occurring the previous day. Nocturnal seizures also reduced the amount of stage II and IV sleep and increased the amount of stage I sleep [21]. This was associated with reduced sleep efficiency and increased drowsiness the day after. Thus, not surprisingly, nocturnal seizures have an impact on sleep architecture, but, more surprisingly, daytime seizures can also have an impact.

Importantly, epilepsy can also have a detrimental effect on sleep physiology. There is increasing evidence that sleep is crucial for memory formation [23], and sleep spindles play an important role in this process. IEDs in the hippocampus during sleep induce aberrant hippocampal-cortical coupling and anomalous sleep spindles [24]. This has a deleterious effect on memory consolidation [24]. Thus, IEDs alter normal sleep physiology, which could compound cognitive problems in people with epilepsy.

Lastly, it is not just seizures and epileptiform discharges that can affect sleep but also antiepileptic drugs. Antiepileptic drugs can have a beneficial effect on sleep and sleep architecture by increasing sleep efficiency and deep sleep (observed with phenobarbital, gabapentin, and pregabalin) or can be associated with decreased deep sleep

Table 2 Effects of some antiepileptic drugs on sleep

	Sleep efficiency	1	2	SWS	REM	Arousal
CBZ	+				+	
ETH		+		−	+	
GBP				+	+	−
LTG			+	−	+	
LEV			+	−		
PB	+		+		−	−
PGB				+		−
PHT		+	+	−		
TGB	+			+	−	
TPM						
VPA		+	−			
ZS						

+ increase, − decreases, red is a negative effect and green is a positive effect.
CBZ, carbamazepine; ETH, ethosuximide; GBP, gabapentin; LTG, lamotrigine; LEV, levetiracetam; PB, phenobarbital; PGB, pregabalin; PHT, phenytoin; TGB, tiagabine; TPM, topiramate; VPA, valproate; ZS: zonisamide.

(e.g., lamotrigine, levetiracetam, phenytoin, and ethosuximide) and even insomnia (e.g., lamotrigine) [25, 26]. However, most antiepileptic drugs do not usually have a clinically relevant impact on sleep (Table 2).

3. Insomnia

Insomnia is defined as a report of problems with sleep initiation or maintenance when there are adequate opportunities and circumstances to sleep and that this problem with sleep has daytime consequences, which can consist of sleepiness or feelings of fatigue [27]. Typically, however, people with insomnia do not complain of falling asleep during the day. Chronic insomnia is when insomnia lasts 3 months or more and is occurring at least three times per week.

Insomnia is more common in people with epilepsy than the general population [28]. Insomnia (predominantly sleep maintenance) affects about 40%–70% of people with epilepsy [28], which is more than twice the prevalence in the general population. The most common insomnia symptom in people with epilepsy is sleep maintenance. Risk factors consist of poor seizure control, nocturnal seizures, treatment with lamotrigine and post-traumatic epilepsy [28]. As with all sleep disorders, the diagnosis of insomnia in epilepsy is critical because of the marked impact that it has on quality of life, and psychosocial health [29]. Insomnia is often underdiagnosed because of the low worth that health care professionals attribute to such a diagnosis despite its well-documented impact and high societal costs [30].

First-line treatment should consist of cognitive behavioral therapy of insomnia (CBT-I) [31], an effective version of which is also available online [32]. There are also many pharmacological approaches that can be used to treat insomnia [31], but these should be used second line. Those treatments with potential antiseizure effects, such as benzodiazepines, should be favored, or, if coexisting depression/anxiety is present, then antidepressant drugs should perhaps be the preferred options.

4. Sleep apnea

Complaints of snoring and even brief apneas are very common in the general population, and, in themselves, are not sufficient for a diagnosis of OSA. The criteria that have been used for the diagnosis of OSA have varied from study to study, resulting in different estimates of prevalence and severity. The present criteria require either signs/symptoms (such as sleepiness or fatigue) or associated medical or psychiatric disorders (such as hypertension, cognitive dysfunction, or mood disorders) along with five or more obstructive respiratory events per hour [27]. If there are no associated symptoms or disorders, then a frequency of obstructive events of >15 per hour satisfies the criteria. Obstructive respiratory events include apnea, hypopneas, and respiratory effort-related arousals.

Estimates of the prevalence of sleep apnea in epilepsy have varied depending on population studied and definitions used. Sleep apnea has been found to affect approximately 10% of people with epilepsy referred to an Italian epilepsy center [33]. The sleep apnea was moderate or severe in one third of patients (i.e., ~3%) [33]. Not surprisingly, the risks factors for developing sleep apnea were similar to those in the general population: older age, heavier weight, and male gender [33, 34]. In patients who are candidates for epilepsy surgery, the prevalence of sleep of apnea is even higher [35]. These prevalences are higher than would be expected in the general population in which 3%–7% of people have sleep apnea [34]. It is not, however, universally accepted that epilepsy increases the risk of sleep apnea [36]. Importantly, the new definitions of sleep apnea include symptoms of sleepiness or associated psychiatric disorder, and since the risk of these may be independently increased in people with epilepsy, there is a danger of overestimating the prevalence of sleep apnea syndrome in people with epilepsy.

Nevertheless, the higher prevalence of OSA that has been described in people with epilepsy may be due to a tendency of people with epilepsy to have a higher body mass index due to inactivity and medication [37]. Medication can also have a sedative and muscle-relaxant effect that could exacerbate sleep apnea. Even vagal nerve stimulation has been described to exacerbate OSA (possibly through an effect on the upper airway) [38, 39]. Indeed, the possible detrimental effects of epilepsy treatments on OSA need to be taken into account when starting such treatments, especially given the high prevalence of OSA in people with refractory epilepsy.

That seizures may also play a part in OSA is indicated by the observation that a specific risk factor for OSA in people with refractory epilepsy is seizures during sleep [35]. The underlying mechanism of this is not entirely clear. Seizures can disrupt sleep architecture, as previously discussed in this chapter, but this does not provide an adequate explanation of the increased incidence of sleep apnea. Seizures are also associated with central apnea and oxygen desaturation; this is more common with temporal lobe seizures and can persist after the seizure ends [40]. Moreover, central sleep apnea and severe hypoxemia may be the only sign of a seizure [41]. However, seizures (or even interictal activity) may have an impact on the control of the upper airway resistance, as remission of OSA as well as seizures have been reported in a patient following frontal lobe resection [42].

Overall, central, and OSA are almost certainly underrecognized in people with epilepsy [35, 40]. The diagnosis of these is, however, important from a range of different perspectives. Sleep apnea is associated with daytime somnolence, and increased risk of cardiovascular disease, cerebrovascular disease, early death [43] and psychiatric disease [44]. Sleep apnea can also affect cognitive performance and can exacerbate progressive memory decline [45], potentially providing a "double hit" in people with temporal lobe epilepsy. Sleep apnea may also increase the risk of sudden unexpected death in epilepsy (SUDEP) [46]. Although no direct association with SUDEP has been shown and the association described may largely be through shared risk factors (e.g., seizures at night), sleep apnea increases sympathetic tone and, along with respiratory compromise, could directly contribute to the risk of SUDEP.

Therefore, treatment of sleep apnea could potentially have an important impact on cognitive performance and depression, two common complaints of people with epilepsy, and may reduce the risk of SUDEP. OSA fragments sleep and reduces sleep efficiency, leading to relative sleep deprivation, which patients report to have a detrimental effect on seizure control [8]. OSA is associated with seizure exacerbation in the elderly [47], and several studies have demonstrated improved seizure control after treatment of concomitant OSA [8, 48, 49]. In a pilot study in patients with refractory epilepsy and OSA, a 50% or greater reduction in seizure frequency was observed in 28% of treated patients compared to 15% of patients in the sham group, although this did not reach significance [48]. Eighteen percent of patients receiving CPAP treatment became seizure free [48]. Therefore, the identification of those people with epilepsy who are at high risk of having OSA is critical. Although many of the screening tools for OSA are long, there are shorter and more easily administered screening tools such as the STOP-BANG questionnaire that could improve diagnosis (see Table 3) [50, 51].

5. Restless leg syndrome and periodic limb movements of sleep

Restless leg syndrome (RLS) is characterized by an irresistible urge to move the legs, which is often accompanied by discomfort that is worse in the evenings and at night and is relieved by movement [27]. Periodic limb movements of sleep (PLMS) are characterized by repetitive limb movements (usually legs but can involve shoulders, arms, and even head). Periodic limb movement disorder is defined by having >15 of these

Table 3 STOP-BANG questionnaire for obstructive sleep apnea

1. Snoring
Do you snore loudly (loud enough to be heard through closed doors or your bed-partner elbows you for snoring at night)?
2. Tired
Do you often feel tired, fatigued, or sleepy during the daytime?
3. Observed
Has anyone observed you stop breathing or choking/gasping during your sleep?
4. Blood Pressure
Do you have or are you being treated for high blood pressure?
5. Body mass index
BMI $>35\,kg/m^2$?
6. Age
Age over 50 yr old?
7. Neck circumference
Neck circumference $>40\,cm$ (16 in.)?
8. Gender
Gender male?
    Score
    3–4 yes = intermediate risk of OSA
    5–8 yes = high risk of OSA

movements per hour, and is highly prevalent in the general population with almost 30% affected [52]. Most people with RLS also have PLMS. However, the majority of people with PLMS do not have RLS. Both of these conditions can disrupt sleep. RLS may disrupt sleep by preventing people from getting to sleep or, if people rouse in the night, it may contribute to problems getting back to sleep. PLMS can disrupt sleep overnight and decrease sleep efficiency. It is my experience that PLMS can present as daytime somnolence even in situations where the person may not be aware of the limb movements overnight.

RLS in epilepsy is often unrecognized and is a major cause of sleepiness. There have been mixed findings on whether RLS is more prevalent in people with epilepsy, with most studies not finding a significant difference in prevalence from that of the general population [53–55]. However, RLS may be more prevalent in specific epilepsy types. In one study of patients undergoing presurgical assessment, RLS was found in 42% of people with right temporal lobe epilepsy, which was significantly greater than the 15% of people with left temporal lobe epilepsy and 10% of controls [56]. Almost half of the people with RLS had it as a reproducible prodrome prior to a seizure [56], raising the possibility that peri-ictal and possibly interictal activity may generate RLS symptoms.

The relationship of PLMS and epilepsy is even less clear. Again, they are almost certainly underrecognized and may contribute to sleepiness in people with epilepsy.

There may be some specific syndromes in which both epilepsy and periodic limb movements occur, such as Angelman syndrome [57], and certain drugs such as antidepressants may increase PLMS, but whether there is a direct relationship between the two conditions has yet to be established.

There are a variety of treatments that can be particularly successful in RLS and PLMS [58]. Treatment of low ferritin, dopamine agonists, gabapentin/pregabalin, clonazepam, and opioids are all common treatments. From the epilepsy perspective, therapies could be chosen that would treat both the epilepsy and the RLS/PLMS. However, pregabalin/gabapentin has also been described to exacerbate absences and myoclonic seizures and is contraindicated in certain epilepsy syndromes, such as juvenile myoclonic epilepsy [59].

6. Parasomnia

Parasomnias are abnormal behaviors, movements, or perceptions that intrude into sleep. These are divided into those that occur from non-REM sleep (usually deep sleep) and those that occur from REM sleep [60]. There are three main subtypes of non-REM parasomnia: sleep walking (somnambulism), night terrors (pavor nocturnis), and confusional arousal. Adults can often have more elaborate behaviors, including sleep eating and sexsomnia [60]. Although very common in childhood, they also occur frequently in adulthood with 3%–4% of the adult population having had a non-REM parasomnia in the last year [61]. Non-REM parasomnia can be considered dissociated arousal states in which there is arousal of only certain areas of the brain, while other areas, in particular the frontal cortex and associative areas, remain "asleep" [62, 63]. People are probably predisposed to having non-REM parasomnia but require an arousal (for whatever reason) to precipitate the events [61, 64]. These arousals may be due to external factors such as noise or internal factors such as psychiatric disease (e.g., depression, anxiety, obsessive-compulsive disorder), other sleep pathology (e.g., PLMS, OSA), drugs, alcohol, medication, and seizures [61, 64]. People are invariably confused during the event and are often amnesic for the event. They occur usually one to three times per night and mostly in the first third of the night (when deep sleep is occurring).

Because of the amnesia and the poor description of nocturnal events by bed partners, non-REM parasomnias and epilepsy can sometimes be difficult to distinguish. Moreover, there can be a strong association between the two. Over one third of patients with nocturnal frontal lobe epilepsy report a history of parasomnias [65]. This association may be due to misdiagnosis of nocturnal seizures as parasomnia or the precipitation of non-REM parasomnia by seizures. There may, however, be a more direct association. There is an increased frequency of arousal parasomnias in families with nocturnal frontal lobe epilepsy compared to the frequency in control subjects [66]. This raises the possibility that nocturnal frontal lobe epilepsy and parasomnias may share pathophysiological mechanisms, such as a shared disorder of the cholinergic arousal system. Moreover, similar features seen during nocturnal frontal lobe seizures and parasomnias further support the hypothesis that the disorders have a common pathogenic background [67, 68]. The activation of central pattern generators, neuronal networks activating specific sequences of basic motor responses, may occur in both nocturnal seizures and non-REM parasomnia through the release of the control of these generators by the neocortex. This results in common phenomenology, such as oroalimentary automatisms, pedaling, wanderings, and emotional responses (ictal fear, night terrors).

These shared features can result in difficulty distinguishing parasomnias and seizure when they are brief, even with the advantage of video-EEG telemetry (the EEG is often obscured by artifact). There are temporal and, semiological features that can be helpful (see Fig. 2). Stereotypy and dystonic posturing are commoner features in seizures, while yawning, waxing and waning, prolonged duration (>2 min), and indistinct offset are commoner in parasomnia [67]. However, particular difficulty can occur when a seizures leads to a non-REM parasomnia. Non-REM parasomnia responds to clonazepam and certain antidepressants [60]. However, it is important to identify and treat any specific triggers (e.g., OSA, PLMS, and seizures) [64].

REM sleep behavioral disorder in which there is loss of the normal REM atonia resulting in dream enactment occurs in elderly people with epilepsy [69]. REM sleep behavioral disorder in the elderly is commonly associated with neurodegenerative disorders (parkinsonism, multisystem atrophy, Lewy body dementia), and cerebrovascular disease syndrome [70]. It is, therefore, not clear whether the association with epilepsy is a coincidence, a shared underlying etiology, a direct impact of seizures on REM sleep, or an effect of REM sleep behavioral disorder on seizure threshold. The treatment of REM sleep behavioral disorder is usually clonazepam and/or melatonin.

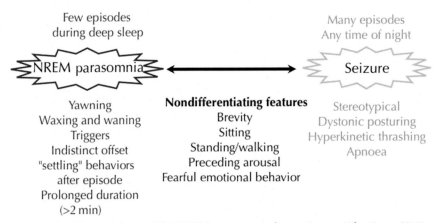

Fig. 2 Features that distinguish non-REM (NREM) parasomnia from seizures. (*After Derry CP, Harvey AS, Walker MC, Duncan JS, Berkovic SF. NREM arousal parasomnias and their distinction from nocturnal frontal lobe epilepsy: a video EEG analysis. Sleep 2009;32:1637–44).*

7. Conclusion

Sleep disturbances are common in epilepsy and may contribute to poor seizure control, deterioration in mental health and increased cognitive difficulties, along with other associations with poor sleep, such as increased risk of accident, increased body mass index, and increased risk of hypertension and cardiovascular disease. The mechanisms by which epilepsy disrupts sleep are not altogether clear. Seizures themselves may play a role but so may epilepsy-related comorbidities. In addition, epilepsy may increase the risk of sleep disorders.

Sleep disorders in people with epilepsy are underrecognized and because of their impact on health and quality of life, greater efforts should be made to diagnose and treat sleep disorders in epilepsy. There are well-established screening tools that can be used to identify patients at risk, but, more importantly, physicians should ask patients with epilepsy about their sleep and should have a low threshold for instigating investigations.

References

[1] Weerd AD, Haas SD, Otte A, Trenité DK-N, Erp GV, Cohen A, Kam MD, Gerven JV. Subjective sleep disturbance in patients with partial epilepsy: a questionnaire-based study on prevalence and impact on quality of life. Epilepsia 2004;45:1397–404. https://doi.org/10.1111/j.0013-9580.2004.46703.x.

[2] Xu X, Brandenburg NA, McDermott AM, Bazil CW. Sleep disturbances reported by refractory partial-onset epilepsy patients receiving Polytherapy. Epilepsia 2006;47:1176–83. https://doi.org/10.1111/j.1528-1167.2006.00591.x.

[3] Kwan P, Yu E, Leung H, Leon T, Mychaskiw MA. Association of subjective anxiety, depression, and sleep disturbance with quality-of-life ratings in adults with epilepsy. Epilepsia 2009;50:1059–66. https://doi.org/10.1111/j.1528-1167.2008.01938.x.

[4] Luyster FS, Choi J, Yeh C-H, Imes CC, Johansson AEE, Chasens ER. Screening and evaluation tools for sleep disorders in older adults. Appl Nurs Res 2015;28:334–40. https://doi.org/10.1016/j.apnr.2014.12.007.

[5] Johns MW. A new method for measuring daytime sleepiness: the Epworth sleepiness scale. Sleep 1991;14:540–5.

[6] Culebras A. Update on disorders of sleep and the sleep-wake cycle. Psychiatr Clin North Am 1992;15:467–89.

[7] Catarino CB, Ng G, Walker MC, Sander JW. A fitful night's sleep. Pract Neurol 2010;10:233–6. https://doi.org/10.1136/jnnp.2010.217810.

[8] Malow BA, Fromes GA, Aldrich MS. Usefulness of polysomnography in epilepsy patients. Neurology 1997;48:1389–94.

[9] Frucht MM, Quigg M, Schwaner C, Fountain NB. Distribution of seizure precipitants among epilepsy syndromes. Epilepsia 2000;41:1534–9. https://doi.org/10.1080/09583150020011717.

[10] Janz D. The grand Mai épilepsies and the sleeping-waking cycle. Epilepsia 1962;3:69–109. https://doi.org/10.1111/j.1528-1157.1962.tb05235.x.

[11] Gibberd FB, Bateson MC. Sleep epilepsy: its pattern and prognosis. Br Med J 1974;2:403–5.

[12] D'Alessandro R, Guarino M, Greco G, Bassein L. Emilia-Romagna study group on clinical and epidemiological problems in neurology. Risk of seizures while awake in pure sleep epilepsies: a prospective study. Neurology 2004;62:254–7.

[13] Manford M, Fish DR, Shorvon SD. An analysis of clinical seizure patterns and their localizing value in frontal and temporal lobe epilepsies. Brain 1996;119(Pt 1):17–40.

[14] Sinha S, Brady M, Scott CA, Walker MC. Do seizures in patients with refractory epilepsy vary between wakefulness and sleep? J Neurol Neurosurg Psychiatry 2006;77:1076–8. https://doi.org/10.1136/jnnp.2006.088385.

[15] Loiseau P, Beaussart M. The seizures of benign childhood epilepsy with Rolandic paroxysmal discharges. Epilepsia 1973;14:381–9.

[16] Yan Liu X, Wong V. Spectrum of epileptic syndromes with electrical status epilepticus during sleep in children. Pediatr Neurol 2000;22:371–9.

[17] Karoly PJ, Ung H, Grayden DB, Kuhlmann L, Leyde K, Cook MJ, Freestone DR. The circadian profile of epilepsy improves seizure forecasting. Brain 2017;140:2169–82. https://doi.org/10.1093/brain/awx173.

[18] Bagshaw AP, Jacobs J, LeVan P, Dubeau F, Gotman J. Effect of sleep stage on interictal high-frequency oscillations recorded from depth macroelectrodes in patients with focal epilepsy. Epilepsia 2009;50:617–28. https://doi.org/10.1111/j.1528-1167.2008.01784.x.

[19] Sammaritano M, Gigli GL, Gotman J. Interictal spiking during wakefulness and sleep and the localization of foci in temporal lobe epilepsy. Neurology 1991;41:290–7.

[20] Hoeppner JB, Garron DC, Cartwright RD. Self-reported sleep disorder symptoms in epilepsy. Epilepsia 1984;25:434–7.

[21] Bazil CW, Castro LH, Walczak TS. Reduction of rapid eye movement sleep by diurnal and nocturnal seizures in temporal lobe epilepsy. Arch Neurol 2000;57:363–8.

[22] Terzano MG, Parrino L, Anelli S, Boselli M, Clemens B. Effects of generalized interictal EEG discharges on sleep stability: assessment by means of cyclic alternating pattern. Epilepsia 1992;33:317–26.

[23] Abel T, Havekes R, Saletin JM, Walker MP. Sleep, plasticity and memory from molecules to whole-brain networks. Curr Biol 2013;23:R774–88. https://doi.org/10.1016/j.cub.2013.07.025.

[24] Gelinas JN, Khodagholy D, Thesen T, Devinsky O, Buzsáki G. Interictal epileptiform discharges induce hippocampal-cortical coupling in temporal lobe epilepsy. Nat Med 2016;22:641–8. https://doi.org/10.1038/nm.4084.

[25] Foldvary-Schaefer N. Sleep complaints and epilepsy: the role of seizures, antiepileptic drugs and sleep disorders. J Clin Neurophysiol 2002;19:514–21.

[26] Jain SV, Glauser TA. Effects of epilepsy treatments on sleep architecture and daytime sleepiness: an evidence-based review of objective sleep metrics. Epilepsia 2014;55:26–37. https://doi.org/10.1111/epi.12478.

[27] Sateia MJ. International classification of sleep disorders-third edition. CHEST 2014;146:1387–94. https://doi.org/10.1378/chest.14-0970.

[28] Macêdo PJOM, de OPS, Foldvary-Schaefer N, Gomes M da M. Insomnia in people with epilepsy: a review of insomnia prevalence, risk factors and associations with epilepsy-related factors. Epilepsy Res 2017;135:158–67. https://doi.org/10.1016/j.eplepsyres.2017.05.014.

[29] Zammit GK, Weiner J, Damato N, Sillup GP, McMillan CA. Quality of life in people with insomnia. Sleep 1999;22(Suppl 2):S379–85.

[30] Buysse DJ. Insomnia. JAMA 2013;309:706–16. https://doi.org/10.1001/jama.2013.193.

[31] Frase L, Nissen C, Riemann D, Spiegelhalder K. Making sleep easier: pharmacological interventions for insomnia. Expert Opin Pharmacother 2018;19:1465–73. https://doi.org/10.1080/14656566.2018.1511705.

[32] Espie CA, Emsley R, Kyle SD, Gordon C, Drake CL, Siriwardena AN, Cape J, Ong JC, Sheaves B, Foster R, Freeman D, Costa-Font J, Marsden A, Luik AI. Effect of digital cognitive behavioral therapy for insomnia on health, psychological well-being, and sleep-related quality of life: a randomized clinical trial. JAMA Psychiat 2018;https://doi.org/10.1001/jamapsychiatry.2018.2745.

[33] Manni R, Terzaghi M, Arbasino C, Sartori I, Galimberti CA, Tartara A. Obstructive sleep apnea in a clinical series of adult epilepsy patients: frequency and features of the comorbidity. Epilepsia 2003;44:836–40.

[34] Punjabi NM. The epidemiology of adult obstructive sleep apnea. Proc Am Thorac Soc 2008;5:136–43. https://doi.org/10.1513/pats.200709-155MG.

[35] Malow BA, Levy K, Maturen K, Bowes R. Obstructive sleep apnea is common in medically refractory epilepsy patients. Neurology 2000;55:1002–7.

[36] Popkirov S, Stone J, Derry CP. Abnormal sleep in patients with epileptic or dissociative (non-epileptic) seizures: a polysomnography study. Eur J Neurol 2018;https://doi.org/10.1111/ene.13798.

[37] Ben-Menachem E. Weight issues for people with epilepsy—a review. Epilepsia 2007;48(Suppl 9):42–5. https://doi.org/10.1111/j.1528-1167.2007.01402.x.

[38] Malow BA, Edwards J, Marzec M, Sagher O, Fromes G. Effects of vagus nerve stimulation on respiration during sleep: a pilot study. Neurology 2000;55:1450–4.

[39] Ebben MR, Sethi NK, Conte M, Pollak CP, Labar D. Vagus nerve stimulation, sleep apnea, and CPAP titration. J Clin Sleep Med 2008;4:471–3.

[40] Lacuey N, Zonjy B, Hampson JP, Rani MRS, Zaremba A, Sainju RK, Gehlbach BK, Schuele S, Friedman D, Devinsky O, Nei M, Harper RM, Allen L, Diehl B, Millichap JJ, Bateman L, Granner MA, Dragon DN, Richerson GB, Lhatoo SD. The incidence and significance of periictal apnea in epileptic seizures. Epilepsia 2018;59:573–82. https://doi.org/10.1111/epi.14006.

[41] Maglajlija V, Walker MC, Kovac S. Severe ictal hypoxemia following focal, subclinical temporal electrographic scalp seizure activity. Epilepsy Behav 2012;24:143–5. https://doi.org/10.1016/j.yebeh.2012.03.019.

[42] Foldvary-Schaefer N, Stephenson L, Bingaman W. Resolution of obstructive sleep apnea with epilepsy surgery? Expanding the relationship between sleep and epilepsy. Epilepsia 2008;49:1457–9. https://doi.org/10.1111/j.1528-1167.2008.01677.x.

[43] Assessment SC on HT. n.d. Obstructive sleep Apnoea syndrome: a systematic literature review.

[44] Sharafkhaneh A, Giray N, Richardson P, Young T, Hirshkowitz M. Association of psychiatric disorders and sleep apnea in a large cohort. Sleep 2005;28:1405–11.

[45] Kerner NA, Roose SP, Pelton GH, Ciarleglio A, Scodes J, Lentz C, Sneed JR, Devanand DP. Association of obstructive sleep apnea with episodic memory and cerebral microvascular pathology: a preliminary study. Am J Geriatr Psychiatry 2017;25:316–25. https://doi.org/10.1016/j.jagp.2016.11.009.

[46] McCarter AR, Timm PC, Shepard PW, Sandness DJ, Luu T, McCarter SJ, Dueffert L, Dresow M, Feemster JC, Cascino GD, So EL, Worrell GA, Britton JR, Sherif A, Jaliparthy K, Chahal AA, Somers VK, Louis EKS. Obstructive sleep apnea in refractory epilepsy: a pilot study investigating frequency, clinical features, and association with risk of sudden unexpected death in epilepsy. Epilepsia 2018;59:1973–81. https://doi.org/10.1111/epi.14548.

[47] Chihorek AM, Abou-Khalil B, Malow BA. Obstructive sleep apnea is associated with seizure occurrence in older adults with epilepsy. Neurology 2007;69:1823–7. https://doi.org/10.1212/01.wnl.0000279334.78298.d5.

[48] Malow BA, Foldvary-Schaefer N, Vaughn BV, Selwa LM, Chervin RD, Weatherwax KJ, Wang L, Song Y. Treating obstructive sleep apnea in adults with epilepsy: a randomized pilot trial. Neurology 2008;71:572–7. https://doi.org/10.1212/01.wnl.0000323927.13250.54.

[49] Hollinger P, Khatami R, Gugger M, Hess CW, Bassetti CL. Epilepsy and obstructive sleep apnea. Eur Neurol 2006;55:74–9. https://doi.org/10.1159/000092306.

[50] Sharma A, Molano J, Moseley BD. The STOP-BANG questionnaire improves the detection of epilepsy patients at risk for obstructive sleep apnea. Epilepsy Res 2017;129:37–40. https://doi.org/10.1016/j.eplepsyres.2016.11.009.

[51] Chung F, Yegneswaran B, Liao P, Chung SA, Vairavanathan S, Islam S, Khajehdehi A, Shapiro CM. STOP questionnaire: a tool to screen patients for obstructive sleep apnea. Anesthesiology 2008;108:812–21. https://doi.org/10.1097/ALN.0b013e31816d83e4.

[52] Haba-Rubio J, Marti-Soler H, Marques-Vidal P, Tobback N, Andries D, Preisig M, Waeber G, Vollenweider P, Kutalik Z, Tafti M, Heinzer R. Prevalence and determinants of periodic limb movements in the general population. Ann Neurol 2016;79:464–74. https://doi.org/10.1002/ana.24593.

[53] Öztürk İ, Aslan K, Bozdemir H, Foldvary-Schaefer N. Frequency of restless legs syndrome in adults with epilepsy in Turkey. Epilepsy Behav 2016;57:192–5. https://doi.org/10.1016/j.yebeh.2016.02.013.

[54] Khatami R, Zutter D, Siegel A, Mathis J, Donati F, Bassetti CL. Sleep-wake habits and disorders in a series of 100 adult epilepsy patients—a prospective study. Seizure 2006;15:299–306. https://doi.org/10.1016/j.seizure.2006.02.018.

[55] Malow BA, Bowes RJ, Lin X. Predictors of sleepiness in epilepsy patients. Sleep 1997;20:1105–10. https://doi.org/10.1093/sleep/20.12.1105.

[56] Geyer JD, Geyer EE, Fetterman Z, Carney PR. Epilepsy and restless legs syndrome. Epilepsy Behav 2017;68:41–4. https://doi.org/10.1016/j.yebeh.2016.12.010.

[57] Miano S, Bruni O, Elia M, Musumeci SA, Verrillo E, Ferri R. Sleep breathing and periodic leg movement pattern in Angelman syndrome: a polysomnographic study. Clin Neurophysiol 2005;116:2685–92. https://doi.org/10.1016/j.clinph.2005.08.005.

[58] Wijemanne S, Ondo W. Restless legs syndrome: clinical features, diagnosis and a practical approach to management. Pract Neurol 2017;17:444–52. https://doi.org/10.1136/practneurol-2017-001762.

[59] Mantoan L, Walker M. Treatment options in juvenile myoclonic epilepsy. Curr Treat Options Neurol 2011;13:355–70. https://doi.org/10.1007/s11940-011-0131-z.

[60] Mahowald MW, Bornemann MC, Schenck CH. Parasomnias. Semin Neurol 2004;24:283–92. https://doi.org/10.1055/s-2004-835064.

[61] Ohayon MM, Mahowald MW, Dauvilliers Y, Krystal AD, Léger D. Prevalence and comorbidity of nocturnal wandering in the US adult general population. Neurology 2012;78:1583–9. https://doi.org/10.1212/WNL.0b013e3182563be5.

[62] Terzaghi M, Sartori I, Tassi L, Didato G, Rustioni V, LoRusso G, Manni R, Nobili L. Evidence of dissociated arousal states during NREM Parasomnia from an Intracerebral neurophysiological study. Sleep 2009;32:409–12.

[63] Bassetti C, Vella S, Donati F, Wielepp P, Weder B. SPECT during sleepwalking. Lancet 2000;356:484–5. https://doi.org/10.1016/S0140-6736(00)02561-7.

[64] Fois C, Wright M-AS, Sechi G, Walker MC, Eriksson SH. The utility of polysomnography for the diagnosis of NREM parasomnias: an observational study over 4 years of clinical practice. J Neurol 2015;262:385–93. https://doi.org/10.1007/s00415-014-7578-2.

[65] Provini F, Plazzi G, Tinuper P, Vandi S, Lugaresi E, Montagna P. Nocturnal frontal lobe epilepsy a clinical and polygraphic overview of 100 consecutive cases. Brain 1999;122:1017–31. https://doi.org/10.1093/brain/122.6.1017.

[66] Bisulli F, Vignatelli L, Naldi I, Licchetta L, Provini F, Plazzi G, Di Vito L, Ferioli S, Montagna P, Tinuper P. Increased frequency of arousal parasomnias in families with nocturnal frontal lobe epilepsy: a common mechanism? Epilepsia 2010;51:1852–60. https://doi.org/10.1111/j.1528-1167.2010.02581.x.

[67] Derry CP, Harvey AS, Walker MC, Duncan JS, Berkovic SF. NREM arousal parasomnias and their distinction from nocturnal frontal lobe epilepsy: a video EEG analysis. Sleep 2009;32:1637–44.

[68] Tassinari CA, Rubboli G, Gardella E, Cantalupo G, Calandra-Buonaura G, Vedovello M, Alessandria M, Gandini G, Cinotti S, Zamponi N, Meletti S. Central pattern generators for a common semiology in fronto-limbic seizures and in parasomnias. A neuroethologic approach. Neurol Sci 2005;26(Suppl 3):s225–32. https://doi.org/10.1007/s10072-005-0492-8.

[69] Manni R, Terzaghi M, Zambrelli E. REM sleep behaviour disorder in elderly subjects with epilepsy: frequency and clinical aspects of the comorbidity. Epilepsy Res 2007;77:128–33. https://doi.org/10.1016/j.eplepsyres.2007.09.007.

[70] Postuma RB, Gagnon J-F, Montplaisir J. Rapid eye movement sleep behavior disorder as a biomarker for neurodegeneration: the past 10 years. Sleep Med 2013;14:763–7. https://doi.org/10.1016/j.sleep.2012.09.001.

CHAPTER 12

Epilepsy and other neurological disorders

Gaetano Zaccara*, Filippo Sean Giorgi†, Fabio Giovannelli‡
*Regional Health Agency of Tuscany, Florence, Italy
†Department of Clinical and Experimental Medicine, Section of Neurology, University of Pisa and Pisa University Hospital, Pisa, Italy
‡Department of Neuroscience, Psychology, Pharmacology and Child Health (NEUROFARBA), University of Florence, Firenze, Italy

Contents

Abbreviations

AEDs	antiepileptic drug
AD	Alzheimer's disease
ARV	antiretroviral
CNS	central nervous system
CFS	cerebrospinal fluid
DRESS	drug-related rash with eosinophilia and systemic symptoms

The Comorbidities of Epilepsy
https://doi.org/10.1016/B978-0-12-814877-8.00012-X

FTD   frontotemporal lobe degeneration
HD   Huntington's disease
LBD   Lewy body disease
MRI   magnetic resonance imaging
MCI   mild cognitive impairment
PD   Parkinson's disease
PET   positron emission tomography
VaD   vascular dementia

1. Introduction

Comorbidity is a greater than coincidental association of two condition in the same individual [1]. In the case of neurologic conditions that occur in association with epilepsy, these may be a cause or a consequence of epilepsy and may precede, co-occur, or follow the diagnosis of epilepsy [2].

There are several explanations for the coexistence of epilepsy with other neurological diseases: (1) the association between epilepsy and the comorbid condition is a result of a bias, and there is not a true causal relationship (chance and artifactual comorbidity); (2) comorbid condition causes epilepsy via direct or indirect causal mechanisms (causative mechanisms); (3) mechanism of association is similar to the causative model, but the temporal sequence is reversed (epilepsy may start before the comorbid condition); (4) a confounding factor is a common cause both for epilepsy and the comorbid condition (shared risk factors); and (5) the two conditions can each cause the other (bidirectional effects) [3].

Recently, it has been suggested that in several conditions comorbid with epilepsy, a systemic dysfunction is in some way responsible for both diseases [4]. As a consequence of this hypothesis, a correct treatment of epilepsy should also include treatment of those dysfunctions that also cause comorbidities.

In this chapter, the most important neurological diseases comorbid with epilepsy are described.

2. Cerebrovascular diseases

In elderly people, cerebrovascular diseases constitute the most frequent cause of epilepsy [2], and several data indicate a complex relationship between these two diseases. Two, not mutually excluding, hypotheses have been proposed: both diseases are caused by a common factor and/or they are each a risk factor of the other (bidirectional effect).

According to the time of their appearance after a stroke, there are two different types of seizures with very different pathophysiological mechanisms and prognosis. Early seizures, also called acute symptomatic seizures, occur within 7 days after stroke onset and are consequent to local metabolic disturbances associated with acute infarction. Late seizures, also called remote symptomatic or unprovoked seizures [3], occur after a silent period, which usually varies from a few months to several years [5], and originate from some injured brain areas where neuronal networks, due to structural modifications, have acquired the new property of becoming persistently hyperexcitable [6].

These different kinds of seizures are associated with different risks of seizure recurrence and require different treatment strategies.

Overall, incidence of acute seizures in different studies varies between 3% and 13% [7] and is probably underestimated [8]. In addition, they are highly dependent on the characteristics of stroke with their prevalence being 2.4% and 4.8% after ischemic or hemorrhagic stroke, respectively. Among ischemic strokes, cardioembolic strokes have a higher risk compared to those associated with small or large vessel disease. The highest risk of early seizures is reported in patients with subarachnoid hemorrhage and venous cerebral thrombosis [7]. In a meta-analysis, intracerebral hemorrhage, cerebral infarction with hemorrhagic transformation, stroke severity, and alcoholism resulted significantly associated with a greater probability of early seizure occurrence [9].

Status epilepticus can be a relatively frequent acute complication of a stroke and is often underdiagnosed, although a closer EEG and clinical monitoring of such patients improve diagnosis. In a retrospective population study of patients admitted for intracerebral hemorrhage, it has been found that prevalence of diagnosis of status epilepticus increased from 1999 to 2011 [10].

As far as late or unprovoked poststroke seizures are concerned, it has been shown that cumulative risk of their appearance, in a large population-based study conducted over a period of 12 years following vascular episode, was 1.5% at 3 months, 3.5% at 1 year, 9% at 5 years, and 12.4% at 10 years [11]. Although risk of late seizures was also influenced by age, being higher in patients below 65 years of age, its main determinant was constituted by the anatomical characteristics of cerebral damage. Total anterior circulation infarct was associated with the greatest risk of poststroke epilepsy, while a progressive lower risk was observed with subarachnoid hemorrhage, primary intracerebral hemorrhage, partial anterior circulation infarct, lacunar infarct, and posterior circulation infarct. Two metaanalyses indicate that risk factors associated with late seizures following a stroke are cortical involvement and stroke severity [9, 12]. Small vessel diseases that may lead to deep infarcts and leukoaraiosis (white matter rarefaction) are also associated with an increased risk of late seizures [13].

While all these data show that vascular diseases are a strong risk factor for epilepsy, epilepsy may be a risk factor for stroke. In fact, it has been shown that epilepsy that starts in the elderly [14] as well as in adulthood [15] is associated with higher incidence of stroke. The explanation for these findings may be that both epilepsy and cerebrovascular diseases share similar risk factors. In fact, heart disease, hypertension, hyperlipidemia, diabetes, smoking, and lower rates of exercise [14] are known risk factors both for stroke and epilepsy. In addition, epilepsy seems to predispose to venous thromboembolism, which is three times more frequent in patients with epilepsy than that among people with migraine [16].

2.1 Treatment of seizures in cerebrovascular disorders

Several evidences indicate that, in patients with cerebrovascular diseases, antiepileptic drug (AED) treatment, mainly with first-generation AEDs, may be associated with a poor rehabilitation outcome and may also worsen progression of atherosclerosis. Typical dose-dependent motor or cognitive adverse effects of several AEDs are more frequently observed in patients with stroke. In addition, early generation AEDs cause subtle metabolic alterations, which may constitute a predisposing factor for atherosclerosis [17]. These agents may have negative effects on lipids and other metabolic parameters associated with a higher risk of cerebrovascular diseases. Cholesterol (HDL, LDL, and VLDL), triglycerides, and lipoproteins can be affected by carbamazepine and phenobarbital [17]. Homocysteine concentration, an independent risk factor for atherosclerosis, as a consequence of enzyme induction, has been found increased in adult epileptic patients treated with phenytoin or phenobarbital.

A symptomatic carbamazepine or oxcarbazepine-induced hyponatremia is more frequent in patients with vascular diseases who are often elderly and receiving several other sodium level-decreasing drugs. Finally, some AEDs (especially gabapentin, pregabalin, vigabatrin, and valproate) may cause an increase in body weight, which is an important risk factor for cardiovascular and cerebrovascular diseases [17].

A further negative effect of several first-generation AEDs in patients with cerebrovascular diseases is the induction of metabolism of many drugs used for treatment of atherosclerosis and prevention of thrombosis [18, 19]. For example, new anticoagulants apixaban, dabigatran, edoxaban, and rivaroxaban may be ineffective or less effective when associated with enzyme-inducing drugs with severe possible consequences, such as cardiac emboli and stroke.

In Table 1, most relevant drug interactions between AEDs and drugs pertaining to the ATC coding system as class B (blood and blood-forming organs) and class C (cardiovascular system) are reported.

The effect of cardio and cerebrovascular agents on epilepsy should also be considered. Recently, concerns have been raised that treatment of acute stroke with recombinant tissue plasminogen activator, which is the only approved thrombolytic agent, might increase the risk of seizures (including early and late seizures). However, in a systematic review of 792 patients with ischemic stroke who received this treatment, rates of seizures were similar in patients treated or not treated with this agent [20].

Based on all these considerations, the decision of starting or not starting a treatment for seizures is of strategic importance. Since there is no clinical evidence of an antiepileptogenic effect for any AED, all guidelines do not recommend primary prevention of

Table 1 Relevant drug interactions between agents pertaining to ATC code B (blood and blood-forming organs) and C (cardiovascular system) and antiepileptic drugs

Kind of interaction	Drug-altering metabolism	Drug whose metabolism is altered
Induction of metabolism of drugs coded B (blood and blood-forming organs agents) in the ATC classification system	Phenobarbital, carbamazepine, phenytoin	Apixaban, bemiparin, bivalirudin, clopidogrel, dabigatran, dalteparin, edoxaban, enoxaparin, heparin, rivaroxaban, ticagrelor, warfarin
Induction of metabolism of drugs coded C in the ATC (cardiovasvular agents)	Phenobarbital, carbamazepine, phenytoin	Amiodarone, amlodipine, atenolol, atorvastatina, bisoprolol, bosentan, digoxin, diltiazem, disopyramide, dopamine, dronedarone, eplerenone, felodipine, fluvastatine, isradipine, ivabradine, labetalol, lacidipine, lercanidipine, losartan, lovastatine, macitentan, metoprolol, mexiletine, nebivolol, nicardipine, nifedipine, nimodipine, nisoldipine, nitrendipine, propafenone, ranolazine, rosuvastatine, simvastatine, tolvaptan, valsartan, verapamil
Inhibition of the serum concentration of AEDs	Diltiazem, ticlopidine, verapamil	Carbamazepine, phenytoin
Induction of P-gp	Levetiracetam	Dabigatran, apixaban, edoxaban, rivaroxaban

This list should not be regarded as exhaustive. Only those interactions considered clinically significant are reported.
From References Zaccara G, Perucca E. Interactions between antiepileptic drugs, and between antiepileptic drugs and other drugs. Epileptic Disord 2014;16(4):409–31 and Medscape. Available from: https://reference.medscape.com/drug-interactionchecker [last accessed 18 April 2018].

epilepsy in patients with stroke or other vascular diseases [21, 22]. Interestingly, experimental studies show that several drugs used for the treatment of vascular diseases might have the property to interfere with the process of epileptogenesis. Statins for example, have been found to reduce the risk of late seizures due to antiinflammatory effects and prevention of blood-brain barrier injury [23].

In a few cases, although high-quality evidence for routine anticonvulsant use in subarachnoid hemorrhage or cerebral venous thrombosis is lacking, short-term prophylactic antiepileptic therapy in the immediate posthemorrhagic period is sometimes used [24, 25], based on the argument that seizures or status epilepticus in such acutely ill patients could lead to additional injury [21, 26].

After a seizure, drug treatment may be indicated for prevention of further seizures, although different treatment strategies should be planned for early or late seizures.

In the case of early seizures, a treatment can be administered to reduce the risk of seizure relapse in the short term and should be discontinued shortly [27] while, after a late seizure, a long-term antiepileptic treatment is required [6].

Patient with vascular diseases are often elderly and with typical age-related pharmacokinetic changes (reduction in hepatic and renal clearance and lower protein binding) that may lead to higher brain concentration and toxicity of some drugs. Hence, in those cases in which AED treatment is appropriate, low starting doses and a slow titration should be adopted.

As large clinical studies have not yet been carried out in this special population of patients, there is no consensus regarding the most appropriate AED that should be used as a first-line drug. However, old generation AEDs have an unfavorable kinetic profile, a potential harmful impact on motor and cognitive functions and negative effects on progression of atherosclerosis. Levetiracetam, lamotrigine, lacosamide, and also topiramate and zonisamide should have a similar efficacy but should be safer than traditional AEDs and should be preferred.

3. Infections of the central nervous system

Central nervous system (CNS) infections and infestations, particularly in resource-poor settings, are among the most common preventable risk factors for acute seizures and symptomatic epilepsy worldwide [28]. They include viral, bacterial, protozoan, fungal, and prion disease (Creutzfeldt-Jakob).

Seizures may occur during all these acute CNS infections, may be the only presenting symptom of infection such as neurocysticercosis, or may appear after a period of latency.

Even in this case, similarly to vascular diseases, early seizures, which may occur in up to 30% of CNS infections soon after the time of a systemic insult, are not considered spontaneous seizures and are thought to be mechanistically different from consequential chronic epilepsy. Early seizures may lead to status epilepticus, which in this case has often a worse prognosis than that due to other etiologies.

Spontaneous recurrent late seizures result from neuronal loss and gliosis, molecular and structural reorganization, and epigenetic reprogramming, which are related to the infectious agent, the severity of brain injury, age, and several other factors. Risk of these late seizures in developed countries is between 6.8% and 8.3%, while it is higher in resource-poor settings [29].

Some antimicrobials may have a proconvulsant effect. In the general population, evidence for the association between antibiotic drugs and seizures as adverse events is low to very low [30]. However, in patients with CNS infections, this risk may be much higher, even though, in such cases, it is almost impossible to establish a cause-effect relationship because of the concomitant effect of the concurrent disease [31]. Antimicrobials considered most often proconvulsant are: antimalarials, carbapenems, cephalosporins, unsubstituted penicillins, and ciprofloxacin in combination. Also, isoniazid overdose has been associated with seizures [18, 30]. Therefore, some precautions should be taken for the selection of the appropriate antimicrobial in patients with CNS infections. A drug with the lowest epileptogenic potential should be selected, dosage should be adjusted according to the degree of possible renal impairment for drugs eliminated by kidneys, and in patients with special predispositions, monitoring of serum antimicrobial levels may be advocated. It should be noted that seizures observed during cephalosporin treatment are often reported to be nonconvulsive, and EEG may be necessary for diagnosis of such complications [30].

There are also interactions between AEDs and infectious diseases. In patients with these diseases, some idiosyncratic adverse drug reactions are more frequently observed. There is evidence for a complex relationship between viral infections and a serious adverse drug reaction, namely drug-related rash with eosinophilia and systemic symptoms (DRESS), which has been associated with aromatic AEDs (phenytoin, phenobarbital, carbamazepine, lamotrigine, oxcarbazepine, eslicarbazepine) [32]. In fact, in the serum of patients with AED-induced DRESS, 2–3 weeks after the onset of the idiosyncratic reaction, a rise has been observed in human herpes virus (HHV)-6 DNA levels, and it has been suggested that this virus might play a pathogenic role in this condition. Reactivation of HHV-7, cytomegalovirus, and/or Epstein-Barr virus may also play a role in such adverse drug reactions [33].

On the other hand, several AEDs have anti-inflammatory properties and, for this reason, might affect immune defense. Recently, in a metaanalysis of 127 randomized clinical trials with 16 AEDs, a mild increased risk of infection has been reported for topiramate and for levetiracetam and brivaracetam when pooled together [34]. It may be reasonable to hypothesize that these AEDs might have a weak facilitating effect for infectious diseases.

Finally, drug interactions between antimicrobials and AEDs are frequent. For example, serum concentration of itraconazole can be reduced more than tenfold by enzyme-inducing AEDs. Macrolide antibiotics increase drug levels of carbamazepine with

Table 2 Most relevant drug interactions between ATC drugs coded J (antiinfectives for systemic use) and antiepileptic dugs

	Drugs that alter drug levels	Drug whose metabolism is altered
Antimicrobials whose metabolism can be stimulated by AEDs	Enzyme-inducing AEDs, most notably carbamazepine, phenytoin, phenobarbital, and primidone	Albendazole, chloramphenicol, doxycycline, efavirenz, indinavir, itraconazole, lopinavir, metronidazole, nevirapine, posiconazole, praziquantel, rifampicin, ritonavir, saquinavir, voriconazole
Antimicrobials that may increase the serum concentration of AEDs	Clarithromycin, erythromycin, fluconazole, isoniazid, itraconazole, ketoconazole, metronidazole, ritonavir, troleandomycin, voriconazole	Carbamazepine
	Chloramphenicol, fluconazole, isoniazid, miconazole, sulfaphenazole	Phenytoin
	Chloramphenicol	Phenobarbital
	Erythromycin, isoniazid	Valproate
	Ketoconazole	Clobazam
	Clarithromycin	Oxcarbazepine
Antimicrobials that may reduce serum levels of AEDs	Imipenem, meropenem, ertapenem, doripenem	Valproic acid
	Rifampicin	Lamotrigine

See legend of Table 1.

consequent toxicity. Meropenem or other carbapenem antibiotics induce metabolism of valproate with consequent loss of efficacy and withdrawal seizures [18].

In Table 2, most relevant drug interactions between AEDs and antimicrobials are reported.

3.1 Neurological complications of HIV infection

HIV prevalence is increasing worldwide mostly because people on antiretroviral therapy are living longer, although new infections are decreasing [35]. Evidence of neurologic involvement has been observed as early as 3 months after HIV infection and extends across all the course of the disease. Prevalence of HIV-associated neurocognitive disorder increases with disease progression and includes asymptomatic neurocognitive impairment, mild neurocognitive disorder, and an advanced form of HIV-associated dementia. Seizures are frequently observed in people affected by this infective disease and may be consequent to a variety of mechanisms, including vulnerability to CNS opportunistic infections, neuronal damage induced by HIV replication within the CNS, and metabolic disturbances [35]. However, after the introduction of a combination of antiretroviral therapy for treatment of the disease, their prevalence has declined from 17% to 6%, which testify that seizures are generally a consequence of the progression of the disease [35].

Also in the case of HIV infection, as in other viral diseases, aromatic AEDs are associated with a higher risk of immunomediated adverse reaction when administrated in such patients [33]. For example, skin rash caused by phenytoin is more common in HIV-infected patients even though such patients are typically anergic and expected to be less prone to immune-mediated adverse reactions. For this reason, special attention should be paid when using aromatic AEDs in these patients. It has also been suggested that valproate may increase viral replication in HIV-infected patients [36].

Since effective HIV treatment requires lifelong treatment with at least three antiretroviral (ARV) drugs, possible interactions between these agents and coadministered AEDs are very important. It should be considered that in these patients, AEDs are also used for conditions other than epilepsy, such as painful neuropathies and psychiatric conditions.

Interactions of greatest concern relate to the P450 system enzyme induction effects of the old-generation AEDs. Phenobarbital, carbamazepine, and phenytoin, which are still most often used in low- and middle-income countries where drug options may be limited, are expected to induce metabolism of nonnucleotide reverse transcriptase inhibitors and protease inhibitors, which are also metabolized by the P450 system. This interaction may lead to clinical disease progression and development of ARV drug resistance. Additional interactions of ARV drugs with AEDs are those characterized by induction of metabolism of AEDs by ARV drugs and inhibition of metabolism of ARV drugs by valproate or stiripentol.

The most important examples of these interactions are a lopinavir/ritonavir plasma level decrease induced by phenytoin, a dramatic 16-fold reduction in blood levels of indinavir induced by carbamazepine, inhibition of zidovuline metabolism by valproate, and a 50% decrease in lamotrigine levels by ritonavir/atazanavir [35].

In several developing countries where phenobarbital is the only available antiepileptic treatment, these interactions are a critical problem. Risk of failure of HIV antiretroviral therapy and the consequent increase in HIV resistance to antiretroviral drugs often lead to the decision of avoiding treatment of seizures [37].

3.2 Treatment of seizures in infectious diseases of the CNS

In patients with infective disease of CNS, epilepsy may present with several acute seizures or even status epilepticus. In these patients, intravenous administration of a benzodiazepine may be required, and especially in patients with established status epilepticus, AEDs must be administered through intravenous route. Formulations for intravenous use are available for four AEDs (phenytoin, phenobarbital, levetiracetam, lacosamide). Although phenytoin is the only AED whose summary of product characteristics reports the indication for treatment of status epilepticus, this drug is not easy to use and is a strong enzymatic inducer, which may interact with several drugs used for treatment of patients with status epilepticus [38]. Levetiracetam, valproic acid, or even lacosamide may be preferable.

In regards to oral treatment, special attention should be given for the selection of AEDs not interacting with antimicrobial drugs and with a low risk of idiosyncratic adverse reactions [18, 33].

4. Inflammatory diseases of the central nervous system

In the case of comorbidity between epilepsy and inflammatory diseases of CNS, inflammation causes acute seizures and epilepsy via direct or indirect causal mechanisms. However, there are also some bidirectional mechanisms in this case.

4.1 Immune-mediated encephalitis

Awareness is growing that immune-mediated epilepsy may constitute a common cause of refractory, apparently cryptogenic epilepsy. Between 11% and 35% of all refractory epilepsies of undefined etiology may have an autoimmune etiology [39]. Unfortunately, epilepsy associated with autoimmune encephalitis remains underdiagnosed, mainly because these patients do not present with a well-defined clinical syndrome. Autoimmune epilepsy should be suspected when epilepsy begins with acute or subacute highly frequent seizures with variable semiologies (particularly after the third decade of life), presence of multifocal seizures on EEG, initial presentation with status epilepticus, or history of autoimmunity or neoplasm. Evidence in support of diagnosis includes inflammatory cerebrospinal fluid (CSF) findings (pleocytosis, elevated IgG index, and/or oligoclonal bands) and magnetic resonance imaging (MRI) findings suggestive of inflammation (typically, T2 hyperintensity in the mesial temporal structures often with a bilateral involvement).

Simultaneous testing of both serum and CSF for the presence of antibodies targeting intracellular antigens or neuronal cell surface proteins is essential for diagnosis, although a negative result does not exclude a case of autoimmune epilepsy [39]. Diagnosis of possible autoimmune epilepsy can still be done if there is a clinical response to immunotherapy [40].

4.2 Treatment of seizures in patients with immune-mediated encephalitis

Seizures associated with autoimmune encephalitis are characteristically refractory to treatment with AEDs.

Seizure freedom can be achieved only in 10% of patients on AED monotherapy, while <15% will have a $\geq$50% reduction in seizure frequency [41]. In addition, specific antibody syndromes may strongly predispose patients to the development of particular adverse drug reactions. For example, oxcarbazepine and carbamazepine may more frequently cause or aggravate hyponatremia in patients with antibodies to the voltage-gated potassium channel complex, and cutaneous adverse effects of aromatic AEDs are observed in up to 50% of patients with LG1 antibodies [40].

No single AED is specifically recommended for the treatment of autoimmune epilepsy. It has been alleged that sodium channel blockers (e.g., carbamazepine, oxcarbazepine, lacosamide, lamotrigine, and phenytoin) are of a certain efficacy [42]. It has also been speculated that some AEDs may exert some positive immunomodulatory effects altering serum levels of interleukins and tumor necrosis factor-α [43]. Experimental findings show that levetiracetam and the newest brivaracetam may have protective and anti-inflammatory effects, modulating production of plasma TNF-α and antioxidant capacity [44]. Mechanism of action of these agents seems to be related with their binding with SV2A protein, which is expressed in neurons but also in other cell types including human CD8 + T lymphocytes. It has been shown that levetiracetam has inhibitory effects on the function of these lymphocytes [45].

However, AEDs are not the mainstay of therapy for treatment of autoimmune encephalitis. Corticosteroids, intravenous immunoglobulin, and plasmapheresis are considered first-line agent immunotherapies for treatment of patients with autoimmune epilepsy, whereas more specific immunosuppressive agents, such as monoclonal antibodies (mainly rituximab), are considered second-line agents [40]. Some patients may need immunosuppressant agents (cyclophosphamide mycophenolate).

Also in this case, it should be remembered that metabolism of corticosteroids and of several immunosuppressive agents is strongly induced by phenobarbital, phenytoin, and carbamazepine. Therefore, enzyme-inducing AEDs should be avoided [18].

4.3 Multiple sclerosis

Multiple sclerosis, the most common chronic immune-mediated disorder affecting CNS, is characterized by inflammation and destruction of myelin sheaths of neurons and has a wide range of signs and symptoms. About 2.3 million people are affected by this disease in the world, with rates varying widely in different regions and among different populations [46].

The occurrence of epilepsy during the course of multiple sclerosis has an annual incidence of 2.28% and a prevalence of 3.09% and suggests that the association of epilepsy and multiple sclerosis is more common than expected by chance [46].

Seizures can occur at any time during the disease and have also been described as the presenting symptom of the disease. Since epileptogenesis must necessarily involve the cortex, a special role in the pathogenesis of epilepsy in such disease should be played by pure intracortical lesions [47]. Interferons, which are used in the treatment of this disease, have been considered proconvulsant [48].

With regard to treatment of seizures, in the context of an acute relapse, seizures are generally self-limiting and do not require treatment, whereas recurrence of seizures unrelated to relapse should be treated.

Clinically important drug interactions between drugs used for chronic treatment of multiple sclerosis and AEDs have not been observed [19]. Impact on motor and cognitive functions, such as fatigue, vertigo, ataxia, diplopia, and cognitive slowing, which are typical of several AEDs, might worsen symptoms of the disease and also mimic disease activity. Although no treatment guidelines are available for treatment of epilepsy in patients with multiple sclerosis, new-generation AEDs with less severe specific motor and cognitive adverse effects should be preferred.

5. Cerebral tumors

Comorbidity between epilepsy and cancer are discussed in detail in Chapter 9. Although the incidence of brain tumors as a cause of epilepsy accounts for only 4% of patients with epilepsy, seizures are relatively frequent in both primary and metastatic tumors. Approximately 30%–50% of patients with cerebral tumors will have seizures as a first sign of tumor and an additional 10%–30% will experience a seizure during the course of disease [49].

Seizure risk depends on type and location of tumor [50]. As a general rule, slow-growing tumors, particularly gangliogliomas and dysembryoplastic neuroepithelial tumors, are associated with the highest rates of seizures while high-grade tumors have lower risk. Patients with metastatic brain lesions experience seizures less frequently than those with primary tumors. Incidence of seizures also varies among different metastatic masses being as high as 67% in metastatic melanoma. In addition, cortical involvement is more frequently associated with seizures while white matter, infratentorial, and sellar tumors are less often associated with seizures [51].

In regards to location, frontal, parietal, and temporal tumors, particularly those involving the mesial temporal lobe, insula, and other paralimbic structures are associated with higher rates of seizures than occipital tumors [51].

Mechanisms of epileptogenesis vary among different tumor types. While in low-grade lesions this process is consequent to slowly developing focal abnormalities by vascular or mechanical changes that may isolate brain regions, in high-grade lesions tissue damage is mainly consequent to necrosis and hemosiderin deposition. In general, epileptic foci do originate from that portion of altered tissue that is between lesional and adjacent normal cortex and can also be at a certain distance from the tumor border. Peritumoral changes alter the permeability of vascular supply leading to breakdown of the blood-brain barrier and possible edema. Loss of balance between excitatory and inhibitory transmission [52], such as alteration of glutamate extracellular concentrations in astrocytes, dysfunction of adenosine-mediated neurotransmission, and alterations of gap junctions, take place in this area and have been found more compromised in low-grade gliomas than in high-grade gliomas [53].

Finally, seizures may not only be the direct consequence of tumor but can also be secondary to infection of the brain, which may result from immunosuppressive effects of chemotherapy or radiation necrosis [17].

5.1 Treatment of seizures in patients with CNS tumors

In patients who have never had seizures, routine prophylactic use of AEDs is not recommended. Several systematic analyses of literature and clinical studies have shown that a prophylactic treatment with phenytoin, phenobarbital, or valproate does not reduce risk of a first seizure but significantly increases risk of adverse effects [54, 55]. Furthermore, AEDs should be withdrawn 1 week after surgery in those patients who received such drugs for prevention of acute symptomatic seizures [56].

After a first unprovoked seizure, a patient with brain tumor should be treated with AEDs [57] although in this case, the choice of the first AED is critical because of a series of concerns. Idiosyncratic adverse effects of AEDs are more frequently observed in this population of patients. For example, risk of carbamazepine-induced aplastic anemia is increased in patients receiving chemotherapy, which depresses the bone marrow, and radiotherapy facilitates the appearance of serious and life-threatening cutaneous adverse reactions caused by aromatic AEDs [51].

Epilepsies caused by brain tumors are more often drug resistant. Seizure freedom after a first AED treatment is observed in about 40% of patients, which is lower than that found in the overall population of epileptic patients. This finding has been explained by overexpression of proteins involved in multidrug resistance, reduced receptor sensitivity, or a wide epileptogenic area [55]. Concerning drug tolerability, it should be considered that patients with brain tumors and consequent neurological damages may be more prone to both motor and cognitive drug-induced adverse effects [56].

However, by far the most important issue is the effect of the coadministered AED on antineoplastic drug efficacy and disease progression. There is increasing awareness that pharmacokinetic interactions between antineoplastic agents and AEDs may have important clinical consequences. Enzyme-inducing AEDs, such as carbamazepine, phenytoin, and barbiturates, enhance the metabolic clearance and make less effective or even ineffective many concomitantly administered anticancer medications and also corticosteroids, which are often prescribed in these patients. Some studies show that overall survival of patients with glioblastoma multiforme is shorter in those patients receiving enzyme-inducing AEDs and this finding has been attributed to a lower efficacy of antineoplastic drugs [58]. With regards to valproic acid, which is an enzymatic inhibitor, it has been reported that coadministration of this agent with temozolomide and other anticancer agents may lead to an increased survival but also to more frequent adverse effects, such as thrombocytopenia and leukopenia [59, 60]. The improved prognosis in such patients has been explained by valproic acid's ability to exert a mild inhibition of clearance of these drugs but also by a direct anticancer effect of valproate, which inhibits angiogenesis and induces cell differentiation and growth arrest of tumor cells through inhibition of histone deacetylase [60].

Increased hematologic toxicity observed with valproate in these patients can be consequent to an increased toxic effect on platelet function exerted by both valproate and antineoplastic agents or to metabolic inhibition of anticancer with consequent toxic levels of these agents [60]. A number of interactions whereby anticancer agents can increase or decrease the serum concentrations of AEDs have also been reported [60].

In Table 3 are reported the most important pharmacokinetic interactions between AEDs and drugs used in patients with brain tumors.

All studies aimed at assessing AED efficacy in patients with brain tumors typically consist of retrospective or small prospective case series, which are heterogeneous concerning tumor histology, disease phase, kind of anticancer treatment, and seizure frequency.

Therefore, treatment choices are largely determined by physicians' opinions and by individual patient characteristics. AEDs that are frequently selected as first-line therapy include second-generation nonenzyme-inducing AEDs lamotrigine, lacosamide levetiracetam, oxcarbazepine, topiramate, and zonisamide, all of which are approved as initial monotherapy for focal seizures. Polytherapy with more than an AED can be considered in those patients who have an unsatisfactory response to the initially prescribed drug at full doses, although there are cases in which persistence of some minor seizures can be inevitable and should be accepted instead as causing intolerable adverse effects.

Surgical resection of the tumor, radiotherapy, and chemotherapy, which are treatment modalities for control of tumor growth, are also generally associated with seizure improvement. On the contrary, seizure recurrence in a patient with previously well-controlled seizures may be caused by recurrence or progression of the tumor, side effects of cancer therapy (radionecrosis), or infectious or metabolic encephalopathy [60].

6. Neurodegenerative disorders

6.1 Dementia

The comorbidity between epilepsy and dementia is quite common among the elderly. The reason for such coexistence may be that both neurological conditions are frequent, although several lines of evidence support higher incidence of epilepsy among demented patients and especially in patients with Alzheimer's disease (AD).

The main causes of dementia are degenerative and vascular, and the two conditions often coexist in the same subject [61]. Strategic infarcts are a frequent cause of vascular dementia (VaD), and these lesions also represent a major cause of acquired epilepsy in the elderly.

Table 3 Relevant drug interactions between antineoplastic and immunosuppressant agents and AEDs

Kind of interaction	Drugs that alter drug levels	Drug whose metabolism is altered
Induction of metabolism of antineoplastic and immunosuppressant agents	Phenobarbital, carbamazepine, phenytoin	Abiraterone, afatinib, axitinib, bendamustine, bexarotene, bleomicine, bortezomib, bosutinib, busulfan, cabazitaxel, capecitabine, carboplatin, carmustine, cisplatin, crizotinib, cyclophosphamide, cyclosporine, dabrafenib, dasatinib, docetaxel, doxorubicin, erlotinib, etoposide, everolimus, fluorouracil, gefitinib, ifosfamide, imatinib, irinotecan, exemestan, lapatinib, methotrexate, mitoxantrone, mycophenolate, nilotinib, pazopanib, pirfenidon, pomalidomide, praclitaxel, procarbazin, regorafenib, sirolimus, sorafenib, sunitinib, tacrolimus, tamoxifen, temsirolimus, teniposide, thiotepa, topotecan, toremifen, trabectedin, vandetanib, vemurafenib, vinblastine, vincristine, vindesine, vinorelbine[a]
Induction of metabolism of steroids that may be used in patients with brain tumor	Phenobarbital, carbamazepine, phenytoin	Cortisol, dexamethasone, hydrocortisone, methylprednisolone, prednisone, prednisolone[a]
Inhibition of metabolism of antineoplastic and immunosuppressant agents by AEDs	Valproate	Cisplatinum, etoposide, nitrosoureas, temozolomide, temsirolimus
Inhibition of metabolism of AEDs	5-Fluorouracil, tacrolimus, tamoxifen	Phenytoin

See legend of Table 1.
[a]In this list, metabolism of each drug was induced by at least one of enzyme-inducing antiepileptic drug.

The link between VaD and epilepsy has been explored trough a population-based nested case-control analysis from a large database of UK general practitioners. It has been shown that incidence rate of epilepsy diagnosis within 2 years from the diagnosis of VaD was more than nine folds higher than among age-matched controls and also higher than in AD (where it was 7.1 folds higher than controls). In the nested analysis, prevalence of dementia (mainly VaD), among a sample of patients with incident epilepsy after 65 years, was one third of the sample [62].

6.1.1 Alzheimer's disease

The main forms of neurodegenerative dementia are represented by (AD), frontotemporal lobe degeneration (FTD) and Lewy body disease (LBD). Among them, AD is by far the most prevalent, especially in patients above 65 years of age [63]. Higher incidence of myoclonus among demented patients, especially in those with a more advanced disease, has been emphasized in old studies [64, 65]. Concerning other seizure types, their precise incidence has not yet been established, as it varies dramatically among different studies [66, 67]. A reason for such discrepancy may be that in earlier studies in which epilepsy was evaluated in AD patients, diagnostic criteria of dementia were different from the ones currently in use. In fact, nowadays the diagnosis of AD is based not only on clinical but also on objective criteria, such as MRI and fluoro-desoxyglucose positron emission tomography (PET), and, more recently, it is supported by biomarkers, such as amyloid levels (either assessed by PET or by CSF analysis) or Tau and Phospho-Tau (at present only in CSF) [68]. Another main limitation of several analyses, those from both clinic-based databases [69] and large community public datasets [70], is that they were retrospective. In all cases, the database from which epilepsy data were extracted had not been designed to specifically evaluate the occurrence of seizures. Thus, only clear, previous tonic-clonic seizures were likely to be reported by relatives of the patients, while more subtle phenomena were easily missed. Complex partial seizures, which are represented by definition by consciousness impairment, can be very difficult to identify in these patients, unless they are also accompanied by a clear motor behavior. Even in the latter scenario, however, repetitive stereotyped behaviors accompanying complex partial seizures can be difficult to discriminate from repetitive behaviors often occurring in demented patients, especially at late dementia stages.

The reasons listed in the previous paragraph concur to underestimate the occurrence of seizures in patients with dementia/cognitive impairment. In any case, in an interesting recent retrospective analysis it was observed that earlier onset of AD is associated with higher incidence of concomitant epilepsy [71]. Furthermore, most seizures in these patients were complex partial and nonconvulsive.

In most of the studies on seizures and AD, EEG data were generally not available or available only in few patients [72]. In one study, performed in a memory clinic, EEG was consecutively collected in a very large cohort of patients (almost 1700) affected by either mild cognitive impairment (MCI), AD, or "other dementia," and evaluated for the occurrence of epileptiform discharges. These were present in approximately 2% of patients with AD or MCI and in 1% of patients with other forms of dementia; in approximately 20% of patients with epileptiform activity, new seizures occurred at follow up; finally, epileptiform activity was more often present in younger patients [72]. A consistently higher percentage of subclinical discharges (>40% of AD patients without prior history of seizures, which was significantly higher than in the group of age-matched controls) was found in a prospective study on 33 patients with more sophisticated techniques of analysis [73].

In conclusion, it is widely accepted that the occurrence of epilepsy among AD is significantly higher than in the normal population and that it might be particularly prevalent in patients with early AD (and especially familial AD) and younger age; seizures are more frequently focal limbic and, at later stages, myoclonic.

Interesting data on the relationship between neuropathogical alterations observed in AD and seizures come from studies in preclinical AD models. Mice transgenic for amyloid pathogenic mutation show a significantly reduced threshold to electrographic seizures before the onset of the AD-related pathologic changes [74]. More recently, it has been also observed that early administration of AEDs in these mice significantly attenuates interictal activity [75] and attenuate cognitive and pathological alterations [76].

Degeneration of the noradrenergic nucleus locus coeruleus seems also to be involved in the pathogenesis of dementia and seizures. Degeneration of such brain nucleus may precede by decades the onset of dementia and seems to play a pathogenic role in the development dementia [76]. On the other hand, noradrenaline has anticonvulsant effects in almost all epilepsy model tested [77].

6.1.1.1 Treatment of epilepsy in Alzheimer's disease

The choice of the best treatment of epilepsy in patients with dementia shares several aspects with treatment indications in elderly, in general, and, concerning VaD, the same principles for cerebrovascular diseases (paragraph 2 of this chapter) can be applied.

For treatment of epilepsy in AD, there are also other specific potential aspects to consider [78].

It has been shown that valproate may worsen cognitive functions, and data show that, in rare cases, it may increase brain atrophy rate [79]. For these reasons, this agent should not be a first-line choice even though it has been used for control of some behavioral disturbances in patients with dementia [80].

Evidences from uncontrolled studies suggest a potential significant efficacy of levetiracetam [81]. Similarly, lamotrigine has also been shown to be similarly effective in demented patients with epilepsy as confirmed by retrospective studies [71]. Despite the potential positive cognitive effects concerning levetiracetam, one should keep in mind the potential psychiatric effects (including agitation), which have been repeatedly described for this drug. However, in favor of levetiracetam and lamotrigine choice, among MCI or patients at early stages of AD, are also the promising recent observations in experimental models of AD (as previously described in this chapter).

Finally, epileptic subjects with dementia are at risk of drug-induced seizures, as they are often exposed to antipsychotics, some of which are significantly proconvulsant [82]. Interactions between antidepressant and antipsychotic drugs are described in other sections of this book (see Chapters 16 and 17).

Some interactions are described between acetylcholinesterase inhibitors, used to improve cognition in demented patients, and AEDs. Metabolism of both donepezil and galantamine is induced by old generation AEDs (phenobarbital, phenytoin, carbamazepine), which often require a dose increase. Instead, rivastigmine, which is without hepatic metabolism by the CYP-450 system, and memantine have no interactions with AEDs.

6.1.2 Other forms of degenerative dementias

There are only rough estimates of epilepsy incidence in LBD, which are based mainly on retrospective analyses; a higher incidence of seizures among patients with LBD than in the general population has been estimated, almost similar to AD [83] or even higher [84]. Furthermore, cortical myoclonus might be particularly frequent in these subjects, affecting >20% of them [85], and its occurrence might be related to specific cortical pathological features. Even though detailed analysis of the most prevalent types of seizures among LBD patients is not available, one should keep in mind that one of the core diagnostic features of LBD is the fluctuation of vigilance during the day, which is often quite abrupt and might make difficult to identify focal seizures that also might be featured mainly by attention/vigilance reduction. It has been documented by several studies that EEG often shows focal sharp waves [85].

There are no specific studies assessing the effects of specific AEDs in LBD patients with seizures. Interestingly, a recent controlled clinical trial provided some evidences of a good profile in terms of cognitive profile and tolerability of zonisamide administered together with L-DOPA in patients with LBD, with even an additive effect on parkinsonism as compared with L-DOPA [86].

FTD is a term describing dementia involving mainly the frontal and temporal lobe, asymmetrically, but under this term different causes of dementia as well as different etiologies are included [87]; thus, coexistence of FTD with other disorders is likely to vary significantly depending on the subtype. A recent retrospective study in a relatively large series of patients showed that FTD is less associated to new-onset seizures than AD and LBD but more than the general population [84].

6.2 Parkinson's disease

Epilepsy and Parkinson's disease (PD) have been considered, in general, nonrelated. Actually, the two conditions have been considered by several neurologists even reciprocally exclusive, that is, the occurrence of one condition associated with a lower incidence of the other. This opinion dates back to the early decades of the last century, after a few observations of patients with postinfective parkinsonism in which development of PD signs was associated with a decrease of seizure frequency [88]. However, postencephalitic syndrome does not correspond neuropathologically to idiopathic parkinsonism (i.e., PD), and even the opposite has been claimed to occur, namely an improvement of PD signs after seizure onset [87]. In any case, both scenarios were merely based on anecdotal reports and have not been studied in large population-based studies. There are, however, interesting data obtained in patients' cohorts, such as the large analysis in a group of PD patients assessed in a tertiary neurology center [89]. In this study, it has been shown that, among 1215 PD patients, the incidence of epilepsy was lower than expected in age-matched general population samples. Of incidental interest for the present review, (but nonetheless intriguing), it has also been assessed that the occurrence of status epilepticus occurred in PD twice as frequently as in the general population.

However, a large epidemiological analysis [2] suggested a slightly increased coexistence of PD among patients with epilepsy. The latter study was based on part of the large patients' UK General Practice Research Database, which included data on more than one million people. Among those with a coded diagnosis of epilepsy, 4% had a coexistent diagnosis of PD. However, several biases may weaken these data. In particular diagnosis of PD, which is mainly based on clinical judgment, was not confirmed by a specialist.

Experimental data do not bring more evidences to the link between epilepsy and PD. In a model of PD in mice, changes as to seizure incidence or threshold of different types of experimental seizures have not been found [90].

Moderate interactions characterized by induction of metabolism of drugs used for treatment of PD are described between L-DOPA, ropinirole, rasagiline, and phenytoin, while selegiline and ropinirole are induced by carbamazepine [19]. Finally, valproate in elderly patients often has a tremorigen effect [91], which might further complicate its use, especially in PD patients.

6.3 Other neurodegenerative disorders

Concerning Huntington's disease (HD), there are several evidences for a high incidence of seizures in patients with early-onset HD [91], while recent data confirm the common belief that prevalence of seizures in patients with adult-onset HD is similar to that of age-matched population [92]. It should be noted that patients with HD are often treated with antipsychotics, which have potential proconvulsant effects [82].

Finally, no information on seizures has been reported in large casistics of subjects with corticobasal degeneration [93] or progressive sopranuclear palsy, although early reports signaled seizures in a nonnegligible percentage of patients [94].

7. Conclusions

Today, much more than in the past, epilepsy is comorbid with several neurological diseases, and all these diseases may be caused by a common etiologic factor [4] or can reciprocally influence each the other. In all cases, therapeutic strategy should carefully consider these aspects.

References

[1] Feinstein AR. The pretherapeutic classification of comorbidity in chronic disease. J Chronic Dis 1970;23:455–68.

[2] Gaitatzis A, Carroll K, Majeed A, et al. The epidemiology of the comorbidity of epilepsy in the general population. Epilepsia 2004;45(12):1613–22.

[3] Beghi E, Carpio A, Forsgren L, Hesdorffer DC, Malmgren K, Sander JW, Tomson T, Hauser WA. Recommendation for a definition of acute symptomatic seizure. Epilepsia 2010;51(4):671–5.

[4] Keezer MR, Sander JW. Comorbidity as an epidemiological construct. Lancet Neurol 2016;15(1):32.

[5] Bladin CF, Alexandrov AV, Bellavance A, Bornstein N, Chambers B, Coté R, Lebrun L, Pirisi A, Norris JW. Seizures after stroke: a prospective multicenter study. Arch Neurol 2000;57(11):1617–22.

[6] Fisher RS, Acevedo C, Arzimanoglou A, Bogacz A, Cross JH, Elger CE, Engel Jr. J, Forsgren L, French JA, Glynn M, Hesdorffer DC, Lee BI, Mathern GW, Moshé SL, Perucca E, Scheffer IE, Tomson T, Watanabe M, Wiebe S. ILAE official report: a practical clinical definition of epilepsy. Epilepsia 2014;55(4):475–82.

[7] Szaflarski JP, Rackley AY, Kleindorfer DO, Khoury J, Woo D, Miller R, Alwell K, Broderick JP, Kissela BM. Incidence of seizures in the acute phase of stroke: a population-based study. Epilepsia 2008;49(6):974–81.

[8] Bentes C, Martins H, Peralta AR, Casimiro C, Morgado C, Franco AC, Fonseca AC, Geraldes R, Canhão P, Pinho E, Melo T, Paiva T, Ferro JM. Post-stroke seizures are clinically underestimated. J Neurol 2017;264(9):1978–85.

[9] Zhang C, Wang X, Wang Y, Zhang JG, Hu W, Ge M, Zhang K, Shao X. Risk factors for post-stroke seizures: a systematic review and meta-analysis. Epilepsy Res 2014;108(10):1806–16.

[10] Mehta A, Zusman BE, Shutter LA, Choxi R, Yassin A, Antony A, Thirumala PD. The prevalence and impact of status epilepticus secondary to intracerebral hemorrhage: results from the US nationwide inpatient sample. Neurocrit Care 2018;11.

[11] Graham NS, Crichton S, Koutroumanidis M, Wolfe CD, Rudd AG. Incidence and associations of poststroke epilepsy: the prospective South London stroke register. Stroke 2013;44(3):605–11.

[12] Ferlazzo E, Gasparini S, Beghi E, Sueri C, Russo E, Leo A, Labate A, Gambardella A, Belcastro V, Striano P, Paciaroni M, Pisani LR, Aguglia U, Epilepsy Study Group of the Italian Neurological Society. Epilepsy in cerebrovascular diseases: review of experimental and clinical data with meta-analysis of risk factors. Epilepsia 2016;57(8):1205–14.

[13] De Reuck J, Nagy E, Van Maele G. Seizures and epilepsy in patients with lacunar strokes. J Neurol Sci 2007;263:75–8.

[14] Cleary P, Shorvon S, Tallis R. Late-onset seizures as a predictor of subsequent stroke. Lancet 2004;363:1184–6.

[15] Shinton RA, Gill JS, Zezulka AV, Beevers DG. The frequency of epilepsy preceding stroke. Case-control study in 230 patients. Lancet 1987;1:11–3.

[16] Martz GU, Wilson DA, Malek AM, Selassie AW. Risk of venous thromboembolism in people with epilepsy. Epilepsia 2014;55(11):1800–7.

[17] Zaccara G. Neurological comorbidity and epilepsy: implications for treatment. Acta Neurol Scand 2009;120(1):1–15.

[18] Zaccara G, Perucca E. Interactions between antiepileptic drugs, and between antiepileptic drugs and other drugs. Epileptic Disord 2014;16(4):409–31.

[19] Medscape. Available from: https://reference.medscape.com/drug-interactionchecker. Accessed 18 April 2018.

[20] Lekoubou A, Awoumou JJ, Kengne AP. Incidence of seizure in stroke patients treated with recombinant tissue plasminogen activator: a systematic review and meta-analysis. Int J Stroke 2017;12(9):923–31.

[21] Connolly Jr. ES, Rabinstein AA, Carhuapoma JR, Derdeyn CP, Dion J, Higashida RT, Hoh BL, Kirkness CJ, Naidech AM, Ogilvy CS, Patel AB, Thompson BG, Vespa P, American Heart Association Stroke Council; Council on Cardiovascular Radiology and Intervention; Council on Cardiovascular Nursing; Council on Cardiovascular Surgery and Anesthesia; Council on Clinical Cardiology. Guidelines for the management of aneurysmal subarachnoid hemorrhage: a guideline for healthcare professionals from the American Heart Association/american Stroke Association. Stroke 2012;43(6):1711–37.

[22] Price M, Günther A, Kwan JS. Antiepileptic drugs for the primary and secondary prevention of seizures after intracranial venous thrombosis. Cochrane Database Syst Rev 2014;8.

[23] Guo J, Guo J, Li J, Zhou M, Qin F, Zhang S, Wu B, He L, Zhou D. Statin treatment reduces the risk of poststroke seizures. Neurology 2015;85:701–7.

[24] Choi KS, Chun HJ, Yi HJ, Ko Y, Kim YS, Kim JM. Seizures and epilepsy following aneurysmal subarachnoid hemorrhage: Incidence and risk factors. J Korean Neurosurg Soc 2009;46:93–8.

[25] Deutschman CS, Haines SJ. Anticonvulsant prophylaxis in neurological surgery. Neurosurgery 1985;17:510–7.

[26] Ferro JM, Bousser MG, Canhão P, Coutinho JM, Crassard I, Dentali F, di Minno M, Maino A, Martinelli I, Masuhr F, Aguiar de Sousa D, Stam J, European Stroke Organization. European stroke organization guideline for the diagnosis and treatment of cerebral venous thrombosis—endorsed by the European Academy of Neurology. Eur J Neurol 2017;24(10):1203–13.

[27] Sykes L, Wood E, Kwan J. Antiepileptic drugs for the primary and secondary prevention of seizures after stroke. Cochrane Database Syst Rev 2014;24(1):CD005398. https://doi.org/10.1002/14651858. CD005398.pub3.

[28] Annegers JF, Hauser WA, Beghi E, Nicolosi A, Kurland LT. The risk of unprovoked seizures after encephalitis and meningitis. Neurology 1988;38:1407–10.

[29] Vezzani A, Fujinami RS, White HS, Preux PM, Blümcke I, Sander JW, Löscher W. Infections, inflammation and epilepsy. Acta Neuropathol 2016;131(2):211–34.

[30] Sutter R, Rüegg S, Tschudin-Sutter. Seizures as adverse events of antibiotic drugs: a systematic review. Neurology 2015;85(15):1332–41.

[31] Sander JW, Perucca E. Epilepsy and comorbidity: infections and antimicrobials usage in relation to epilepsy management. Acta Neurol Scand 2003;108:16–22.

[32] Tohiama M, Hashimoto K, Yasukawa M, et al. Association of human herpesvirus-6 reactivation with the flaring and severity of drug-induced hypersensitivity syndrome. Clin Lab Invest 2007;157:934–40.

[33] Zaccara G, Franciotta D, Perucca E. Idiosyncratic adverse reactions to antiepileptic drugs. Epilepsia 2007;48(7):1223–44.

[34] Zaccara G, Giovannelli F, Giorgi FS, Franco V, Gasparini S, Tacconi FM. Do antiepileptic drugs increase the risk of infectious diseases? A meta-analysis of placebo-controlled studies. Br J Clin Pharmacol 2017;83(9):1873–9.

[35] Birbeck GL, French JA, Perucca E, Simpson DM, Fraimow H, George JM, Okulicz JF, Clifford DB, Hachad H, Levy RH, Quality Standards Subcommittee of the American Academy of Neurology, Ad Hoc Task Force of the Commission on Therapeutic Strategies of the International League Against Epilepsy. Antiepileptic drug selection for people with HIV/AIDS: evidence-based guidelines from the ILAE and AAN. Epilepsia 2012;53(1):207–14.

[36] Bearden D, Steenhoff AP, Dlugos DJ, Kolson D, Mehta P, Kessler S, Lowenthal E, Monokwane B, Anabwani G, Bisson GP. Early antiretroviral therapy is protective against epilepsy in children with human immunodeficiency virus infection in botswana. J Acquir Immune Defic Syndr 2015; 69(2):193–9.

[37] Jennings HR, Romanelli F. The use of valproic acid in HIV positive patients. Ann Pharmacother 1999;33:1113–6 Epilepsy and HIV—a dangerous combination. Lancet Neurol 2007;6:747.

[38] Zaccara G, Giorgi FS, Amantini A, Giannasi G, Campostrini R, Giovannelli F, Paganini M, Nazerian P. Tuscany study group on seizures in the emergency department and status epilepticus in adults. Why we prefer levetiracetam over phenytoin for treatment of status epilepticus. Acta Neurol Scand 2018; https://doi.org/10.1111/ane.12928.

[39] Brenner T, Sills GJ, Hart Y, Howell S, Waters P, Brodie MJ, et al. Prevalence of neurologic autoantibodies in cohorts of patients with new and established epilepsy. Epilepsia 2013;54(6):1028–35.

[40] Bhatia S, Schmitt SE. Treating immune-related epilepsy. Curr Neurol Neurosci Rep 2018;18(3):10.

[41] Feyissa AM, López Chiriboga AS, Britton JW. Antiepileptic drug therapy in patients with autoimmune epilepsy. Neurol Neuroimmunol Neuroinflamm 2017;4(4).

[42] Suleiman J, Brilot F, Lang B, Vincent A, Dale RC. Autoimmune epilepsy in children: case series and proposed guidelines for identification. Epilepsia 2013;6:1036–45.

[43] Himmerich H, Bartsch S, Hamer H, Mergl R, Schönherr J, Petersein C, et al. Modulation of cytokine production by drugs with antiepileptic or mood stabilizer properties in anti-CD3- and anti-Cd40-stimulated blood in vitro. Oxid Med Cell Longev 2014;2014:8061–2.

[44] Erbaş O, Yeniel AÖ, Akdemir A, Ergenoğlu AM, Yilmaz M, Taskiran D, et al. The beneficial effects of levetiracetam on polyneuropathy in the early stage of sepsis in rats: electrophysiological and biochemical evidence. J Invest Surg 2013;26:312–8.

[45] Nowak M, Bauer S, Schlegel K, Stei S, Allenhöfer L, Waschbisch A. Levetiracetam but not valproate inhibits function of CD8+ T lymphocytes. Seizure 2013;22:462–6.

[46] World Health Organization. Atlas: multiple sclerosis resources in the World 2008 (PDF). Geneva: World Health Organization; 2008. p.15–6. ISBN 92-4-156375-315-6.

[47] Koch M, Uyttenboogaart M, Polman S, De Keyser J. Seizures in multiple sclerosis. Epilepsia 2008;49:948–53.

[48] Ruffmann C, Bogliun G, Beghi E. Epileptogenic drugs: a systematic review. Expert Rev Neurother 2006;6:575–89.

[49] Moots PL, Maciunas RJ, Eisert DR, Parker RA, Laporte K, Abou-Khalil B. The course of seizure disorders in patients with malignant gliomas. Arch Neurol 1995;52:717–24.

[50] van Breemen MS, Wilms EB, Vecht CJ. Epilepsy in patients with brain tumours: epidemiology, mechanisms, and management. Lancet Neurol 2007;6:421–30.

[51] Ertürk Çetin Ö, İşler C, Uzan M, Özkara Ç. Epilepsy-related brain tumors. Seizure 2017;44:93–7.

[52] Wolf HK, Roos D, Blümcke I, Pietsch T, Wiestler OD. Perilesional neurochemical changes in focal epilepsies. Acta Neuropathol 1996;91:376–84.

[53] Aronica E, Gorter JA, Jansen GH, Leenstra S, Yankaya B, Troost D. Expression of connexin 43 and connexin 32 gap-junction proteins in epilepsy-associated brain tumors and in the perilesional epileptic cortex. Acta Neuropathol 2001;101:449–59.

[54] Tremont-Lukats IW, Ratilal BO, Armstrong T, Gilbert MR. Antiepileptic drugs for preventing seizures in people with brain tumours. Cochrane Database Syst Rev 2008;16(2).

[55] Politsky JM. Brain tumor-related epilepsy: a current review of the etiologic basis and diagnostic and treatment approaches. Curr Neurol Neurosci Rep 2017;17(9):70.

[56] Glantz MJ, Cole BF, Forsyth PA, et al. Practice parameter: anticonvulsant prophylaxis in patients with newly diagnosed brain tumors. Report of the Quality Standards Subcommitee of the American Academy of Neurology. Neurology 2000;54:1886–93.

[57] Klinger NV, Shah AK, Mittal S. Management of brain tumor-related epilepsy. Neurol India 2017;65 (Suppl):S60–70.

[58] Oberndorfer S, Piribauer M, Marosi C, et al. P450 enzyme-inducing and non-enzyme inducing antiepileptics in glioblastoma patients treated with standard chemotherapy. J Neurooncol 2005;72:255–60.

[59] Weller M, Gorlia T, Cairncross JG, van den Bent MJ, Mason W, Belanger K, Brandes AA, Bogdahn U, Macdonald DR, Forsyth P, Rossetti AO, Lacombe D, Mirimanoff RO, Vecht CJ, Stupp R. Prolonged survival with valproic acid use in the EORTC/NCIC temozolomide trial for glioblastoma. Neurology 2011;77:1156–64.

[60] Perucca E. Optimizing antiepileptic drug treatment in tumoral epilepsy. Epilepsia 2013;54 (Suppl 9):97–104.

[61] Langa KM, Foster NL, Larson EB. Mixed dementia: emerging concepts and therapeutic implications. JAMA 2004;292(23):2901–8.

[62] Imfeld P, Bodmer M, Schuerch M, Jick SS, Meier CR. Seizures in patients with Alzheimer's disease or vascular dementia: a population-based nested case-control analysis. Epilepsia 2013; 54(4):700–7.

[63] Alzheimer's Association. Alzheimer's disease facts and figures. Alzheimers Dement 2016; 12(4):459–509.

[64] Hauser WA, Morris ML, Heston LL, Anderson VE. Seizures and myoclonus in patients with Alzheimer's disease. Neurology 1986;36(9):1226–30.

[65] Chen JY, Stern Y, Sano M, Mayeux R. Cumulative risks of developing extrapyramidal signs, psychosis, or myoclonus in the course of Alzheimer's disease. Arch Neurol 1991;48(11):1141–3.

[66] Friedman D, Honig LS, Scarmeas N. Seizures and epilepsy in Alzheimer's disease. CNS Neurosci Ther 2012;18(4):285–94.

[67] Subota A, Pham T, Jetté N, Sauro K, Lorenzetti D, Holroyd-Leduc J. The association between dementia and epilepsy: a systematic review and meta-analysis. Epilepsia 2017;58(6):962–72.

[68] Dubois B, Feldman HH, Jacova C, Hampel H, Molinuevo JL, Blennow K, DeKosky ST, Gauthier S, Selkoe D, Bateman R, Cappa S, Crutch S, Engelborghs S, Frisoni GB, Fox NC, Galasko D, Habert MO, Jicha GA, Nordberg A, Pasquier F, Rabinovici G, Robert P, Rowe C, Salloway S, Sarazin M, Epelbaum S, de Souza LC, Vellas B, Visser PJ, Schneider L, Stern Y, Scheltens P, Cummings JL. Advancing research diagnostic criteria for Alzheimer's disease: the IWG-2 criteria. Lancet Neurol 2014;13(6):614–29.

[69] Giorgi FS, Baldacci F, Dini E, Tognoni G, Bonuccelli U. Epilepsy occurrence in patients with Alzheimer's disease: clinical experience in a tertiary dementia center. Neurol Sci 2016;37(4):645–7.

[70] Bell JS, Lönnroos E, Koivisto AM, Lavikainen P, Laitinen ML, Soininen H, Hartikainen S. Use of antiepileptic drugs among community-dwelling persons with Alzheimer's disease in Finland. J Alzheimers Dis 2011;26(2):231–7.

[71] Vossel KA, Beagle AJ, Rabinovici GD. Seizures and epileptiform activity in the early stages of Alzheimer disease. JAMA Neurol 2013;70(9):1158–66.

[72] Liedorp M, Stam CJ, van der Flier WM, Pijnenburg YA, Scheltens P. Prevalence and clinical significance of epileptiform EEG discharges in a large memory clinic cohort. Dement Geriatr Cogn Disord 2010;29(5):432–7.

[73] Vossel KA, Ranasinghe KG, Beagle AJ, Mizuiri D, Honma SM, Dowling AF, Darwish SM, Van Berlo V, Barnes DE, Mantle M, Karydas AM, Coppola G, Roberson ED, Miller BL, Garcia PA, Kirsch HE, Mucke L, Nagarajan SS. Incidence and impact of subclinical epileptiform activity in Alzheimer's disease. Ann Neurol 2016;80(6):858–70.

[74] Palop JJ, Chin J, Roberson ED, Wang J, Thwin MT, Bien-Ly N, Yoo J, Ho KO, Yu GQ, Kreitzer A, Finkbeiner S, Noebels JL, Mucke L. Aberrant excitatory neuronal activity and compensatory remodeling of inhibitory hippocampal circuits in mouse models of Alzheimer's disease. Neuron 2007;55(5):697–711.

[75] Zhang MY, Zheng CY, Zou MM, Zhu JW, Zhang Y, Wang J, Liu CF, Li QF, Xiao ZC, Li S, Ma QH, Xu RX. Lamotrigine attenuates deficits in synaptic plasticity and accumulation of amyloid plaques in APP/PS1 transgenic mice. Neurobiol Aging 2014;35(12):2713–25.

[76] Giorgi FS, Ryskalin L, Ruffoli R, Biagioni F, Limanaqi F, Ferrucci M, Busceti CL, Bonuccelli U, Fornai F. The neuroanatomy of the reticular nucleus locus coeruleus in Alzheimer's disease. Front Neuroanat 2017;19(11):80.

[77] Giorgi FS, Pizzanelli C, Biagioni F, Murri L, Fornai F. The role of norepinephrine in epilepsy: from the bench to the bedside. Neurosci Biobehav Rev 2004;28(5):507–24.

[78] Giorgi FS, Guida M, Vergallo A, Bonuccelli U, Zaccara G. Treatment of epilepsy in patients with Alzheimer's disease. Expert Rev Neurother 2017;17(3):309–18.

[79] Fleisher AS, Truran D, Mai JT, et al. For Alzheimer's disease cooperative study, chronic divalproex sodium use and brain atrophy in Alzheimer disease. Neurology 2011;77(13):1263–71.

[80] Tariot PN, Schneider LS, Cummings J, Thomas RG, Raman R, Jakimovich LJ, Loy R, Bartocci B, Fleisher A, Ismail MS, Porsteinsson A, Weiner M, Jack Jr. CR, Thal L, Aisen PS, Alzheimer's Disease Cooperative Study Group. Chronic divalproex sodium to attenuate agitation and clinical progression of Alzheimer disease. Arch Gen Psychiatry 2011;68(8):853–61.

[81] Belcastro V, Costa C, Galletti F, Pisani F, Calabresi P, Parnetti L. Levetiracetam monotherapy in Alzheimer patients with late-onset seizures: a prospective observational study. Eur J Neurol 2007;14(10):1176–8.

[82] Mula M, Monaco F, Trimble MR. Use of psychotropic drugs in patients with epilepsy: interactions and seizure risk. Expert Rev Neurother 2004;4(6):953–64.

[83] Morris M, Sanchez PE, Verret L, Beagle AJ, Guo W, Dubal D, Ranasinghe KG, Koyama A, Ho K, Yu GQ, Vossel KA, Mucke L. Network dysfunction in α-synuclein transgenic mice and human Lewy body dementia. Ann Clin Transl Neurol 2015;2(11):1012–28.

[84] Beagle AJ, Darwish SM, Ranasinghe KG, La AL, Karageorgiou E, Vossel KA. Relative incidence of seizures and myoclonus in Alzheimer's disease, dementia with Lewy bodies, and frontotemporal dementia. J Alzheimers Dis 2017;60(1):211–23.

[85] Barber PA, Varma AR, Lloyd JJ, Haworth B, Haworth JSS, Neary D. The electroencephalogram in dementia with Lewy bodies. Acta Neurol Scand 2000;101:53–6.

[86] Murata M, Odawara T, Hasegawa K, Iiyama S, Nakamura M, Tagawa M, Kosaka K. Adjunct zonisamide to levodopa for DLB parkinsonism: a randomized double-blind phase 2 study. Neurology 2018;90(8):e664–72.

[87] Vercueil L. Parkinsonism and epilepsy: case report and reappraisal of an old question. Epilepsy Behav 2000;1:128–30.

[88] Yakovlev P. Epilepsy and Parkinsonism. N Engl J Med 1928;198:629–38.

[89] Feddersen B, Rémi J, Einhellig M, Stoyke C, Krauss P, Noachtar S. Parkinson's disease: less epileptic seizures, more status epilepticus. Epilepsy Res 2014;108(2):349–54.

[90] Bonuccelli U, Fariello RG. Evidence for an epileptogenic action of 1-methyl-4-phenyl-1,2,3,6,-tetrahydropyridine. Neuropharmacology 1989;28(12):1419–22.

[91] Barker RA, Squitieri F. The clinical phenotype of juvenile Huntington's disease. In: OWJ Q, Brewer HM, Squitieri F, Barker RA, Nance MA, Landwehrmeyer GB, editors. Juvenile Huntington's disease and other trinucleotide repeat disorders. Oxford: Oxford University Press; 2009. p. 39–50.

[92] Sipilä JO, Soilu-Hänninen M, Majamaa K. Comorbid epilepsy in Finnish patients with adult-onset Huntington's disease. BMC Neurol 2016;16:24.

[93] Kompoliti K, Goetz CG, Boeve BF, Maraganore DM, Ahlskog JE, Marsden CD, Bhatia KP, Greene PE, Przedborski S, Seal EC, Burns RS, Hauser RA, Gauger LL, Factor SA, Molho ES, Riley DE. Clinical presentation and pharmacological therapy in corticobasal degeneration. Arch Neurol 1998;55(7):957–61.

[94] Duvoisin RC, Golbe LI, Lepore FE. Progressive supranuclear palsy. Can J Neurol Sci 1987;14 (3 Suppl):547–54.

Further reading

[95] Warren JD, Rohrer JD, Rossor MN. Clinical review. Frontotemporal dementia. BMJ 2013;347:f4827.

[96] Easterford K, Clough P, Kellett M, Fallon K, Duncan S. Reversible parkinsonism with normal beta-CIT-SPECT in patients exposed to sodium valproate. Neurology 2004;62(8):1435–7.

CHAPTER 13

Epilepsy and cognition

Rachel Friefeld Kesselmayer, Gloria M. Morel, Jessica M. Bordenave, Jana Jones, Bruce Hermann
Department of Neurology, University of Wisconsin School of Medicine and Public Health, Madison, WI, United States

Contents

Abbreviations

ABM	autobiographical memory
AED	antiepileptic drug
ALF	accelerated long-term forgetting
BECTS	benign partial epilepsy of childhood with centrotemporal spikes
CWE	children with epilepsy
DRS	Dementia Rating Scale
FSIQ	full scale intelligence quotient
GGE	genetic generalized epilepsy
GTCS	generalized tonic-clonic seizure
IQ	intelligence quotient
JME	juvenile myoclonic epilepsy
LRE	localization-related epilepsy
RCFT	Rey Complex Figure Test
RE	rolandic epilepsy
RMT	Warrington Recognition Memory Test
SI	seizures improved group
SU	seizures unimproved group
TEA	transient epileptic amnesia
TLE	temporal lobe epilepsy

The Comorbidities of Epilepsy
https://doi.org/10.1016/B978-0-12-814877-8.00013-1

T2	time two
VIQ	verbal intelligence quotient
WAIS	Wechsler Adult Intelligence Scale
WAIS-R	Wechsler Adult Intelligence Scale—Revised
WAIS-III	Wechsler Adult Intelligence Scale—Third Edition
WISC	Wechsler Intelligence Scale for Children
WMS-III	Wechsler Memory Scale—Third Edition

1. Introduction

According to the current definition of epilepsy put forth by the International League Against Epilepsy [1], "epilepsy is a disease characterized by an enduring predisposition to generate epileptic seizures and by the neurobiological, cognitive, psychological, and social consequences of this condition." Researchers and clinicians have been concerned about the effects of epilepsy—to various degrees of medico-theoretical understanding—on cognition, mental status, and psychiatric status for several hundred years. Commentaries recognizing the impact of epilepsy on cognitive abilities can be found in the 18th-century literature, for example, by Tissot (1770), who recognized diminished memory and judgment, especially with severe and frequent seizures (as cited in Berrios [2]). More "modern" understanding and observation emerged in the early 19th century by Esquirol [3], who reported cognitive impairment (dementia with memory impairment) and mental disorder in a cohort of female child patients with epilepsy and remarked on the gradual decline in intelligence, perception, and memory, and Bouchet and Cazauvieilh [4], who reported on the development of dementia and insanity in epilepsy. Gowers [5] also postulated more frequent cooccurrence of dementia with epilepsy, "The mental state of epileptics, as is well known, frequently presents deterioration," and inferred that dementia and epilepsy may represent a shared underlying etiology rather than one leading to the other.

The advent of the field of neuropsychology and its psychometric measurement of cognition has allowed for objective quantification of discrete cognitive abilities and their change over time in epilepsy. It was not until 2004 that Carl Dodrill published the first review of the literature focusing specifically on longitudinal change in cognition in people with epilepsy [6]. In that review he examined publications in which formal objective psychological assessment was performed on at least two occasions and were not meant to assess treatment effects (e.g., drug, surgery). Dodrill [6] identified 22 papers that met his criteria (9 involving children and 13 with adolescents and adults), and the review concluded that there were "mild but definite relationships" between epilepsy and cognitive decline over time. This conclusion was tempered by the fact that multiple studies indicated mixed or uncertain results, as well as several studies demonstrating no relationship between seizures and deterioration of cognition. An updated review of the literature was published by Seidenberg et al. [7] using the same study inclusion criteria articulated by Dodrill [6], focusing on the longitudinal studies published in the interim, in order to extend Dodrill's monitoring of studies examining prospective cognitive change. They reported ongoing evidence of cognitive progression in a subset of adults with epilepsy and a complicated pattern of prospective cognitive course in children. Further details regarding the specific findings contained in these reviews will be summarized in the respective pediatric and adult sections to follow.

This review updates the prior reviews by Dodrill [6] and Seidenberg et al. [7], examining the totality of longitudinal research assessing cognitive change in adults and youth with epilepsy published to date. That said, it should be made clear that we take a fresh view and initially considered all published longitudinal cognitive investigations, including those contained in the prior reviews, plus others that we were able to locate in diverse sources, including book chapters. Consistent with Dodrill [6] and Seidenberg et al. [7], only studies that included objective measures of cognition on at least two evaluations were considered. Given the limitations of comparison and generalizability put forth by Seidenberg et al. when discussing studies without control subjects, this review includes only research that utilized a comparison group (healthy or other medical conditions). Additional inclusion criteria included formal neuropsychological assessments conducted with at least two time points, and in regard to the pediatric literature, only studies examining children who were school-aged were included for review.

In essence, we take a fresh view and reexamine the prospective epilepsy-neuropsychology literature, adding important additional selection criteria, finding new studies not previously included, and moving some papers reviewed in the Dodrill and Seidenberg et al. papers to uncontrolled status, which is not a primary focus here. While our focus is squarely on controlled prospective investigations, we have included tables that list and summarize findings from published uncontrolled pediatric and adult investigations, thereby compiling the prospective cognitive literature in a comprehensive manner. Cross-sectional investigations and analyses are neither considered nor tabled.

2. The prospective epilepsy-neuropsychology literature: A quick synopsis

Table 1 provides an overall summary of core features of the published literature that is reflected in detail in Table 2 (controlled studies—children) and Table 3 (controlled studies—adults), which represent the focus of this chapter. Tables 4 and 5 provide additional information on uncontrolled pediatric (Table 4) and adult (Table 5) studies. These tables are not reviewed in this chapter and can be located in the Appendix.

Taking a summary look at the prospective literature (Table 1), in terms of controlled studies it can be appreciated that this is a modestly sized literature, containing only 11 pediatric and 9 adult studies. Some of the published studies come from the same cohort, and when this is considered, the controlled literature is composed of seven independent pediatric and eight independent adult cohorts—the limited nature of this literature notable given the longstanding interest in this clinical issue. The total number of participants in the controlled pediatric and adult studies is modest as well, including less

Table 1 Synopsis of prospective literature

	Pediatric	Adults
Controlled studies		
Earliest study	Bourgeois et al. [8]	Dodrill and Wilensky [9]
Most recent study	Rathouz et al. [10]	Savage et al. [11]
Number of studies	10	9
Number of independent cohorts	6	8
Test-retest intervals	3 months–6 years	1–10 years
Total epilepsy subjects	658 (652 at follow-up)	543
Total control subjects	497 (503 at follow-up)	422
Studies without controls		
Earliest study	Fox [12]	Barnes and Fetterman [13]
Most recent study	Reuner et al. [14]	Mameniškienė et al. [15]
Number of studies	14	16
Number of independent cohorts	14	14
Test-retest intervals	1 month–9 years	1–13 years
Total epilepsy subjects	1423	1271

than 700 pediatric epilepsy patients and 550 adult patients in studies that began in 1983 and 1990, respectively. All but three studies involved only two test-retest sessions.

The structure of the uncontrolled literature is interesting as well. It can be seen that interest in this topic is longstanding with the first pediatric and adult studies appearing in 1924 and 1938, respectively. The most recent uncontrolled studies appeared recently (2016), but again with a total number of epilepsy participants under 1500 in the pediatric and adult literature.

In summary, the important clinical concern of the prospective course of cognition was addressed empirically for the first time in 1924, with both controlled and uncontrolled studies ongoing over the decades with publications appearing up to the present time. Despite this longstanding interest and the important clinical implications of this research, the degree of investigation (especially reflected in controlled studies) is modest in terms of the number of studies, number of participants, and number of controlled investigations.

We now turn to a review of the controlled pediatric and adult studies (Tables 2 and 3) and begin with a brief summary provided in the prior reviews followed by critical examination of the target literature as described.

3. Child and adolescent studies

3.1 Summary of previously reviewed child and adolescent literature

Dodrill [6] and Seidenberg et al. [7] provided discussions of controlled and uncontrolled prospective child and adolescent studies. Of the controlled studies, the earliest reviewed

Table 2 Controlled prospective pediatric studies

Study	(N) Seizure type	Control group	Age	Mean retest interval	Cognitive domains examined	Key results
Bourgeois et al. [8]	72 generalized motor, generalized absence, mixed, simple febrile	45 siblings without epilepsy	21 months–15.9 years	4 years	IQ	Baseline: cognitive domains not significantly different compared to controls. No prospective decline: across all cognitive domains
Bailet and Turk [16]	74 idiopathic epilepsy	23 siblings without epilepsy	8–13 years	≥3 years	IQ, psychomotor speed, memory (verbal and visual), academic achievement	Baseline: all cognitive domains significantly lower compared to controls. No prospective decline: across all cognitive domains
Oostrom et al. [17]	51 idiopathic or cryptogenic epilepsy	48 sex-matched classmates	7–16 years	3 and 12 months	General cognition, memory, sustained attention, academic achievement	Baseline: attention, reaction times, location learning, academic skills significantly lower compared to controls. Prospective decline: academic achievement. No prospective decline: general cognition, memory, sustained attention
Lindgren et al. [18]	32 initial, 26 follow-up rolandic epilepsy (RE)	25 healthy classmates	7–15 years	2.5–3 years	Memory (verbal and visual), executive function	Baseline: memory and learning of auditory-visual material, delayed recall, measures of executive functioning and word comprehension significantly lower compared to controls. No prospective decline: across all cognitive domains

Continued

Table 2 Controlled prospective pediatric studies—cont'd

Study	(N) Seizure type	Control group	Age	Mean retest interval	Cognitive domains examined	Key results
Oostrom et al. [19]	42 idiopathic or cryptogenic epilepsy	30 gender-matched healthy classmates	7–16 years	3, 12, 42 months	IQ, attention, memory, processing speed, academic linguistic skills	Baseline: all cognitive domains significantly lower compared to controls. No prospective decline: across all cognitive domains
Hermann et al. [20]	52 idiopathic generalized, localization-related epilepsy (LRE)	48 healthy first-degree cousins	8–18 years	2 years	IQ, academic achievement, language, memory, executive function, motor function	Baseline: cognitive domains of CWE with *neurobehavioral comorbidities* significantly lower compared to controls. Prospective decline: across all cognitive domains for CWE with *neurobehavioral comorbidities*
Dunn et al. [21]	197 mixed epilepsy (generalized and LRE)	131 siblings (13 not at baseline, 7 not at follow-up)	6–14 years	36 months	Academic achievement (reading, writing, math)	Baseline: writing significantly lower compared to controls. Prospective decline: across all cognitive domains
Almane et al. [22]	50 focal and generalized	41 healthy first-degree cousins	8–18 years	2 and 5 years	Academic achievement (reading, spelling, math)	Baseline: all cognitive domains significantly lower compared to controls for CWE with *academic problems*. Prospective decline: across all cognitive domains for CWE with *academic problems* across all domains

Lin et al. [23]	19 juvenile myoclonic epilepsy (JME)	57 healthy first-degree cousins	8–18 years	2 years	IQ, executive function, response inhibition, cognitive/psychomotor processing speed	Baseline: IQ, response inhibition and psychomotor speed significantly lower compared to controls. Prospective decline: IQ. No prospective decline: response inhibition, psychomotor speed, problem-solving abilities
Rathouz et al. [10]	69 idiopathic and focal epilepsy	62 healthy first-degree cousins	8–18 years	2, 5, 6 years	Academic achievement (reading, spelling, math), IQ, language, executive function, motor function	Baseline: arithmetic computation, response inhibition, attention, fine motor dexterity, and psychomotor speed significantly lower than controls. No prospective decline: across all cognitive domains

Table 3 Controlled prospective adult studies

Study	(N) Seizure type	Control group	Age	Mean retest interval	Cognitive domains examined	Key results
Dodrill and Wilensky [9]	143 chronic unspecified epilepsy syndrome	105 without status epilepticus	Mean age 22 years	5 years	IQ	Baseline: IQ insignificantly lower compared to controls. Prospective decline: IQ
Aikiä et al. [24]	39 new-onset, previously untreated left temporal lobe epilepsy (TLE), 16 chronic left TLE	46 healthy controls	Mean age newly diagnosed: 5; chronic: 42; controls: 31	5 years	IQ, verbal memory	Baseline: among *newly diagnosed LTLE* total immediate recall, delayed recall, and % retained significantly lower than controls; among *chronic LTLE* total immediate recall, recency, delayed recall, % retained, and delayed recognition significantly lower than controls. No prospective decline: verbal memory
Dodrill [25]	35 localization related epilepsy (LRE)	35 controls with no history of medical problems	Mean age 30 years at study onset	10 years (±6 months)	IQ, academic achievement, memory, motor function	Baseline: not provided. Prospective decline: visual memory loss noted across both groups; significance not indicated. *Notes greater improvement in control group on 3 of 20 variables; comparison to baseline or significance not provided

Study	Subjects	Controls	Age	Follow-up	Cognitive domains	Results
Hermann et al. [26]	46 LRE	65 controls	14–59 years	4 years	IQ, language, visuoperceptual/spatial skills, memory, executive function, psychomotor processing, fine motor	Baseline: all cognitive domains significantly lower compared to controls. Prospective decline: indicated among a subset of LRE; 40% confrontation naming; 27% delayed visual memory; 38% delayed verbal memory; 64% bilateral motor speed
Piazzini et al. [27]	50 LRE	50 healthy controls	18–60 years	Over 5 years	IQ, attention, psychomotor speed, language, memory (verbal and visual)	Baseline: no significant differences across cognitive domains compared to controls. Prospective decline: attention; psychomotor speed. No prospective decline: IQ; language; memory (verbal and visual)
Andersson-Roswall et al. [28]	36 LRE, half with secondarily generalized tonic–clonic seizures	25 healthy controls	Mean age subjects: 33 years; controls: 36	4.8 years (epilepsy); 3.1 years (controls)	Verbal memory, verbal cognition, attention/processing speed	Baseline: all cognitive domains significantly lower compared to controls. Prospective decline: 2 verbal memory variables; 3 attention/processing speed variables. No prospective decline: verbal cognition

Continued

Table 3 Controlled prospective adult studies—cont'd

Study	(N) Seizure type	Control group	Age	Mean retest interval	Cognitive domains examined	Key results
Griffith et al. [29]	17 epilepsy older adults with LRE and generalized epilepsy	17 healthy older adults	Mean age subjects: 65; controls: 64	2–3 years	Verbal memory, attention, visuospatial/constructional, executive function, language	Baseline: overall cognitive and verbal memory significantly lower than controls. Prospective decline: executive control. No prospective decline: verbal memory, attention, visuospatial/constructional and language
Baker et al. [30]	147 new-onset, unspecified epilepsy syndromes	69 healthy controls	Mean age subjects: 40; controls: 29	12 months	Memory, executive function, psychomotor speed, information processing, mood	Baseline: psychomotor speed, memory, mental flexibility, information processing significantly lower than controls. Prospective decline: psychomotor speed, higher executive functioning, memory
Savage et al. [11]	14 patients with transient epileptic amnesia (TEA) in TLE	12 healthy age-matched controls	Mean age at follow-up: 78; no baseline info	10 years	IQ, visuospatial/constructional, memory (verbal and visual), executive function	Baseline: no significant differences across cognitive domains compared to controls. Prospective decline: memory. No prospective decline: visual recall, object naming, visuoconstructional skills, executive functioning

case-control prospective investigation compared the intelligence of children with active epilepsies and nonepileptic sibling controls to determine the stability of intelligence quotient (IQ) over time and found no significant differences between groups at baseline and follow-up [8]. Differences in intelligence were recognizable within groups; children with symptomatic epilepsy having a significantly lower IQ than children with idiopathic epilepsy. The authors noted a decrease in IQ in a minority of children with epilepsy (CWE, 11%) associated with a decrease of IQ by 10 or more points attributable to earlier age of onset of epilepsy, frequent seizures, and drug toxicity. Further drug toxicity, specifically phenobarbital, predicted decreases in IQ better than poor seizure control [8].

Lindgren et al. [18] found that general IQ did not differ between children with rolandic epilepsy (RE) and healthy classmate controls. Children with RE also did not differ from controls across measures of immediate memory, reading comprehension, reading speed, and spelling. At the initial evaluation, children with RE had greater difficulties with memory and learning of auditory-verbal material, delayed recall, measures of executive functioning, and word comprehension; however, these differences did not persist at follow-up leading investigators to conclude at nearly 5 years post-onset, that children with RE do not have major cognitive declines compared to controls.

Also extending beyond a focus on only intelligence and aiming to understand educational predicaments of CWE, Oostrom et al. [17] compared CWE to healthy classmate controls across various components of cognition. CWE obtained significantly lower scores across measures of attention, reaction time, location learning, and academic skills at all follow-up time points (3 and 12 months). Contrary to findings by Bourgeois et al. [8], these findings could not be explained by epilepsy features within group.

3.2 Present review of child and adolescent literature

The present primer reviews seven case-control longitudinal studies identified since reviews by Dodrill [6] and Seidenberg and colleagues [7]. Of these seven studies, four utilized the same cohort [10,20,22,23]. As such, the most recent and encompassing article from each will be included in this chapter as part of the review [10]. What proceeds is a discussion of domain-specific findings in five articles new to this literature. Significant findings were noted across a number of cognitive domains, including intelligence, academic achievement, executive function, and motor function. Full summation of these studies is presented in Table 3.

Child and adolescent cognitive abilities were evaluated using a wide variety of domains and related tests including: intelligence (Wechsler Intelligence Scale for Children [WISC]—Revised, Coloured Progressive Matrices, Standard Progressive Matrices, WISC—Revised [Dutch edition], Wechsler Abbreviated Scale of Intelligence [vocabulary, matrix reasoning], Kaufman Brief Intelligence Test); academic achievement (Wide Range Achievement Test); executive function (Delis-Kaplan Executive Function System [Confirmed Correct Sorts, Color-Word Interference Test-Inhibition], Connors

Continuous Performance Test-II, Colour Trails I and II, Balloon Piercing); memory (word span forward and backward, learning locations, Everyday Memory Questionnaire, WISC [Fourth Edition], Wide Range Assessment of Memory and Learning [Second Edition], Detroit Tests of Learning Aptitude-Revised, Benton Revised Visual Retention Test); motor function (WISC—Revised [coding subtest], Reaction Time [Vienna Test System], Grooved Pegboard, WISC [Third Edition, digit symbol-coding]).

3.2.1 Intelligence

Three of the four newly reviewed studies included measures of intelligence across test-retest intervals ranging from 3 months to 6 years 10,16,19]. Two of these studies found children with idiopathic and genetic generalized epilepsies to perform significantly worse than sibling and healthy children controls in direct case-control comparison [16] and stand in contrast to previously reviewed studies indicating no prospective differences between groups in IQ [8,18]. Bailet and Turk [16] assessed children across three test sessions with an unspecified amount of time between sessions. The epilepsy-control group effects on IQ were noted to be significantly lower than siblings for the first two sessions only. These comparisons, though concluded to indicate pervasive cognitive deficits, are not formal prospective changes. Investigations have found epilepsy severity, earlier age of onset and seizure type to be insignificant predictors poor performance across domains of intelligence [16]. Rathouz et al. [10] did not find significant differences or prospective changes in IQ across time. The remaining study did not explicitly report findings from intelligence measures [19].

3.2.2 Academic achievement

Across three testing sessions administered by Bailet and Turk [16], CWE performed worse than controls across all three sessions on measures of reading and spelling and only performed worse than controls at the third session on measures of arithmetic, suggesting variable group differences at individual time points, leading the authors to conclude persistent academic difficulties were present. Dunn et al. [21] found baseline reading and math scores to be comparable with follow-up at 36 months indicating deteriorating performance. Writing performance was significantly worse at baseline and follow-up with prospective decline. Consistent with Bourgeois et al. [8], earlier age of epilepsy onset and symptomatic/cryptogenic etiology were identified as risk factors for worse performance [21].

Rathouz et al. [10] found statistically significant differences only across measures of arithmetic computation while elemental academic skills, including word reading and spelling, were less affected. Further, these impairments, though present at baseline, remained stable with no progressive decline up to 6 years following baseline evaluation. General trends across these three studies measuring academic achievement indicate that CWE performed worse than control participants at the various time points but with no significant change over time. These findings are in the context of different populations of epilepsy examined and different measures of academic performance.

3.2.3 Executive function

Recent studies continue to examine executive abilities of CWE. Though previously reviewed studies [18] suggest positive and comparable performance across executive functioning between CWE and controls, others find sustained attention and response inhibition to be vulnerable domains [10,19]. While Oostrom and colleagues [19] found CWE to maintain poor attentional abilities throughout follow-up, Rathouz et al. [10] only recognized differences in response inhibition and attention at baseline. The baseline impairments remained stable over time and did not appear to worsen or decline across subsequent evaluations.

3.2.4 Memory

Two studies found CWE to have deficits compared to control participants across measures of verbal, visual, everyday, working, and short-term memory [16,19]. One of these studies recognized static group differences at two of three assessment points over the course of 3 or more years, finding CWE to have worse immediate verbal and visual recall [16]. Progressive decline was also found in memory span for words [19]. These findings occur in the context of test-retest intervals ranging from 3 months to 3.5 years and varying assessments across studies. Poorer performance at follow-up was associated with pre-diagnostic learning history [19].

3.2.5 Motor function

Additionally, findings suggest impairments in motor and psychomotor function among CWE that persist over time but are not progressive. Bailet and Turk [16] found CWE to have worse psychomotor speed than controls at test sessions one and two, but not at the third, indicating no progressive decline. Rathouz et al. [10] found fine motor dexterity and psychomotor speed to be vulnerable areas of cognitive development at baseline with abnormalities that persisted, but stable and not progressively worsening over time.

In summary, across these investigations, CWE tended to perform worse than control participants at their initial assessments, sometimes but not always assessed near the onset of their epilepsy, across the areas of intelligence, academic achievement, executive function, memory, and motor function. These impairments are noted across varying retest intervals (3 months–6 years), assessment measures, and types of epilepsy. Frank declines were observed in intelligence [20,23], executive function [19], and academic achievement [17,20–22]. Otherwise, nonprogressive cognitive abnormalities predominated.

4. Adult studies

4.1 Summary of previously reviewed adolescent and adult literature

In Dodrill's [6] initial review, he found that, compared to the pediatric literature, adult studies included and examined a more diverse group of cognitive domains and tests (8 of 13 studies examined other cognitive domains in addition to IQ) with longer test-retest intervals (1–10 years). Similar to studies assessing cognition in childhood epilepsy, the adult studies examined by Dodrill often did not provide specific details with regard to seizure type or frequency, with limited exceptions. Taken together, the findings were felt to be mixed, demonstrating a mild correlation between epilepsy and cognitive decline. For the studies reporting seizure frequency, seizures were related to adverse effects on verbal and visual memory, attention, executive function, and intellectual function (with gain in IQ associated with improved seizure control).

In the Seidenberg et al. review [7] it was noted that, overall, the pattern of cognitive change exhibited by the epilepsy group could be described as "a lack of or less improvement compared to the controls [lack of practice effect from test-retest], rather than an absolute level of decline." However, several studies reported objective decline in multiple cognitive domains, which were found to be most dramatic for verbal memory, attention, and psychomotor speed.

4.2 Present review of adult literature

Results from nine longitudinal investigations with adults (Table 3) revealed progressive changes in verbal memory, attention, processing speed, and higher order executive functions. Five hundred twenty-seven individuals with epilepsy (e.g., partial, generalized, and mixed) and their controls (410) were followed and measured cognitive changes between 1- to 10-year periods.

Cognitive abilities were evaluated using various assessments divided into specific cognitive domains including: IQ (Wechsler Adult Intelligence Scale [WAIS], WAIS-Revised, WAIS-III, Wechsler Abbreviated Scale of Intelligence, Wechsler Test of Adult Reading, Raven's Progressive Matrices); achievement (Wide Range Achievement Test), global cognitive status (Dementia Rating Scale, DRS); attention/psychomotor speed (WAIS-R, Digit Span, Digit Symbol, Trail Making Test [Parts A and B], Binary Choice Reaction Time, and Computerized Visual Search Task); memory (Wechsler Memory Scale [WMS], WMS-III, Rey Auditory Verbal Learning Task, Claeson-Dahl Learning and Retention test, Cronholm-Molander Memory Test, Adult Memory and Information Processing Battery, Auditory Verbal Learning Test, Rey Complex Figure Test [RCFT] Delayed Recall, and the Warrington Recognition Memory Test [RMT]—Words and RMT-Faces); visuospatial/constructional abilities (RCFT); executive functions (Wisconsin Card Sorting Test, Stroop-Interference Test, WMS-III, Working Memory, and Executive Interview Test); language (Graded Naming Test, Graded Faces Test, Boston Naming Test, Controlled Oral Word Accentuation Test,

FAS, animal fluency, and Token Test), and motor abilities (Grooved Pegboard). The Halsted-Reitan Neuropsychological Battery was utilized in only one study [25].

4.2.1 Memory

Five studies involving individuals with partial, generalized, and mixed epilepsy were followed for a period between 1 and 10 years demonstrating prospective declines in verbal memory [25,26,28–30]. Stable verbal memory performance was noted in four studies [11,24,27,29]. Andersson-Roswall [28] considered verbal memory declines to be the strongest association of epilepsy in a partial epilepsy cohort. Lower levels of verbal memory performance were also evident at baseline [28]. Worse verbal memory performance was associated with early onset in newly diagnosed and chronic left temporal lobe epilepsy individuals with secondary generalizations, but without noted decline over time [24]. Griffith et al. [29] found older adults with chronic partial epilepsy to perform lower on verbal memory measures than controls at baseline, but without evidence of a progressive verbal memory decline. Another cohort with transient epileptic amnesia demonstrated evidence of accelerated forgetting at baseline, with most individuals demonstrating improvements in recent autobiographical memory, but not in remote memory [11]. Two prospective studies (total of 81 subjects) with localization-related epilepsy were followed between 4 and 10 years demonstrating an association of status epilepticus with prospective changes in visual memory scores [25,26]. Two other cohorts demonstrated stability in visual memory performances [11,27].

4.2.2 Intelligence

Differences in IQ scores in individuals with status epilepticus have also been found in the literature. Two studies found changes in IQ scores over time [9,25]. One study found prospective changes in verbal IQ [9] and another in overall intelligence (e.g., WAIS FSIQ) [25].

4.2.3 Attention/processing speed

Attention and processing speed are domains particularly associated with progressive declines in individuals with epilepsy. Two studies demonstrated declines in attention [27,28], psychomotor speed [28,30], and processing speed [28]. Conversely, Griffith et al. [29] found no progressive changes in attentional measures (e.g., DRS) in a cohort of older adults over time. Attentional measures in this study were part of a cognitive screener, which may not be sensitive to more subtle cognitive changes.

4.2.4 Executive functions

Declines in executive functions were evident in three longitudinal studies of epilepsy [26,29,30]. A study with older adults revealed lower performance in cognitive function at baseline, but these declines were not considered progressive. Declines were evident in executive control [29]. Baker et al. [30] found declines in mental flexibility.

Hermann et al. [26] reported changes in aspects of executive functions over a 4-year interval. In this study, 12%–25% of individuals exhibited adverse cognitive outcomes, with declines associated with abnormalities in baseline quantitative magnetic resonance volumetrics, lower intellectual capacity, longer duration of epilepsy, and older chronological age [26].

Overall, results of these nine studies are indicative of longitudinal changes (1–10 years) in individuals with epilepsy, particularly in verbal memory, attention, processing speed, and higher order executive functions.

4.2.5 Limitations

The current review focused on controlled prospective studies, which examined the cognitive trajectory of adults and adolescents with epilepsy. Though previous concerns regarding lack of control groups and, in turn, the ability to speak to conclusions about cognitive progression [7] were addressed, this compilation of studies is considered in the context of several methodological limitations identified the literature. First, the utilization of multiple and varied assessments to measure similar domains across studies serves to limit direct comparison of findings. While a standardized assessment battery across centers would certainly prove difficult to implement, it would certainly facilitate comparison of results across studies, particularly in long-term follow-up. Second, modest test–retest intervals continue to be seen in the reviewed articles. Several researchers [6,10,21,26] have acknowledged that perhaps longer durations of time must pass in order to fully characterize the possible extent of adverse effects of epilepsy on cognitive function. Third, with the exception of two studies [9,21], participant group sizes tend to be less than 100 individuals, perhaps limiting generalizability of findings outside the research context and across epilepsy types. Accounting for these limitations is essential in looking towards future directions of prospective studies on neuropsychological functioning of adults and CWE.

We remain with the general view that cognitive decline does occur in some patients with epilepsy; this is the exception rather than the rule. More common are static abnormalities over time, lack of practice effects, or lack of normal development in pediatric patients. Compared to other fields of investigation (aging, preclinical Alzheimer's disease, schizophrenia), controlled prospective neuropsychological research in epilepsy remains arguably rudimentary. Those fields show the importance of multiple assessments (>2) to rule out chance and transient declines of uncertain etiology, longer follow-up intervals, greater consideration of other important predictor variables (e.g., baseline health status, neuroimaging status), and use of advanced metrics to identify reliable change. Research of this type is complicated and expensive and requires the dedicated participation of persons with epilepsy. This is clearly an important clinical issue requiring substantial economic investment and collaboration across investigators and centers to undertake a big data approach to conclusively answer an empirical question first addressed in 1924 and of clinical concern far before that time.

Appendix

Table 4 Uncontrolled prospective pediatric studies

Study	(N) Seizure type	Age	Mean retest interval	Cognitive domains examined	Key results
Fox [12]	130 unspecified epilepsy syndrome	5–17	1 year (1922 vs. 1923)	IQ	General tendency toward deterioration
Patterson and Fonner [31]	128 unspecified epilepsy syndrome		98 cases (51 boys, 47 girls) were tested twice; 30 cases (12 boys, 18 girls) tested three times	IQ	IQ variable over time (in either positive or negative direction)
Fetterman and Barnes [32]	46 unspecified epilepsy syndrome	Not provided	21 months	IQ	No decided trend. Conjectured changes no different than those that would be found in healthy individuals
Sullivan and Gahagan [33]	103 organic (definite or questionable), idiopathic (undifferentiated or psychogenic), or unspecified epilepsy syndrome		1 month–4 years 11 months (average interval 14 months)	IQ	IQ scores varied in positive or negative direction
Kugelmass et al. [34]	129 idiopathic epilepsy		Varied from 3 months to 3 years	IQ	Trend toward deterioration in unimproved group
Tenny [35]	284 unspecified epilepsy syndrome	Not provided	Not provided	IQ	IQ scores varied in positive or negative direction. The negative change

Continued

Table 4 Uncontrolled prospective pediatric studies—cont'd

Study	(N) Seizure type	Age	Mean retest interval	Cognitive domains examined	Key results
Rodin et al. [36]	64 unspecified epilepsy syndrome	Initially between ages 5 and 16	At least 5 years (mean 9.6 years, range 5–33 years)	IQ	in IQ was somewhat more marked in pupils whose seizures were increased in frequency than for those whose seizures were unchanged, decreased, or controlled Verbal, performance, and FSIQ scores slightly lower but insignificant at follow-up. IQ insignificantly rose in children with controlled seizures, while IQ insignificantly fell in children with uncontrolled seizures
Aldenkamp et al. [37]	45 generalized epilepsy, partial (left or right), or multifocal epilepsy	Assessed at mean ages of 9.3, 10.5 (only 20), and 13.5 years	Mean follow-up 4.2 years (range from 2.1 to 9.8 years)	IQ	Stable pattern of cognitive performance—mean full scale, verbal, and performance IQs did not yield significant increase or decrease. Following subtests consistently yielded lower scores: information, coding, digit span, vocabulary

Study	Epilepsy type	Age at onset	Assessment interval	Cognitive domains	Findings
Metz-Lutz and Filippini [38]	44 rolandic epilepsy (RE)	Onset between 4 and 7 years	Twice yearly; WISC every 18 months	Language, visuospatial/constructional, memory, executive function	Atypical group had significantly lower FSIQ and verbal IQ than typical group. Slower reaction times
Northcott et al. [39]	42 RE	3–15 years	Varied: 17 between 12 and 18 months; 8 between 18 and 24 months; 3 at longer intervals (2+, 3+, 5+ years)	IQ, memory, academic achievement, processing speed, language, executive function	Improvement in verbal memory, receptive language ability, and phonemic manipulation. No change in visual memory and aspects of phonologic awareness. Improvements were not related to the clinical variables
Prevost et al. [40]	21 frontal lobe epilepsy	Mean age of onset 6.7 (+/− 3.9)	9.4+/− 3.5 years	Not specified	No clear outcome data provided
Berg et al. [41]	198 West syndrome, benign partial epilepsy of childhood with centrotemporal spikes (BECTS), childhood absence epilepsy, myoclonic-atonic, nonsyndromic with focal features, generalized or mixed epilepsy, and unspecified epilepsy syndrome	Onset <8	8–9 years	IQ	Pharmacoresistance associated with 11.4 point lower FSIQ. IQ correlated with age of onset in pharmacoresistant group

Continued

Table 4 Uncontrolled prospective pediatric studies—cont'd

Study	(N) Seizure type	Age	Mean retest interval	Cognitive domains examined	Key results
van Iterson et al. [42]	113 generalized, focal, bilateral or multifocal, and unspecified epilepsy syndrome	4–15 years	Varied based on need for reassessment	IQ	Downward progression. Later age of onset associated with greater decline in verbal performance at follow-up
Reuner et al. [14]	76 idiopathic epilepsy	6–17 years	3 months	Attention, executive function (EpiTrack Junior®)	Children with new onset epilepsy have prospective impaired performance compared to controls but better performance than children with chronic epilepsy. Unknown etiology or unclassified is predictor for prospective decline incognitive functions even before antiepileptic treatment

Table 5 Uncontrolled prospective adult studies

Adult studies without controls

Study	(N) Seizure type	Age	Mean retest interval	Cognitive domains examined	Key results
Barnes and Fetterman [13]	35 idiopathic, organic, birth trauma, postencephalitic, alcoholic, glandular, hysterical epilepsy	15–52 years	1 year	IQ, verbal memory	Duration of epilepsy, with chronological age and number of attacks held constant, was determined to be a significant factor in "loss of efficiency," in people with epilepsy
Somerfeld-Ziskind and Ziskind [43]	100 unspecified epilepsy syndrome	3–58 years	1 year	IQ	No impairment noted in cognition after one year. No perceptible difference in IQ
Arieff and Yacorzynski [44]	27 nonorganic epilepsy	16–68 years	1–10 years	IQ, verbal memory	Patients with organic epilepsy as a group show definite deterioration by 6 IQ points between first and last test
Yacorzynski and Arieff [45]	63 mixed epilepsy	10–57 years	1–7 years	IQ	Eight patients showed a significant increase in IQ between the first and final tests. One patient showed a significant decrease in IQ. No relationship between reduction in number or severity of seizures and the changes in IQ
Falk et al. [46]	85 mixed epilepsy	23–63 years	9–14 years	IQ	No evidence of cognitive deterioration was found except in the case of three psychotic patients

Continued

Table 5 Uncontrolled prospective adult studies—cont'd

Adult studies without controls

Study	(N) Seizure type	Age	Mean retest interval	Cognitive domains examined	Key results
Hilkevitch [47]	66 idiopathic epilepsy	8–53 years	Not reported	IQ	Negligible degree of deterioration and much variability during institutionalization. Difference in IQ approximately 4 points between test 1 and 2 means. 17 (65.4%) individuals had a stable or improved IQ on retest. Average of 19–point drop in IQ in 9 (34%) deteriorated cases. Tendency for lower IQ to be related to more frequent attacks; seizure frequency related to change in IQ
Seidenberg et al. [48]	58 partial elementary, partial complex, partial secondarily generalized, absence, tonic-clonic	Mean age 22	18.6 months for seizures improved group (SI); 19.4 months for seizures unimproved group (SU)	IQ, motor speed, processing speed, memory	Retest revealed that 9 of 14 WAIS scores of SI were significantly higher than the SU. Changes in seizure frequency were associated with changes on the test–retest scores. Decrease more likely to be found on VIQ

Study	Epilepsy type	Age	Follow-up	Cognitive domains	Findings
Trimble [49]	240 tonic-clonic, complex partial, spike-wave, unspecified epilepsy syndrome	20–57 years	Not reported	IQ	Decline in IQ (15%), mean fall was 21.3. IQ deterioration related to medication use—phenytoin and serum folic acid. 21 (70%) of 30 demonstrated IQ deterioration greater than 15 points. Seizure type, head injury, and AED linked to deterioration
Dodrill and Wilensky [50]	198 unspecified epilepsy syndrome	16+ years	5 years	IQ, attention, executive function, memory, processing speed, language	For performance IQ, no statistically significant difference could be found with respect to any single group over time using the student t statistic. This study did not find evidence that sustained administration of AEDs was associated with cognitive losses over time
Selwa et al. [51]	47 temporal lobe epilepsy (TLE)	Mean age surgical group: 31; nonsurgical group: 30	1–8 years	IQ, memory (verbal and visual)	Little change occurs in measurable memory or IQ of medically managed TLE patients over relatively long time
Holmes et al. [52]	35 intractable complex partial epilepsy	16–59 years	10 years	IQ, attention, executive function, memory,	For most adults with medically intractable complex partial epilepsy, there were no general changes in IQ

Continued

Table 5 Uncontrolled prospective adult studies—cont'd

Adult studies without controls

Study	(N) Seizure type	Age	Mean retest interval	Cognitive domains examined	Key results
				processing speed, language	or neuropsychological functioning after 10 years. Neuropsychological test scores remain reasonably stable over the decade
Bjornaes et al. [53]	34 mixed epilepsy (17 children, 17 adults)	Mean age children: 10; adults: 24	3.5 years (children) and 6.0 years (adults)	IQ	In the children, there was a decline in mean IQ scores during the test-retest interval, while the IQ scores increased in the adult group. Recurrent seizures may represent a considerable risk for intellectual decline in children, while intellectual functioning seem to be less vulnerable in adults with early onset epilepsy
Pai and Tsai [54]	64 partial and nonpartial, symptomatic and idiopathic/ cryptogenic	Mean age high education: 32; low education: 45	1 year	Memory, attention, executive function, language, visuospatial/ constructional	Decline: attention, mental manipulation Improvement: verbal fluency. No change: memory, language, abstract thinking, orientation, drawing

Thompson and Duncan [55]	136 mixed epilepsy	Mean age baseline: 31; follow-up: 44	10 years	IQ, memory, language, executive function	Decline: all domains Frequency of GTCS was strongest predictor of decline. Complex partial seizure frequency was associated with decline in memory and executive skills but not in IQ. Periods of remission were associated with better cognitive outcome
Taylor and Baker [56]	50 newly diagnosed and previously untreated partial, generalized, and unspecified epilepsy syndrome	Baseline: 15–78 years; follow-up: 21–84 years	5 years	Psychomotor speed, memory, executive function, mood, subjective report of cognitive complaints	Decline: reaction time, verbal memory. Trend for worse performance on serial recognition of words, information processing, and computerized visual search. Trend toward improvement on serial recognition of figures and inhibition
Mameniškienė et al. [15]	33 TLE	30–66 years	13 years	Psychomotor speed, attention, verbal (verbal and visual)	No significant change in most domains. Nonverbal memory declined

References

[1] Scheffer IE, Berkovic S, Capovilla G, Connolly MB, French J, Guilhoto L, Hirsch E, Jain S, Mathern GW, Moshe SE, Nordli DR, Perucca E, Tomson T, Wiebe S, Zhang YH, Zuberi SM. ILAE classification of the epilepsies: position paper of the ILAE commission for classification and terminology. Epilepsia 2017;58(4):512–21.

[2] Berrios GE. Memory disorders and epilepsy during the nineteenth century. In: Zeman A, Kapur N, Jones-Gotman M, editors. Epilepsy and memory. United Kingdom: Oxford University Press; 2012. p. 51–9.

[3] Esquirol PE. Des maladies mentales: considérées sous les rapports médical, hygiénique et médico-legal. Paris: Chez J.B. Baillière; 1838.

[4] Bouchet C, Cazauvieilh G. De la epilepsie considérée dans ses rapports avec l'alienation mentale: recherches sur la nature et le siège de ces deux maladies. Arch Gen Med 1825;9:510–42.

[5] Gowers WR. Epilepsy and other chronic convulsive disorders: their causes, symptoms, & treatment. London: J & A Churchill; 1881.

[6] Dodrill CB. Neuropsychological effects of seizures. Epilepsy Behav 2004;5:S21–4.

[7] Seidenberg M, Pulsipher DT, Hermann BP. Cognitive progression in epilepsy. Neuropsychol Rev 2007;17:445–54.

[8] Bourgeois BFD, Prensky AL, Palkes HS, Talent BK, Busch SG. Intelligence in epilepsy: a prospective study in children. Ann Neurol 1983;14(4):438–44.

[9] Dodrill C, Wilensky A. Intellectual impairment as an outcome of status epilepticus. Neurology 1990;40 (Suppl. 2):23–7.

[10] Rathouz PJ, Zhao Q, Jones JE, Jackson DC, Hsu DA, Stafstrom CE, Seidenberg M, Hermann BP. Cognitive development in children with new onset epilepsy. Dev Med Child Neurol 2014;56 (7):635–41.

[11] Savage S, Hoefeijzers S, Milton F, Streatfield C, Dewar M, Zeman A. The evolution of accelerated long-term forgetting: evidence from the TIME study, Cortex 2017;1–21. [cited 2017 June 25], https://doi.org/10.1016/j.cortex.2017.09.007.

[12] Fox JT. The response of epileptic children to mental and educational tests. Br J Med Psychol 1924;4 (3):235–48.

[13] Barnes MR, Fetterman JL. Mentality of dispensary epileptic patients. Arch Neurol Psychiatr 1938;40 (5):903–10.

[14] Reuner G, Kadish NE, Doering JH, Balke D, Schubert-Bast S. Attention and executive functions in the early course of pediatric epilepsy. Epilepsy Behav 2016;60:42–9.

[15] Mameniškienė R, Rimšienė J, Puronaitė R. Cognitive changes in people with temporal lobe epilepsy over a 13-year period. Epilepsy Behav 2016;63:89–97.

[16] Bailet LL, Turk WR. The impact of childhood epilepsy on neurocognitive and behavioral performance: a prospective longitudinal study. Epilepsia 2000;41(4):426–31.

[17] Oostrom KJ, Smeets-Schouten A, Kruitwagen CLJJ, Boudewyn Peters AC, Jennekens-Schinkel A. Not only a matter of epilepsy: early problems of cognition and behavior in children with "epilepsy only"—a prospective, longitudinal, controlled study starting at diagnosis. Pediatrics 2003;112 (6):1338–44.

[18] Lindgren Å, Kihlgren M, Melin L, Croona C, Lundberg S, Eeg-Olofsson O. Development of cognitive functions in children with rolandic epilepsy. Epilepsy Behav 2004;5(6):903–10.

[19] Oostrom KJ, van Teeseling H, Smeets-Schouten A, Peters ACB, Jennekens-Schinkel A. Three to four years after diagnosis: cognition and behaviour in children with 'epilepsy only'. A prospective, controlled study. Brain 2005;128(7):1546–55.

[20] Hermann BP, Jones JE, Sheth R, Koehn M, Becker T, Find J, et al. Growing up with epilepsy: a two-year investigation of cognitive development in children with new onset epilepsy. Epilepsia 2008;49 (11):1847–58.

[21] Dunn DW, Johnson CS, Perkins SM, Fastenau PS, Byars AW, deGrauw TJ, Austin JK. Academic problems in children with seizures: relationships with neuropsychological functioning and family variables during the 3 years after onset. Epilepsy Behav 2010;19(3):455–61.

[22] Almane D, Jones JE, Jackson DC, Seidenberg M, Koehn M, Hsu DA, Hermann BP. Brief clinical screening for academic underachievement in new-onset childhood epilepsy: utility and longitudinal results. Epilepsy Behav 2014;43:117–21.

[23] Lin JJ, Dabbs K, Riley JD, Jones JE, Jackson DC, Hsu DA, Stafstrom CE, Seidenberg M, Hermann BP. Neurodevelopment in new-onset juvenile myoclonic epilepsy over the first 2 years. Ann Neurol 2014;76(5):660–8.

[24] Aikia M, Salmenpera T, Partanen K, Kalviainen R. Verbal memory in newly diagnosed patients with chronic left temporal epilepsy. Epilepsy Behav 2001;2:20–7.

[25] Dodrill CB. Progressive cognitive decline in adolescents and adults with epilepsy. Prog Brain Res 2002;135:399–407.

[26] Hermann BP, Seidenberg M, Dow C, Jones J, Rutecki P, Bhattacharya A, et al. Cognitive prognosis in chronic temporal lobe epilepsy. Ann Neurol 2006;60(60):80–7.

[27] Piazzini A, Turner K, Chifari R, Morabito A, Canger R, Canevini MP. Attention and psychomotor speed decline in patients with temporal lobe epilepsy: a longitudinal study. Epilepsy Res 2006;72(2–3): 89–96.

[28] Andersson-Roswall L, Engman E, Malmgren K, Samuelsson H. Verbal cognition and attention deficits do not explain the verbal memory decline associated with pharmacoresistant partial epilepsy. Epilepsy Behav 2007;17(3):413–20.

[29] Griffith R, Martin RC, Bambara JK, Faught E, Vogtle LK, Marson DC. Cognitive functioning over 3 years in community dwelling older adults with chronic partial epilepsy. Epilepsy Res 2007;74(2–3):91–6.

[30] Baker GA, Taylor J, Aldenkamp AP. Newly diagnosed epilepsy: cognitive outcome after 12 months. Epilepsia 2011;52(6):1084–91.

[31] Patterson HA, Fonner D. Some observations on the intelligence quotient in epileptics. Psychiatry Q 1928;2(4):542–8.

[32] Fetterman J, Barnes M. Serial studies of the intelligence of patients with epilepsy. Arch Neurol Psychiatr 1934;32(4):797–801.

[33] Sullivan EB, Gahagan L. On intelligence of epileptic children. Genet Psychol Monogr 1935;17:309–76.

[34] Kugelmass IN, Poull LE, Rudnick J. Mental growth of epileptic children. Am J Dis Child 1938;55 (2):295–303.

[35] Tenny JW. Epileptic children in Detroit's special school program: a study. Except Child 1955;21 (5):162–7.

[36] Rodin EA, Schmaltz S, Twitty G. Intellectual functions of patients with childhood-onset epilepsy. Dev Med Child Neurol 1986;28(1):25–33.

[37] Aldenkamp AP, Alpherts WCJ, De Bruine-Seeder D. Test-retest variability in children with epilepsy— a comparison of WISC-R profiles. Epilepsy Res 1990;7(2):165–72.

[38] Metz-Lutz M-N, Filippini M. Neuropsychological findings in rolandic epilepsy and Landau-Kleffner syndrome. Epilepsia 2006;47(Suppl. 2):71–5.

[39] Northcott E, Connolly AM, McIntyre J, Christie J, Berroya A, Taylor A, Batchelor J, Aaron G, Soe S, Bleasel AF, Lawson JA, Bye AM. Longitudinal assessment of neuropsychologic and language function in children with benign rolandic epilepsy. J Child Neurol 2006;21(6):518–22.

[40] Prevost J, Lortie A, Nguyen D, Lassonde M, Carmant L. Nonlesional frontal lobe epilepsy (FLE) of childhood: clinical presentation, response to treatment and comorbidity. Epilepsia 2006;47 (12):2198–201.

[41] Berg AT, Zelko FA, Levy SR, Testa FM. Age at onset of epilepsy, pharmacoresistance, and cognitive outcomes: a prospective cohort study. Neurology 2012;79(13):1384–91.

[42] van Iterson L, Zijlstra BJH, Augustijn PB, van der Leij A, de Jong PF. Duration of epilepsy and cognitive development in children: a longitudinal study. Neuropsychology 2014;28(2):212–21.

[43] Somerfeld-Ziskind E, Ziskind E. Effect of phenobarbital on mentality of epileptic patients. Arch Neurol Psychiatr 1940;43(1):70–9.

[44] Arieff AJ, Yacorzynski GK. Deterioration of patients with organic epilepsy. J Nerv Ment Dis 1942;96 (1):49–55.

[45] Yacorzynski GK, Arieff AJ. Absence of deterioration in patients with non-organic epilepsy with special reference to bromide therapy. J Nerv Ment Dis 1942;95(6):687–97.

[46] Falk R, Penrose LS, Clark EA. The search for intellectual deterioration among epileptic patients. Am J Ment Defic 1945;49:469–71.

[47] Hilkevitch RR. A study of the intelligence of institutionalized epileptics of the idiopathic type. Am J Orthopsychiatry 1946;16(2):262–70.

[48] Seidenberg M, O'Leary D, Berent S, Boll T. Change in seizure frequency and test-rest scores on the Wechsler Adult Intelligence Scale. Epilepsia 1981;22(1):75–83.

[49] Trimble MR. Cognitive hazards of seizure disorders. Epilepsia 1988;29(1):19–24.

[50] Dodrill C, Wilensky A. Neuropsychological abilities before and after 5 years of stable antiepileptic drug therapy. Epilepsia 1992;33(2):327–34.

[51] Selwa LM, Berent S, Giordano B, Henry TR, Buchtel HA, Ross D. Serial cognitive testing in temporal lobe epilepsy: longitudinal changes with medical and surgical therapies. Epilepsia 1994;35(4):743–9.

[52] Holmes MD, Dodrill C, Wilkus RJ, Ojemann LM, Ojemann GA. Is partial epilepsy progressive? Ten-year follow-up of EEG and neuropsychological changes in adults with partial seizures. Epilepsia 1998;39(11):1193–8.

[53] Bjørnaes H, Stabell K, Henriksen O, Løyning Y. The effects of refractory epilepsy on intellectual functioning in children and adults. A longitudinal study. Seizure 2001;10(4):250–9.

[54] Pai MC, Tsai JJ. Is cognitive reserve applicable to epilepsy? The effect of educational level on the cognitive decline after onset of epilepsy. Epilepsia 2005;46(Suppl. 1):7–10.

[55] Thompson PJ, Duncan JS. Cognitive decline in severe intractable epilepsy. Epilepsia 2005;46(11):1780–7.

[56] Taylor J, Baker GA. Newly diagnosed epilepsy: cognitive outcome at 5 years. Epilepsy Behav 2010;18(4):397–403.

CHAPTER 14

Epilepsy and intellectual disabilities

Christian Brandt
Department of General Epileptology, Bethel Epilepsy Centre, Bielefeld, Germany

Contents

1. Definition of intellectual disability

The DSM–5 defines intellectual disability (ID) as a "disorder with onset during the developmental period that includes both intellectual and adaptive functioning deficits in conceptual, social and practical domains" [1]. Terms and definitions have been subject to change over time with further understanding but certainly also with the intent of avoiding stigmatization. The term "mental retardation" has previously been used. Nowadays, "intellectual and developmental disability" is also in use.

The intelligence quotient (IQ) is measured by intelligence tests. An ID will be diagnosed when the IQ is at least two standard deviations below the mean. See the work of Brue and Wilmshurst [2] for a framework of assessments.

2. Prevalence

The prevalence of epilepsy in the general population is about 1%. It is, however, considerably higher in persons with ID. The prevalence of epilepsy in this group varies

The Comorbidities of Epilepsy
https://doi.org/10.1016/B978-0-12-814877-8.00014-3

according to the degree of ID. Among children with mild ID, 6% also have epilepsy, 24% in severe ID, and 50% in most severe ID [3]. A meta-analysis of 46 studies led to a prevalence estimate of 22.2% in persons with ID [4]. The prevalence of epilepsy varies also according to the complexity of the disability. In adults with cerebral palsy, 13% suffer from epilepsy. It is 25% in persons with autism, 26% in persons with mental retardation, and 40% in those with a coexistence of all three. The prognosis of epilepsy in persons with epilepsy and ID is worse than in those with normal intelligence. Nevertheless, seizure freedom may be achieved. Among 675 persons with epilepsy living in a long-term residential care institution, 36% were seizure-free [5]. Once again, there was an association with the severity of ID; the rate of seizure freedom was 44% in persons with borderline intelligence, 39% in those with mild ID, 33% in moderate ID, 32% in severe ID, and 22% in profound ID. It can be speculated that persons living in residential care have more difficult epilepsies than those living in the community so that prognosis might be better in the latter group. Mortality is already higher in people with epilepsy than in the general population with a standardized mortality ratio (SMR) of 1.6–3, but even higher in those with epilepsy plus ID or cerebral palsy. The SMR ranges from 7 to 50 in this group [6]. Frequent causes of death are pneumonia and seizure-related deaths, such as sudden unexpected death in epilepsy (SUDEP). SUDEP is actually the second most common cause of death in persons with epilepsy and ID after respiratory diseases [7]. There is no clear evidence whether the risk of SUDEP is increased in persons with epilepsy and ID. Among 49 studies assessing risk factors for SUDEP, 23 considered this question, and 14 of those concluded that coexisting ID was a SUDEP risk factor [8]. No study found ID to be a protective factor against SUDEP. The suicide risk, however, seems to be lower in persons with epilepsy and ID as compared to those with epilepsy and normal intelligence. The SMR from suicide was 0.3 in a large study on the causes of death in persons with epilepsy and mild developmental disabilities [9]. Generally, life expectancy has considerably increased over the last years in persons with ID [10]. It is nearly the same as in the general population in persons with milder ID [10].

3. Approach to persons with epilepsy and ID

As with epilepsy, the ID deserves as well accurate diagnostics including assessing its degree and etiology. Patients with this comorbidity demonstrate special needs on encounters with the medical professions. They may have limited verbal skills, behavior disorder (see further in this chapter), and additional physical handicaps. Their capability to adapt to the situation of an appointment at the clinics or even to an inpatient stay may be limited. Health care providers (HCPs) will need more time for a consultation as usual, and interaction with relatives and caregivers is crucial. This applies to history taking as well as to planning and performing diagnostics and to shared decision-making with regard to treatment. Relatives may be medical lay persons but are usually "experts" on the patient's history, disease, personality, and behavior. Nevertheless, it is important to address the patient directly wherever possible. Interactions among different medical specialists, such as neurologists, psychiatrists, and orthopedic surgeons, are necessary. Institutions are quite often not adequately equipped to cater for the needs of persons with ID, and training of doctors may be insufficient. Self-management programs are available for persons with epilepsy and ID and may improve epilepsy-related knowledge, even seizure frequency, and quality of life [11]. Examples of such programs are the German Psycho-Educative Programme about Epilepsy (PEPE; http://www.bethel-regional.de/psycho-edukatives-programm-epilepsie.html) or the English version with the same name (https://www.epilepsysociety.org.uk/pepe-facilitator-training#.WyllwC35yb8).

A consensus group working on the management of adults with epilepsy and an ID prioritized 11 guideline areas using a modified Delphi process [12]. Seven out of these concerned either epilepsy treatment and/or behavioral issues. Two were related to differential diagnosis and access to diagnostic methods, and one was related to comorbidity.

4. Diagnostics

With regard to diagnostics, as always in medicine, careful history-taking is the first step. This is especially important as misdiagnosis of epilepsy as nonepileptic, for instance behavioral events, is frequent among persons with ID [13]. Physical examination is essential in order to identify somatic comorbidities. Neuroimaging is often only possible under general anesthesia. Therefore, the relation between expected benefits and risks has to be assessed. Accurate MRI diagnostics are essential when epilepsy surgery is considered, but it may also be helpful in order to discriminate between an alleged etiology (e.g., "perinatal brain damage" as a diagnosis out of cluelessness) and a structural brain lesion of other cause (e.g., focal cortical dysplasia). In case of unknown etiology, genetic examinations should be considered. Array CGH or panel diagnostics may be helpful in establishing a diagnosis. This may assist with finding an appropriate treatment option (see further in this chapter) or with genetic counseling of the patient or family members. It may also be helpful for families to finally find a diagnosis when long-standing uncertainty about the etiology caused enduring distress. It is important to obtain informed consent from the patient or legal guardian. Besides medical obligation, this may be subject to national law. Considerable scientific progress has been achieved in recent years in medical genetics, and further steps may be expected.

5. Comorbidities

This chapter is about ID as a comorbidity of epilepsy, and now there will be a subchapter of even more comorbidities. On first sight, this may appear to be a contradiction in itself. This is, however, justified and necessary as the combination of epilepsy and ID is associated with special comorbid conditions. Here we have to differentiate between comorbid conditions that may occur in persons with epilepsy and ID, in general, sometimes in interaction with antiepileptic drugs (AEDs), and those associated with specific syndromes. There is an overlap between these domains. Taking another point of view, we have to look at psychiatric/behavioral and somatic comorbidities.

Autism and attention-deficit/hyperactivity disorder have to be mentioned [14]. Challenging behavior is frequent among persons with ID. It occurs in >50% of persons with ID and is severe in about 10% [15–17]. Challenging behavior may have many different appearances. It may be verbal or physical aggression, property damage, self-injury, disruptive behavior, temper tantrums, stereotypies, and noncompliance. It is important to consider the developmental level of a person with ID in order to understand the origin of challenging behavior [18]. The Scale of Emotional Development—Short has been developed for the assessment of the emotional development in adults with ID [19]. Depression may present atypically at least in persons with severe ID.

The coexistence of epileptic and psychogenic nonepileptic seizures (PNES) is generally frequent. Study evidence about this coexistence is sparse. In a recent study among a group of persons with epilepsy and ID living in a care facility, 7.1% were also found to have PNES. Most of them were female and had a mild or moderate level of ID. Compared to persons with epilepsy and ID but no PNES, they had more depressive symptoms and negative life events and, more often, an ID profile where one domain was more impaired than the others [20]. While persons with PNES generally should be treated with psychotherapy, persons with ID may, setting aside the limited psychotherapeutic options in this group, benefit especially from a meticulous analysis of PNES-provoking circumstances and situations. Sociotherapeutic interventions may be more important than psychotherapeutic ones in a narrower sense. It is important to ask about loss of relatives, change of staff in the sheltered workshop, mental overload or underload at work, noisy mates in the residential care facility, and so on.

Physical comorbidities comprise handicaps (e.g., spasticity, CP), obesity, constipation, dental problems, respiratory infections (pneumonia), urinary tract infections, bone fractures, reflux esophagitis, nutritional problems, and so on. Some of these may be explained, at least partially, by interactions with medication effects, such as obesity (may be caused by valproate), constipation (psychotropic drugs), gingival hyperplasia (phenytoin which is, however, more rarely administered than it was years ago), osteoporosis (enzyme-inducing AEDs), and nutritional problems (topiramate, zonisamide).

Persons with epilepsy and ID may have multiple risk factors for osteoporosis [21]. They may have nutritional problems, decreased exposure to sunlight (possibly caused by lack of assistance in leaving the house), and lack of exercise (refraining from sports either because of physical handicaps or because of—often unjustified—prohibitions). Certain syndromes (e.g., Down syndrome) may have an intrinsic risk for osteoporosis. Enzyme-inducing AEDs may increase the risk further. More than 50% of persons with ID are overweight or obese; about 5% are underweight [22,23]. Overweight may be associated with specific, genetically determined syndromes, such as Prader-Willi syndrome and Down syndrome [24]. As previously stated, AED side effects have to be taken into account.

Some syndromes are associated with special constellations of comorbidities. Tuberous sclerosis complex (TSC) is a disease originating from a mutation in the TSC1 or TSC2 genes. These mutations lead to disturbances in the *mechanistic* target of rapamycin (mTOR) signaling pathway [25]. Epilepsy occurs in 80%–90% of individuals with TSC. It is, however, a multiorgan disease that may present with ID, cardiac rhabdomyomas, subependymal giant cell astrocytomas, renal angiomyolipomas, pulmonary lymphangioleiomyomatosis, thyroid nodules, bone fibrous dysplasia, and dental problems [26–29]. Neuropsychiatric comorbidity is frequent in TSC. The term "tuberous-sclerosis associated neuropsychiatric disorders" (TAND) has been coined [30]. It affects almost all persons with TSC and comprises behavioral, intellectual, and psychosocial aspects. Fifty percent of persons with TSC have an ID of varying degree [30]. About 40%–50% of persons with TSC have autism spectrum disorder, and 30%–40% suffer from attention-deficit/hyperactivity disorder [30]. Regular examinations for these comorbid conditions are recommended but are only being done for a certain proportion of patients, according to a recent study in adult patients with TSC in Germany [31]. Interdisciplinary TSC centers may be helpful in improving health care in this group of patients.

Down syndrome may be associated with congenital cardiac anomalies, visual impairment, hearing loss, dental problems, acute neurologic disorders, early-onset Alzheimer's disease (AD), and autoimmune diseases. Persons with Down syndrome may develop epilepsy in early life or—with increasing frequency along with the increasing life-expectancy—in the context of AD [32]. In the latter case, the most frequent seizure types are generalized tonic-clonic seizures and myoclonic seizures [33]. The term "late-onset myoclonic epilepsy in Down syndrome" (LOMEDS) has been coined [34] in regards to senile myoclonic epilepsy by other authors [35]. EEG recordings show generalized epileptiform discharges. Levetiracetam is frequently effective but may be associated with psychiatric side effects.

6. Treatment

6.1 Aims

Epilepsy treatment aims generally at improvement of seizure frequency—seizure freedom at best—with no or at least tolerable side effects. As previously mentioned, the chance of achieving seizure freedom is limited in persons with epilepsy and ID. Some of them will even experience multiple seizures every day. Therefore, adapted outcome criteria may be more useful. Prevention of injury by decreasing the number of drop attacks may be more important than decreasing the number of seizures in general. Improving the frequency of emergency room admissions or of status epilepticus may be equally important. Tolerability of drug treatment is especially important in those not achieving seizure freedom. Decreasing the number of administered AEDs is one way to do this.

Treatment can either be done on an outpatient or inpatient basis. The option to admit a person with epilepsy to hospital for epilepsy diagnostics and treatment is not equally available in different countries. Even in a country like Germany, where inpatient treatment over a period of some weeks is still possible, there is increasing economic pressure to shorten the duration of an inpatient stay or to do just outpatient treatment instead. It could, however, be shown in a prospective controlled study that inpatient treatment in a department with a program dedicated to persons with epilepsy and ID has several benefits, as demonstrated by a caregivers' rating scale [36]. The treatment group showed, in comparison to the control group, a highly significant improvement in the standardized GEOS-43D (total score) and in the subscales "Concerns about Seizures," "Seizure-Related Risks," and "Side Effects/Medical Treatment."

6.2 Standards of AED treatment

Generally, AED treatment in persons with ID follows the same standards and principles as in others. One problem is that persons with ID are excluded from most placebo-controlled trials. This is a measure of protection of persons who are not able to give informed consent by themselves. It means, on the other hand, that there is no real knowledge about the efficacy and safety of a newly licensed AED in this special patient group. A recent Cochrane review looked at randomized controlled trials (RCTs) and quasi-RCTs of pharmacological interventions for people with epilepsy and a learning disability [37]. Only 14 trials with 1116 probands were found. This is a number that can easily be found in a few pivotal AED trials for a given drug in the general epilepsy population. The standards of the trials varied markedly; only four reported on seizure freedom rates and eight on seizure frequency. The authors came to the conclusion that efficacy and safety of AEDs were similar in persons with epilepsy and ID as in the general epilepsy population. Behavioral adverse events (AEs), however, are not adequately assessed for in most of the RCTs. None of the RCTs assessed for cognitive AEs. Behavioral side effects of AEDs in persons with ID have been observed in open studies, sometimes retrospective ones. These were mainly side effects that were already known in persons with normal intelligence but were now more precisely defined.

Behavioral AEs have been reported for a couple of AEDs, and it seems that persons with IDs are more vulnerable in this respect [38,39]. They have even been reported in lamotrigine, which is not notorious for behavioral side effects otherwise [40]. Open studies have demonstrated behavioral AEs also under perampanel and brivaracetam [41,42]. Behavioral tolerability of AED treatment must be monitored. Standardized instruments are helpful. Behavioral changes may be assessed by administration of the Aberrant Behavior Checklist [43]. Cognitive AEs also have to be taken into account. We have shown in a study at our center that persons with ID may experience the same cognitive AEs under topiramate that may occur in persons with normal intelligence [44]. The cognitive tolerability of AED treatment has to be observed carefully. A cognitive decline might otherwise be unnoticed or attributed to the ID or to dementia but not to drug treatment. If a person is not able to undergo a formal neuropsychological examination, careful observation, for instance by occupational therapists, is helpful.

Careful physical examination, lab and imaging examinations, and taking of the history are essential as well as knowledge about possible drug-drug interactions and therapeutic drug monitoring (TDM) [45]. It is not unusual in clinical practice to see a person with loss of appetite, nausea, and vomiting who had repeated gastroscopy but no blood drawn for TDM. The establishment of methods to use other matrices than blood—for instance, saliva—for TDM would make TDM more feasible in persons who have difficulties undergoing blood draws [46]. AEs may also be mistaken as part of the ID rather than as AED side effects. Only few standardized outcome measures designed for use in persons with epilepsy and ID exist. They mainly focus on behavior, impulsiveness, functionality, cognition, and quality of life [47].

In general, as in other persons with epilepsy, enzyme-inducing AEDs should be avoided and nonsedating drugs with a favorable cognitive tolerability profile should be selected.

6.3 Orphan drugs and personalized medicine

A few drugs have been designated orphan drug status, such as stiripentol for the treatment of Dravet syndrome and rufinamide for the treatment of drop attacks in Lennox-Gastaut syndrome (LGS). LGS is a severe epileptic and developmental encephalopathy characterized by multiple seizure types, a typical electroencephalographic pattern, and ID [48]. Epilepsy in the context of LGS is usually difficult to treat, and success rates under AED are quite low [49]. Other drugs are currently under evaluation or have been studied, such as fenfluramine for the treatment of Dravet syndrome [50] and cannabidiol for Dravet syndrome or LGS [51–53]. The advances of genetics in science and clinical practice and an improved knowledge about the pathophysiology of certain syndromes have led to a dawn of personalized medicine in epileptology. This applies mainly for syndromes associated with ID. The significance of the mTOR pathway for TSC has already highlighted above. The knowledge about this pathway has led to the discovery that the mTOR-inhibitor everolimus is of benefit for the treatment of subependymal giant cell astrocytoma and renal angiomyolipoma and also, as recently shown, for epileptic seizures in TSC [54]. The response rate in a recent RCT was significantly higher for everolimus than for placebo [54], both for low-exposure and, even more, high-exposure everolimus. A strong, consistent, and highly significant relationship between everolimus exposure and efficacy has been observed [55]. Ketogenic diet is another example as it is a treatment of choice in glucose-transporter type 1 and pyruvate dehydrogenase deficiency and mitochondrial complex I defects [56].

6.4 Epilepsy surgery

Previously, persons with ID were quite often banned from epilepsy surgery as the diffuse brain damage associated with ID was believed to be an unfavorable prognostic factor. However, the presence of ID does not justify the exclusion of a patient from presurgical monitoring. A retrospective study found a comparable outcome in patients with a verbal IQ <70 and those with normal intelligence. Numbers of persons with low IQ were low in that study [57]. The prognosis of resective epilepsy surgery in persons with ID depends on the level of impairment; the higher the IQ, the better the prognosis, and vice versa. A study showed that 22% (4/18) of persons with IQ <50, 37% (20/54) of persons with IQ between 50 and 69, and 61% (228/376) of persons with IQ ≥70 became seizure-free [58]. Resective surgery is also an option in TSC. According to a meta-analysis, 57% of the included patients became seizure-free, and another 18% experienced a >90% reduction of seizure frequency [59]. Corpus callosotomy is a palliative surgical option in epilepsy patients with drop attacks. This is, for instance, of special importance for persons with LGS who suffer from frequent drop attacks causing serious injury. Corpus callosotomy has been found to be a valuable option in this patient group. Nearly 40% of patients have been reported to be free of disabling seizures (defined as drop attacks and generalized tonic-clonic seizures one year after surgery) in a small series [60]. Vagus nerve stimulation may also be considered [48].

6.5 Health status

Persons with ID display unmet health needs. Some institutional issues have been outlined in this chapter. Besides intrinsic barriers (e.g., lack of ability to adequately cooperate), persons with ID quite often face discrimination and negative attitudes [61]. Efforts have been made to improve the primary health status of persons with ID. Unmet needs may be detected by a formalized screening shown to lead to sustained benefits in health outcome [62]. Primary health care teams, specialized nurses, and other organizational matters have been introduced in the United Kingdom [63,64]. Along with the increasing life expectancy in persons with ID (see earlier in this chapter), disorders like cataract, hearing disorder, diabetes, hypertension, osteoarthritis/arthrosis, and osteoporosis are present, as well as a sedentary lifestyle [10]. As stated previously in this chapter, underweight occurs in a considerable number of persons with ID. Tube feeding via a percutaneous endoscopic gastrostomy may help if the underweight is a consequence of difficulties with swallowing. Despite initial skepticism by many relatives, this frequently leads not only to weight gain but also to more relaxed behavior of the affected person.

7. Conclusion and perspectives

ID is a frequent comorbidity of epilepsy. Epileptologists and other HCPs must be aware of the special needs of this group of patients. Epilepsy and ID presents with a special constellation of medical and psychosocial needs. There is no standard approach to this patient group. Diagnostics and treatment have to be tailored to the different forms of epilepsy, the degrees of ID, and the characteristics of defined syndromes. This may be the field where the most important advances can be expected within the next years: to find a way from a "one-fits-all" approach to personalized medicine.

References

[1] AP Association. Diagnostic and statistical manual of mental disorders (DSM-5®). American Psychiatric Pub; 2013.

[2] Brue AW, Wilmshurst L. Essentials of intellectual disability assessment and identification. John Wiley & Sons; 2016.

[3] Lhatoo SD, Sander JW. The epidemiology of epilepsy and learning disability. Epilepsia 2001;42 Suppl 1:6–9; discussion 19–20. PubMed PMID: 11422344. Epub 2001/06/26.

[4] Robertson J, Hatton C, Emerson E, Baines S. Prevalence of epilepsy among people with intellectual disabilities: a systematic review. Seizure 2015;29:46–62. PubMed PMID: 26076844.

[5] Huber B, Hauser I, Horstmann V, Jokeit G, Liem S, Meinert T, et al. Seizure freedom with different therapeutic regimens in intellectually disabled epileptic patients. Seizure 2005;14(6):381–6. PubMed PMID: 15985376. Epub 2005/06/30.

[6] Fauser S, Essang C, Altenmuller DM, Staack AM, Steinhoff BJ, Strobl K, et al. Long-term seizure outcome in 211 patients with focal cortical dysplasia. Epilepsia 2015;56(1):66–76. PubMed PMID: 25495786.

[7] Kiani R, Tyrer F, Jesu A, Bhaumik S, Gangavati S, Walker G, et al. Mortality from sudden unexpected death in epilepsy (SUDEP) in a cohort of adults with intellectual disability. J Intellect Disabil Res 2014;58(6):508–20. PubMed PMID: 23647577.

[8] Young C, Shankar R, Palmer J, Craig J, Hargreaves C, McLean B, et al. Does intellectual disability increase sudden unexpected death in epilepsy (SUDEP) risk?. Seizure, 2015;25:112–6. PubMed PMID: 25457453.

[9] Day SM, Wu YW, Strauss DJ, Shavelle RM, Reynolds RJ. Causes of death in remote symptomatic epilepsy. Neurology 2005;65(2):216–22. PubMed PMID: 16043789.

[10] Haveman M, Perry J, Salvador-Carulla L, Walsh PN, Kerr M, Van Schrojenstein Lantman-de Valk H, et al., Ageing and health status in adults with intellectual disabilities: results of the European POMONA II study. J Intellect Dev Disabil 2011;36(1):49–60. PubMed PMID: 21314593.

[11] Dannenberg M, Mengoni SE, Gates B, Durand MA. Self-management interventions for epilepsy in people with intellectual disabilities: a scoping review. Seizure 2016;41:16–25. PubMed PMID: 27447692.

[12] Kerr M, Scheepers M, Arvio M, Beavis J, Brandt C, Brown S, et al. Consensus guidelines into the management of epilepsy in adults with an intellectual disability. J Intellect Disabil Res 2009;53 (8):687–94. PubMed PMID: 19527434.

[13] Chapman M, Iddon P, Atkinson K, Brodie C, Mitchell D, Parvin G, et al. The misdiagnosis of epilepsy in people with intellectual disabilities: a systematic review. Seizure 2011;20(2):101–6. PubMed PMID: 21123090. Epub 2010/12/03.

[14] Depositario-Cabacar DF, Zelleke TG. Treatment of epilepsy in children with developmental disabilities. Dev Disabil Res Rev 2010;16(3):239–47. PubMed PMID: 20981762. Epub 2010/10/29.

[15] Kay SR, Wolkenfeld F, Murrill LM. Profiles of aggression among psychiatric patients. II. Covariates and predictors. J Nerv Ment Dis 1988;176(9):547–57. PubMed PMID: 3418328.

[16] Lowe K, Allen D, Jones E, Brophy S, Moore K, James W. Challenging behaviours: prevalence and topographies. J Intellect Disabil Res 2007;51(Pt 8):625–36. PubMed PMID: 17598876.

[17] Emerson E, Kiernan C, Alborz A, Reeves D, Mason H, Swarbrick R, et al. The prevalence of challenging behaviors: a total population study. Res Dev Disabil 2001;22(1):77–93. PubMed PMID: 11263632.

[18] Dosen A. Applying the developmental perspective in the psychiatric assessment and diagnosis of persons with intellectual disability: part I—assessment. J Intellect Disabil Res 2004;49(1):1–8. 2005/01/01.

[19] Sappok T, Barrett BF, Vandevelde S, Heinrich M, Poppe L, Sterkenburg P, et al. Scale of emotional development—short. Res Dev Disabil 2016;59:166–75. PubMed PMID: 27614275. Epub 2016/09/11.

[20] van Ool JS, Haenen AI, Snoeijen-Schouwenaars FM, Aldenkamp AP, Hendriksen JGM, Schelhaas HJ, et al. Psychogenic nonepileptic seizures in adults with epilepsy and intellectual disability: a neglected area. Seizure 2018;59:67–71. PubMed PMID: 29754013. Epub 2018/05/14.

[21] Mayer T. Besondere Bedeutung von Knochenstoffwechselstörungen bei mehrfach–behinderten Menschen mit Epilepsie. Z Epileptol 2005;18(3):178–83. 2005/08/01.

[22] Krause S, Ware R, McPherson L, Lennox N, O'Callaghan M. Obesity in adolescents with intellectual disability: prevalence and associated characteristics. Obes Res Clin Pract. 2016;10(5):520–30. PubMed PMID: 26559898. Epub 2015/11/13.

[23] Temple VA, Foley JT, Lloyd M. Body mass index of adults with intellectual disability participating in Special Olympics by world region. J Intellect Disabil Res 2014;58(3):277–84. PubMed PMID: 23331860. Epub 2013/01/22.

[24] Melville CA, Cooper SA, McGrother CW, Thorp CF, Collacott R. Obesity in adults with Down syndrome: a case-control study. J Intellect Disabil Res 2005;49(Pt 2):125–33. PubMed PMID: 15634321. Epub 2005/01/07.

[25] Curatolo P. Mechanistic target of rapamycin (mTOR) in tuberous sclerosis complex-associated epilepsy. Pediatr Neurol 2015;52(3):281–9. PubMed PMID: 25591831.

[26] Thiele EA, Granata T, Matricardi S, Chugani HT. Transition into adulthood: tuberous sclerosis complex, Sturge-Weber syndrome, and Rasmussen encephalitis. Epilepsia 2014;55 Suppl 3:29–33. PubMed PMID: 25209083.

[27] Auladell M, Boronat S, Barber I, Thiele EA. Thyroid nodules on chest CT of patients with tuberous sclerosis complex. Am J Med Genet A 2015;167A(12):2992–7. PubMed PMID: 26332136.

[28] Li P, Boronat S, Geffrey Alexandra L, Barber I, Grottkau Brian E, Thiele Elizabeth A. Rib and vertebral bone fibrous dysplasia in a child with tuberous sclerosis complex. Am J Med Genet A 2015;167 (11):2755–7. 2015/11/01.

[29] Purwar P, Sareen S, Sheel V, Gupta A, Ansari U, Becharbhai PU, et al. Gingival overgrowth leading to the diagnosis of familial tuberous sclerosis complex. Case Rep Dent 2016;2016:8195321. PubMed PMID: 26885413. Pubmed Central PMCID: PMC4738710.

[30] Curatolo P, Moavero R, de Vries PJ. Neurological and neuropsychiatric aspects of tuberous sclerosis complex. Lancet Neurol 2015;14(7):733–45.

[31] Hamer HM, Pfafflin M, Baier H, Bosebeck F, Franz M, Holtkamp M, et al. Characteristics and health-care situation of adult patients with tuberous sclerosis complex in German epilepsy centers. Epilepsy Behav 2018;82:64–7. PubMed PMID: 29587187.

[32] Pueschel SM, Louis S, McKnight P. Seizure disorders in Down syndrome. Arch Neurol 1991;48 (3):318–20. PubMed PMID: 1825777. Epub 1991/03/01.

[33] Gholipour T, Mitchell S, Sarkis RA, Chemali Z. The clinical and neurobehavioral course of Down syndrome and dementia with or without new-onset epilepsy. Epilepsy Behav 2017;68:11–6. PubMed PMID: 28109983. Epub 2017/01/23.

[34] Moller JC, Hamer HM, Oertel WH, Rosenow F. Late-onset myoclonic epilepsy in Down's syndrome (LOMEDS). Seizure 2001;10(4):303–6. PubMed PMID: 11466028. Epub 2001/07/24.

[35] De Simone R, Puig XS, Gelisse P, Crespel A, Genton P. Senile myoclonic epilepsy: delineation of a common condition associated with Alzheimer's disease in Down syndrome. Seizure 2010;19(7):383–9. PubMed PMID: 20598585. Epub 2010/07/06.

[36] Brandt C, Mueffelmann B, May T, Thorbecke R, Hopf L, Ottenottebrock H, et al. Effects of a specialized inpatient treatment program on epilepsy related impairments of patients with epilepsy and intellectual disability as rated by relatives and carers. Epilepsia 2017;58(Suppl. 5):S5–S199.

[37] Jackson CF, Makin SM, Marson AG, Kerr M. Pharmacological interventions for epilepsy in people with intellectual disabilities. Cochrane Database Syst Rev 2015 03(9):CD005399. PubMed PMID: 26333428.

[38] Helmstaedter C, Fritz NE, Kockelmann E, Kosanetzky N, Elger CE. Positive and negative psychotropic effects of levetiracetam. Epilepsy Behav 2008;13(3):535–41. PubMed PMID: 18583196. Epub 2008/06/28.

[39] Harbord MG. Significant anticonvulsant side-effects in children and adolescents. J Clin Neurosci 2000;7(3):213–6. PubMed PMID: 10833618.

[40] Beran RG, Gibson RJ. Aggressive behaviour in intellectually challenged patients with epilepsy treated with lamotrigine. Epilepsia 1998;39(3):280–2.

[41] Andres E, Kerling F, Hamer H, Kasper B, Winterholler M. Behavioural changes in patients with intellectual disability treated with perampanel. Acta Neurol Scand 2017;136(6):645–53. PubMed PMID: 28568478.

[42] Andres E, Kerling F, Hamer H, Winterholler M. Behavioural changes in patients with intellectual disability treated with brivaracetam. Acta Neurol Scand. 2018. 138(3): 195–202 PubMed PMID: 29658982. Epub 2018/04/17.

[43] Aman MG, Singh NN, Stewart AW, Field CJ. The aberrant behavior checklist: a behavior rating scale for the assessment of treatment effects. Am J Ment Defic 1985;89(5):485–91. PubMed PMID: 3993694.

[44] Brandt C, Lahr D, May TW. Cognitive adverse events of topiramate in patients with epilepsy and intellectual disability. Epilepsy Behav 2015;45:261–4. PubMed PMID: 25843340.

[45] Brandt C, May TW. Therapeutic drug monitoring of newer antiepileptic drugs. LaboratoriumsMedizin. 2011;35(3):161–9. PubMed PMID: WOS:000293164300005.

[46] Brandt C, Bien CG, Helmer R, May TW. Assessment of the correlations of lacosamide concentrations in saliva and serum in patients with epilepsy. Epilepsia 2018;59(4):e34–e9. PubMed PMID: 29450894. Epub 2018/02/17.

[47] Copeland L, Meek A, Kerr M, Robling M, Hood K, McNamara R. Measurement of side effects of anti-epileptic drugs (AEDs) in adults with intellectual disability: a systematic review. Seizure 2017;51:61–73. PubMed PMID: 28806588. Epub 2017/08/15.

[48] Cross JH, Auvin S, Falip M, Striano P, Arzimanoglou A. Expert opinion on the management of Lennox-Gastaut syndrome: treatment algorithms and practical considerations. Front Neurol 2017;8:.

[49] Nikanorova M, Brandt C, Auvin S, McMurray R. Real-world data on rufinamide treatment in patients with Lennox-Gastaut syndrome: results from a European noninterventional registry study. Epilepsy Behav 2017;76:63–70. PubMed PMID: 28927712.

[50] Ceulemans B, Boel M, Leyssens K, Van Rossem C, Neels P, Jorens PG, et al. Successful use of fenfluramine as an add-on treatment for Dravet syndrome. Epilepsia 2012;53(7):1131–9. PubMed PMID: 22554283. Epub 2012/05/05.

[51] Devinsky O, Cross JH, Laux L, Marsh E, Miller I, Nabbout R, et al. Trial of cannabidiol for drug-resistant seizures in the Dravet syndrome. N Engl J Med 2017;376(21):2011–20. PubMed PMID: 28538134.

[52] Devinsky O, Patel AD, Cross JH, Villanueva V, Wirrell EC, Privitera M, et al. Effect of cannabidiol on drop seizures in the Lennox-Gastaut syndrome. N Engl J Med 2018;378(20):1888–97. 2018/05/17.

[53] Thiele EA, Marsh ED, French JA, Mazurkiewicz-Beldzinska M, Benbadis SR, Joshi C, et al. Cannabidiol in patients with seizures associated with Lennox-Gastaut syndrome (GWPCARE4): a randomised, double-blind, placebo-controlled phase 3 trial. Lancet 2018;391:1085–96.

[54] French JA, Lawson JA, Yapici Z, Ikeda H, Polster T, Nabbout R, et al. Adjunctive everolimus therapy for treatment-resistant focal-onset seizures associated with tuberous sclerosis (EXIST-3): a phase 3, randomised, double-blind, placebo-controlled study. Lancet 2016;388(10056):2153–63. PubMed PMID: 27613521.

[55] Franz DN, Lawson JA, Yapici Z, Brandt C, Kohrman MH, Wong M, et al. Everolimus dosing recommendations for tuberous sclerosis complex-associated refractory seizures. Epilepsia 2018;59 (6):1188–97. PubMed PMID: 29727013. Epub 2018/05/05.

[56] Elia M, Klepper J, Leiendecker B, Hartmann H. Ketogenic diets in the treatment of epilepsy. Curr Pharm Des 2017;23(37):5691–701. PubMed PMID: 28799513. Epub 2017/08/12.

[57] Davies R, Baxendale S, Thompson P, Duncan JS. Epilepsy surgery for people with a low IQ. Seizure 2009;18(2):150–2. PubMed PMID: 18657450. Epub 2008/07/29.

[58] Malmgren K, Olsson I, Engman E, Flink R, Rydenhag B. Seizure outcome after resective epilepsy surgery in patients with low IQ. Brain 2008;131(Pt 2):535–42. PubMed PMID: 18063587.

[59] Jansen FE, van Huffelen AC, Algra A, van Nieuwenhuizen O. Epilepsy surgery in tuberous sclerosis: a systematic review. Epilepsia 2007;48(8):1477–84. PubMed PMID: 17484753. Epub 2007/05/09.

[60] Asadi-Pooya AA, Malekmohamadi Z, Kamgarpour A, Rakei SM, Taghipour M, Ashjazadeh N, et al. Corpus callosotomy is a valuable therapeutic option for patients with Lennox-Gastaut syndrome and

medically refractory seizures. Epilepsy Behav 2013;29(2):285–8. PubMed PMID: 24012506. Epub 2013/09/10.

[61] Ali A, Scior K, Ratti V, Strydom A, King M, Hassiotis A. Discrimination and other barriers to accessing health care: perspectives of patients with mild and moderate intellectual disability and their carers. PLoS One 2013;8(8):e70855. PubMed PMID: 23951026. Pubmed Central PMCID: PMC3741324.

[62] Cooper SA, Morrison J, Melville C, Finlayson J, Allan L, Martin G, et al. Improving the health of people with intellectual disabilities: outcomes of a health screening programme after 1 year. J Intellect Disabil Res 2006;50(Pt 9):667–77. PubMed PMID: 16901294.

[63] Melville CA, Finlayson J, Cooper SA, Allan L, Robinson N, Burns E, et al. Enhancing primary health care services for adults with intellectual disabilities. J Intellect Disabil Res 2005;49(Pt 3):190–8. PubMed PMID: 15713194.

[64] Balogh R, McMorris CA, Lunsky Y, Ouellette-Kuntz H, Bourne L, Colantonio A, et al. Organising healthcare services for persons with an intellectual disability. Cochrane Database Syst Rev 2016;4: CD007492. PubMed PMID: 27065018.

CHAPTER 15

Epilepsy and autistic spectrum disorder: Diagnostic challenges and treatment consideration

Stéphane Auvin, Blandine Dozières-Puyravel, Anna Loussouarn
Pediatric Neurology Department, Robert-Debré University Hospital, Paris, France

Contents

1. Introduction

Since Kanner, who first described a patient suffering from both autistic spectrum disorders (ASD) and epilepsy [1], many authors have argued for a strong association between autism and epilepsy [2]. Although there is a large consensus over the comorbidity of ASD and epilepsy, the estimation of the prevalence and incidence of epilepsy in patients suffering from ASD varies a lot according to the different studies. This is indeed not a highly frequent clinical situation. The diagnosis of epilepsy in ASD patients is definitively challenging because of the limits of the usual questions used in a clinical interview, the difficulties to perform electroencephalogram (EEG) recording in this population and the high frequency of abnormalities on EEG recordings.

The Comorbidities of Epilepsy
https://doi.org/10.1016/B978-0-12-814877-8.00015-5

Indeed, EEG registrations are most of the time abnormal in the ASD population, leading sometimes to some complexity in the clinical reasoning. Moreover, patients suffering from ASD are at higher risk for developing epilepsy as compared to the general population, and they are often subjected to EEG recordings. In most of the situations, epileptiform abnormalities are found without seizures. For some authors, EEG abnormalities might be correlated to clinical characteristics such as regression or risk of seizure occurrence. For other authors, these abnormalities are incidental and do not appear to be correlated with any relevant clinical event.

This chapter begins with a review of the actual definitions of epilepsy and ASD according to the International League Against Epilepsy (ILAE) and the Diagnostic and Statistical Manual of Mental Disorders, 5th edition (DSM-V) criteria. The chapter then considers the main epidemiological findings about the relationship between ASD and epilepsy and tries to account for the variability across studies in terms of prevalence and of incidence of epilepsy in patients suffering from ASD. The third section describes the challenges of the electroclinical evaluation of ASDs suspected to have new-onset epilepsy. This chapter will also focus on the debated issue of whether EEG might be considered a biomarker in ASD. The chapter then considers again the variability in the estimations of the prevalence of abnormalities of EEG registrations in patients with ASD. Looking at the recurrence and the location of these EEG abnormalities across various recordings, the chapter then discusses whether EEG might be a useful tool to predict epilepsy in patients with ASD. The last section considers the relationship between clinical regression and epilepsy in patients suffering from ASD and discusses whether there are reasons to think that epilepsy plays a role in early childhood regression, as may be the case in Landau-Kleffner syndrome and epileptic encephalopathy with continuous spike and waves during sleep (EE-CSWS). Finally, we would present some consideration for the treatment of epilepsy in ASD patients.

2. Defining epilepsy and autistic spectrum disorders

2.1 The ILAE definition of epilepsy

According to the ILAE definition of epilepsy [3], epilepsy is a brain disease with an enduring predisposition of the brain to generate epileptic seizures defined by any of the following conditions:

— At least two unprovoked seizures occurring more than 24 h apart.
— One unprovoked (or reflex) seizure and a probability of further seizures similar to the general occurrence risk (60% at least) after two unprovoked seizures, occurring over the next 10 years.
— Diagnosis of an epilepsy syndrome.

The ILAE framework for epilepsy classification distinguishes three levels of classifications [4]. First, seizure types are classified as focal onset, generalized onset, or unknown onset. Second, epilepsies are classified by the seizure type previously identified as focal, generalized, or combining generalized and focal seizure types. A third step consists of characterizing the epilepsy syndromes, when a specific epilepsy syndrome can be pointed out. Along each step, the classification tries to identify one or several etiological factors, according to therapeutic considerations, such as genetic, structural, metabolic, immune, infectious, or unknown etiology [4].

2.2 The DSM-V definition of autism

ASD was first defined by Kanner as a disorder characterized by Wing's "triad of impairments" consisting of: (1) qualitative impairment in social interactions; (2) qualitative impairment in communication; and (3) restricted repetitive and stereotyped patterns of behavior, interests, and activities [1]. The definition of the DSM is actually quite close to Kanner's definition.

According to this definition, the diagnosis of ASD relies on the following criteria:

A. Persistent deficits in social communication and social interaction across contexts, not accounted for by general developmental delays, and manifest by all three of the following:

   1. Deficits in social-emotional reciprocity.

   2. Deficits in nonverbal communicative behaviors used for social interaction.

   3. Deficits in developing and maintaining relationships.

B. Restricted, repetitive patterns of behavior, interests, or activities as manifested by at least two of the following:

   1. Stereotyped or repetitive speech, motor movements, or use of objects.

   2. Excessive adherence to routines, ritualized patterns of verbal or nonverbal behavior, or excessive resistance to change.

   3. Highly restricted, fixated interests that are abnormal in intensity or focus.

   4. Hyper- or hyporeactivity to sensory input or unusual interest in sensory aspects of environment.

C. Symptoms must be present in early childhood (but may not become fully manifest until social demands exceed limited capacities).

D. Symptoms together limit and impair everyday functioning.

3. Epilepsy and ASD: Epidemiological considerations

3.1 Prevalence of epilepsy in ASD patients

Although there is an important variability in the estimation of the degree at which the risk of epilepsy is increased for patients suffering from ASD [5], there is a large consensus over the fact that the prevalence of epilepsy in ASD is more important than in the general population. Indeed, whereas the prevalence of epilepsy in the general population is about

1%, it tends to be of 6%–30% in the population suffering from ASDs [2, 6]. It is estimated at 7% in preschoolers with ASD and have been reported to increase up to 20%–35% in adulthood [2].

This variability in the estimation of prevalence of epilepsy in ASD patients can be explained by several methodological considerations. Some studies included secondary autism in addition to primary autism, whereas others focused only on primary autism [5]. This is a possible major bias since the prevalence of epilepsy in primary and secondary autism ranges from 12% to 61%, the latter having thus a 5 to 1 relative risk for developing epilepsy [7]. This difference in terms of prevalence even lead Pavone et al. to relativize the influence of autism on the risk of developing epilepsy, suggesting that this risk might be more related to associated comorbidities and brain dysfunctions of autistic patients than to autism itself. Furthermore, some studies included febrile seizures that have an incidence of 3%–5% in the general population resulting in a risk of overestimating the prevalence of epilepsy [5]. Finally, different estimations of prevalence might rely on differences in the definition of epileptic seizures themselves and on methodological biases [5, 8]. Indeed, not all studies rely on the current or past ILAE definitions for epilepsy. As a matter of fact, some studies consider that an abnormal EEG following a paroxysmal event is enough to consider the diagnosis of epilepsy. However, the prevalence of epileptiform activities in patients suffering from ASD is high, that is, rising from 15% to 32% and even to 60.7% in studies based on prolonged EEG registrations [9]. It nevertheless has to be disentangled from the prevalence of epilepsy per se, given that abnormal EEGs without seizures are frequently reported [8, 10–13].

Differences in estimations of prevalence might thus rely on false positive diagnosis of epilepsy in ASD patients based on methodological difficulties. They might also rely on the existence of possibly confounding factors that represent risk factors for epilepsy in patients with ASD.

3.2 Risk factors

Three main risk factors to develop epilepsy in ASD have been described in many studies that contribute to the prevalence of epilepsy in patients with ASD. First, there is a positive correlation between age and epilepsy, the prevalence of epilepsy being higher in adolescents or young adults with ASD as compared to younger children [14, 15]. Secondly, the cognitive level is inversely associated with the risk of developing epilepsy, patients with moderate to severe mental retardation being more at risk of developing epilepsy as compared to patients with higher IQ [6, 13, 16]. Third, the degree of language disorders is correlated with the risk of epilepsy, patients with severe language disorders being more at risk [17].

Other more controversial risk factors have been described in the literature. For example, sex has been found to interact with the influence of the cognitive level on the risk of developing epilepsy [18]. In Danielsson et al. epilepsy was found more frequent in women (58% versus 32% in male) [18]. On the contrary, a meta-analysis conducted by Amiet et al. on data extracted from published reports between 1963 and 2006 on autism and epilepsy reported that the male/female ratio of autism in patients suffering from both ASD and epilepsy appeared to be close to 2 to 1, whereas a ratio of 3.5 to 1 was found in patients without epilepsy [6].

Another controversial risk factor is the socio-economical status. It would be inversely correlated to the risk of developing epilepsy according to some authors [19].

3.3 Incidence

Su et al. have run two cohort studies over 10 years, from 1997 to 2008, and analyzed the data of patients newly diagnosed as suffering from ASD or epilepsy, who had no comorbidity with epilepsy and ASD, respectively, at the moment of their diagnosis [20]. On this basis, they estimated the incidence of epilepsy in patients with ASD (and with no prior known epilepsy) of 13.7% (as compared to 1.3% in the control population), with a hazard ratio of 9.4 (95% CI: 5.5–12.7). It is to be noticed that, conversely, the incidence of ASD in patients diagnosed with epilepsy (without prior diagnosis of ASD at the moment of the inclusion again) was 3.4 versus 0.3 in patients who were not suffering from epilepsy, which corresponded to a hazard ratio of 8.4 (95% CI: 6.2–11.4) [20].

Another study to estimate the incidence of epilepsy in patients with primary ASD was also conducted on 130 patients with primary ASD diagnosed in childhood. They ran a 10-year follow-up study based on annual clinical and electrophysiological evaluations of the patients age 18–35 years. Epileptic seizures and epilepsy were defined according to the ILAE criteria. Of the 130 autistic patients screened, 33 (25%) displayed epileptic seizures at one point of their evaluations, with an onset of epilepsy defined from 8 to 26 years old. It is to be noticed that 61% of patients in the group who manifested epilepsy had epileptic discharges without seizures before the onset of epilepsy [16].

Given these confounding factors and methodical difficulties in the estimation of the prevalence and the incidence of epilepsy in ASD patients, there is a need for epidemiological studies to further establish the exact incidence and prevalence. However, the available studies underlie the links between ASD and epilepsy, in particular on the occurrence of epilepsy in patients with ASD.

4. Electroclinical approaches for epilepsy diagnosis in ASD patients

In this context of the higher risk of epilepsy in ASD patients, physicians tend to monitor their patients on an electrophysiological point of view. The problem is that most of the time EEG recordings are abnormal, without necessarily registering seizures. So-called epileptiform abnormalities are very hard to interpret in this context. A significant number of studies have tried to evaluate whether EEG might be a predictor of upcoming epilepsy. The following section considers what is known about the prevalence and incidence of abnormal EEG.

4.1 Prevalence of epileptiform abnormalities and seizures in EEG registrations of ASD patients

In a study on 106 patients with primary ASD only, Rossi et al. found a rate of 18.9% of patients who had paroxysmal epileptiform abnormalities, without any registration of seizures. It is to be noted that such abnormalities are much more important in this population than in the general one in which it is estimated from 1.1% to 6.8% [13] or from 2.4% to 3.5% in the pediatric healthy population [21].

Hara et al. found a similar rate of epileptiform abnormalities on their large 10-year follow-up study of 130 ASD patients. During this follow up, they examined no less than 1165 EEGs, 464 from patients with both ASD and epilepsy and 701 from patients with ASD only. They found 18% of epileptic discharges in the nonepileptic (i.e., ASD only) group. Interestingly, 61% (24/33 individuals) of the patients of the epileptic group had discharges before the onset of epilepsy [16].

The prevalence reported by Akshoomoff et al. on a population of 62 patients (49 with ASD and 11 with pervasive developmental disorders) was even higher, that is, 32% of abnormal EEG, with only 3% of seizures registrations [11]. They explain this higher rate by the fact that the population studied was older.

Those rates based on short EEG registrations might underestimate to a large extent the prevalence of EEGs abnormalities. In a retrospective study conducted from 1996 to 2005, Chez et al. analyzed 24 h ambulatory EEG data recorded from 889 patients suffering from ASD. The patients included had no genetic syndrome, brain malformation, prior medications, or clinical seizures. They found a rate of 60.7% of abnormal epileptiform activity [9]. Similarly, another retrospective study conducted on the basis of 24-h EEGs registrations of 32 patients 2 years old or more with ASD diagnosed according to the DSM-IV reported that 19 out of 32 patients (59%) had interictal epileptiform abnormalities [8]. However, Kim et al. raised attention to the fact that it is important to distinguish epileptiform from nonepileptiform and epileptiform abnormalities from seizures. Among the interictal EEGs analyzed, 31% were normal, 9% had nonepileptiform abnormalities, 22% had interictal epileptiform abnormalities, and 38% combined both nonepileptiform abnormalities and interictal epileptiform abnormalities. Furthermore, they notice that many patients who displayed epileptiform abnormalities did not have seizures during these episodes [8].

4.2 Clinical approach and diagnosis

Coming back to the ILAE definition of epilepsy [3], there are three possibilities to fit in the definition of epilepsy as described in the first section. Regarding the second point (one seizure and a risk of recurrence higher than 60%), there is no study establishing that an ASD patient with epileptiform abnormalities after a single epileptic seizure has such a risk of seizure recurrence. In other words, an ASD with a unique seizure should not be diagnosed with epilepsy regardless of the presence of any interictal abnormalities on the EEG recording.

The diagnosis of epilepsy in a patient with ASD will be made if a patient experienced at least two unprovoked seizures occurring more than 24 h apart or if it is possible to identify an epilepsy syndrome.

The first step is then to determine if the paroxysmal events that occurred in ASD patients are seizures. If the occurrence of generalized onset seizure such as clonic seizure or tonic-clonic seizure is easy to identify by the clinical interview, it might be more difficult for the focal onset seizure with impairment of the awareness. This is particularly true when there is minimal motor involvement. Some repetitive behaviors seen in ASD, such as tic-like movements or unusual stereotypic movements can be troublesome to distinguish clinically from seizures. Video recordings from the caregivers are frequently requested but there are not always helpful. Two studies are probably illustrative of these difficulties. A first study evaluated staring episodes in ASD patients by conducting a retrospective analysis of 92 EEGs of children with ASD that were below 16 years of age, and who were recorded during staring, inattentiveness, or reduced responsiveness [12]. EEG recordings were reanalyzed. No child displayed any absence or focal onset seizures with awareness impairment during these EEG recordings. Twenty-two EEGs considered abnormal by the first electrophysiologist and 70 EEGs reported as normal were analyzed again. The second look reclassified seven so-called abnormal EEG as normal. Finally, abnormalities were found in 80 patients but were most of the time nonepileptiform. Only seven children had typical epileptiform activity. The authors conclude that most of the interictal abnormalities registered are incidental and of no relevance with the clinical problem [12]. Similarly, the second study reported the data of video-EEG telemetry of 32 ASD patients [8]. Twenty-two of the 32 patients were referred for paroxysmal events looking like seizures. Of the 22 patients referred for seizure evaluation, 15 had recorded events but none was an epileptic seizure. The other seven patients had no recorded events. The nonepileptic events recorded were most frequently multiple types (14/15). Quiet staring was the most frequent event in 14/15 followed by transient arousals, limb stiffening/jerks, limb twitches during sleep, and head shaking [8]. Impaired communication, cognitive deficits, and associated repetitive stereotypic behaviors make this diagnosis certainty of seizure a major challenge.

A significant number of studies evaluate the seizure types that could be seen in ASD patients, but very few studies discuss the epilepsy syndromes that are observed. All seizure types have been reported [2]. Looking at the available study, it seems that most of the seizures are focal onset seizures, sometimes becoming bilateral tonic-clonic (formerly called secondary generalization). However, generalized onset seizures could be also observed [13, 16, 18, 22]. In a cohort of 108 young adults with ASD, 43 have been diagnosed with epilepsy; 23 of them (i.e., 55%) have been diagnosed with focal onset seizure [18]. In the younger ages, three fourths of all children with autism and epilepsy also had focal onset seizures only or in combination with other seizure types [16, 22]. Some authors have reported some patients with epilepsy with centrotemporal spikes [13]. This needs to be further studies because the number of patients is limited: 17% (4/23) of the ASD with epilepsy within a cohort of 60 patients [13]. Unfortunately, most of the studies focused only on seizure type, and we don't have a clear study establishing the epilepsy syndromes that are observed and if there is any epilepsy syndrome more specific of ASD. It is then usual to look for underlying etiologies that would consist in a brain MRI that have to be performed under generalized anesthesia in most of the patients. Based on the clinical findings, such as dysmorphic features, malformation, or intellectual disabilities, targeted genetic investigations should be considered. This could include a clinic in a rare epilepsy center, the evaluation for chromosomal duplication or deletion (e.g., CGH-array), and gene panel analysis.

5. The controversial role of epileptiform abnormalities and epilepsy in the regression of ASD patients

During a clinical interview, the regression will be evaluated by doing a list of the loss of already attained intellectual/developmental abilities. Autistic regression can be defined as a loss or significant deterioration in language, behavior, and social communicative skills in children. It occurs in patients with ASD in 30% of children [23]. This occurs most frequently at the age of 18–24 months. In some epilepsy syndromes, such as EE-CSWS and Landau-Kleffner syndrome (LKS), a regression can be also observed [24]. The regression in EE-CSWS can be observed on any cognitive function and on behavior while the regression in LKS consists in an acquired aphasia or an auditory agnosia. The regression in EE-CSWS and in LKS should be distinguished from autistic regression by clinical and paraclinical investigations.

In EE-CSWS, most of the patients have experienced few seizures around 4–5 years of age that have been easily controlled by antiepileptic drugs (AEDs). This is followed by seizure recurrence consisting in frequent multiple seizures preceding the regression around the age of 6–7 years of age. The EEG recordings at the time of the regression consist of continuous generalized spike-wave discharges during sleep [24, 25]. In ASD, the regression is most of the time observed at a younger age and is not preceded by any seizure or seizure worsening. On the behavior component, the regression in ASD involves sociability, and the ASDs patient are more prone to develop rigidity and repetitive behavior [2]. As previously stated, the EEG abnormalities are frequent in ASD and continuous generalized spike-wave discharges could be observed during sleep.

Because of some similarities, a controversial question concerns whether epileptic abnormalities and epilepsy per se might contribute to or even cause autistic regression. Many diverse data have been published about the question of their being a correlation between epilepsy and autistic or neurocognitive regression. Tuchman and Rapin reported more abnormal EEGs in patients with ASD and regression (i.e., 19%) but found no correlation between epileptic seizures per se and regression [10]. Hrdlicka et al. reported the converse result, namely, they found a relation between epilepsy and autistic regression but no correlation between epileptiform abnormalities and autistic regression [26]. By contrast with both converse results, Rossi et al. and Canitano et al. (2005) did not find correlation between clinical regression and the rate of epileptiform abnormalities or the rate of seizures registrations [13, 27]. Akshoomoff et al found no correlation either between the level of neurological dysfunction and EEG abnormalities [11]. These diverging results might rely on differences in the populations studied.

Although results on the correlation between epileptiform abnormalities or seizures and ASD are not very convincing, the idea persists in the literature that epilepsy might cause cognitive and autistic regression in ASD patients. To date, there is no report suggesting any overlap between regression in ASD and the epileptic encephalopathies with cognitive regression (i.e., EE–CSWS and LKS). A cautious clinical reasoning should be helpful to conclude either for a regression for ASD patients or a regression due to epileptic encephalopathies.

6. Treatment consideration

The aim of the treatment is to control the seizure with the medication like in any epilepsy patient. The ideal goal is to obtain total seizure freedom without clinically significant adverse effects due to AEDs. In the epilepsy population, this is achievable in more than two-thirds of the patients. In the case of epilepsy in ASDs, the incidence of pharmacoresistant epilepsy is not yet established. The frequency of seizures differs according to the studies. The seizures were mostly reported not frequent, that is, approximately one per year and controllable by AEDs by Rossi et al. [13], whereas Hara et al. found 73% pharmacoresistant epilepsy [16].

The aim of AED treatment might change over time in particular if the seizures are pharmacoresistant. Then the goal would be mainly to reduce or suppress the seizures that are the most disruptive to daily life, for example, it would be more acceptable that a patient experience two seizures a week with a short loss of awareness without any fall or any consequence than a patient facing one seizure every 2 weeks leading to the call of an ambulance each time. In other words, the aim of the treatment becomes the quality of life of the patient.

In the past 20 years, the evaluation of AEDs in both adults and children has led to the approval of more than 15 AEDs for focal onset seizure and generalized onset seizure [28, 29]. However, there is no study that explores the efficacy and safety of AEDs in the population of patients with ASDs and epilepsy. This results in a lack of evidence on the choice of AED in relation to seizure type, epilepsy syndrome, comedication, and comorbidity. The AED choice is then based on an extrapolation of the efficacy and the safety profile of the AED reported in the epilepsy population.

Despite the paucity of controlled studies, it appears as though children with epilepsy and ASDs may be at an increased risk of psychiatric or behavioral problems. The selection of an AED would then take into an account the possible worsening of psychiatric symptoms. It would also be important to take into consideration the possible role on the cognition. Then we can recommend selecting an AED with the lowest impact on cognition. Some AEDs should also be used when others have failed. Phenobarbital and topiramate would be initially avoided due to the possible impact on cognition [30, 31]. Levetiracetam and perampanel would also be initially avoided due to the risk of worsening aggression or hyperactivity [32–34]. More rarely, other psychiatric side effects, such as psychosis and autistic regression, have been reported with levetiracetam in epilepsy patients [35, 36]. A large online survey might also warn us about the risk of side effects in ASD patients with epilepsy. Although this is not a controlled study, a large number of patients have been involved in this survey (733 with both ASD and epilepsy and 290 with ASD). If the results of the survey reported that AEDs improve the seizure, the occurrence of side effects was also constantly reported with a worsening in sleep, communication, behavior, attention, and mood [37]. This special population of ASD patients with epilepsy might be more sensitive to some side effects. This needs to be further established by well-conducted studies.

AEDs have been also considered in the past as a treatment option for the psychiatric symptoms of ASDs. A meta-analysis has been performed on seven randomized controlled trials (RCTs) using valproate in three RCTs, and one RCT each of lamotrigine, levetiracetam, and topiramate. Some studies might have been underpowered, but no difference between any AED treatment and the placebo has been found for irritability/agitation or for a global behavioral improvement [38].

In conclusion, we should pay particular attention to the behavior and cognition of symptoms of ASD patients after the initiation of any AED to avoid a negative benefit-risk ratio. A full control of seizure with a dramatic change in behavior or cognitive level challenging all the efforts for the daily management is definitely not the goal of an AED treatment in this special population. There is currently evidence for the improvement of some symptoms of ASDs with AEDs. By extension, no data suggest that we should try to modify the EEG abnormalities in order to change any cognitive or behavioral abnormalities.

Some of these patients might also need comedication in particular molecules that might modulate the psychiatric symptoms. The prescription should follow the usual rules to combined drugs based on the pharmacokinetics properties and the possible drug-drug interactions. Some concerns also exist with some drugs based on a possible risk for seizure aggravation. The use of risperidone, an atypical antipsychotic medication, is possible. Despite some initial concerns, there are now several studies that did not find any significant worsening in the seizure frequency in pediatric epilepsy patients [39, 40]. Antipsychotic medications might be associated with sedation, which is not the ultimate goal of any pediatric treatment. It is possible that the combination of antipsychotic medication with an AED regimen might further increase this risk. It is then important to find a good balance between the control of some psychiatric symptoms, such as self-injurious, aggressive, or destructive behavior, the level of seizure control, and the sedation. Achieving a good balance is not always an easy task.

7. Conclusion

It now clearly established that epilepsy is more frequently observed in ASD patients than in the general population. Despite the epidemiological studies linking epilepsy and autism, the exact links between these two entities remains to be fully deciphered. In addition to the complexity of the neurobiological processes leading to the emergence of epilepsy in autism and of autism in epilepsy, it is still a challenge to confirm the diagnosis of epilepsy in ASD patients. The diagnosis of epilepsy should be based on the definition of the ILAE. The clinical interview is frequently difficult. It is then frequently difficult to confirm the nature of repetitive paroxysmal events in ASD patients even with videos of the events. If the seizure types observed in ASD patients are described in the literature, there is almost nothing on the epilepsy syndromes in ASDs, the investigations are then based on the medical history without any recommendation currently. The EEG recordings are most frequently abnormal even in ASD patients without epilepsy. The occurrence of a single seizure with an abnormal EEG recording is not enough to confirm the diagnosis of epilepsy. AED treatment is mostly based on the seizure type. In the absence of studies evaluating AEDs for seizure in ASD patients, we used to extrapolate the efficacy from the data of the general population. Patients with both ASD and epilepsy seem to easily experience cognitive or behavioral side effects of AEDs. A regular and careful evaluation of the benefit-risk ratio is then required for this special group of patients.

This chapter illustrates a lot of gaps. It would be of interest to further understand the links, if any, between the EEG abnormalities and the ASD phenotype. The identification of epilepsy syndrome in ASD would be helpful to analyze the possible underlying etiologies, to choose more appropriately the AED, and to explain the prognosis to the caregivers. Finally, the progress in the understanding of the genetic factors and the related neurobiological changes might be helpful to develop, in the future, personalized medicine treatments for some of these patients.

References

[1] Kanner L, Kanner L. Autistic disturbances of affective contact. Nerv Child 1943;2:217–50.

[2] Tuchman R, Rapin I. Epilepsy in autism. Lancet Neurol 2002;1(6):352–8.

[3] Fisher RS, Acevedo C, Arzimanoglou A, Bogacz A, Cross JH, Elger CE, et al. ILAE official report: a practical clinical definition of epilepsy. Epilepsia 2014;55(4):475–82.

[4] Scheffer IE, Berkovic S, Capovilla G, Connolly MB, French J, Guilhoto L, et al. ILAE classification of the epilepsies: position paper of the ILAE commission for classification and terminology. Epilepsia 2017;58(4):512–21.

[5] McCue LM, Flick LH, Twyman KA, Xian H, Conturo TE. Prevalence of non-febrile seizures in children with idiopathic autism spectrum disorder and their unaffected siblings: a retrospective cohort study. BMC Neurol 2016;16:245.

[6] Amiet C, Gourfinkel-An I, Bouzamondo A, Tordjman S, Baulac M, Lechat P, et al. Epilepsy in autism is associated with intellectual disability and gender: evidence from a meta-analysis. Biol Psychiatry 2008;64(7):577–82.

[7] Pavone P, Incorpora G, Flumara A, Parano E, Trifiletti RR, Ruggieri M. Epilepsy is not a prominent feature of primary autism. Neuropediatrics 2004;35(4):207–10.

[8] Kim HL, Donnelly JH, Tournay AE, Book TM, Filipek P. Absence of seizures despite high prevalence of epileptiform EEG abnormalities in children with autism monitored in a tertiary care center. Epilepsia 2006;47(2):394–8.

[9] Chez MG, Chang M, Krasne V, Coughlan C, Kominsky M, Schwartz A. Frequency of epileptiform EEG abnormalities in a sequential screening of autistic patients with no known clinical epilepsy from 1996 to 2005. Epilepsy Behav 2006;8(1):267–71.

[10] Tuchman RF, Rapin I. Regression in pervasive developmental disorders: seizures and epileptiform electroencephalogram correlates. Pediatrics 1997;99(4):560–6.

[11] Akshoomoff N, Farid N, Courchesne E, Haas R. Abnormalities on the neurological examination and EEG in young children with pervasive developmental disorders. J Autism Dev Disord 2007;37(5):887–93.

[12] Hughes R, Poon WY, Harvey AS. Limited role for routine EEG in the assessment of staring in children with autism spectrum disorder. Arch Dis Child 2015;100(1):30–3.

[13] Rossi PG, Parmeggiani A, Bach V, Santucci M, Visconti P. EEG features and epilepsy in patients with autism. Brain Dev 1995;17(3):169–74.

[14] Viscidi EW, Triche EW, Pescosolido MF, McLean RL, Joseph RM, Spence SJ, et al. Clinical characteristics of children with autism spectrum disorder and co-occurring epilepsy. PLoS One 2013;8(7):e67797.

[15] Rossi PG, Posar A, Parmeggiani A. Epilepsy in adolescents and young adults with autistic disorder. Brain Dev 2000;22(2):102–6.

[16] Hara H. Autism and epilepsy: a retrospective follow-up study. Brain Dev 2007;29(8):486–90.

[17] Ballaban-Gil K, Tuchman R. Epilepsy and epileptiform EEG: association with autism and language disorders. Ment Retard Dev Disabil Res Rev 2000;6(4):300–8.

[18] Danielsson S, Gillberg IC, Billstedt E, Gillberg C, Olsson I. Epilepsy in young adults with autism: a prospective population-based follow-up study of 120 individuals diagnosed in childhood. Epilepsia 2005;46(6):918–23.

[19] Thomas S, Hovinga ME, Rai D, Lee BK. Brief report: prevalence of co-occurring epilepsy and autism spectrum disorder: the US national survey of children's health 2011-2012. J Autism Dev Disord 2017;47(1):224–9.

[20] Su CC, Chi M, Lin SH, Yang YK. Bidirectional association between autism spectrum disorder and epilepsy in child and adolescent patients: a population-based cohort study. Eur Child Adolesc Psychiatry 2016;25(9):979–87.

[21] Cavazzuti GB, Cappella L, Nalin A. Longitudinal-study of epileptiform eeg patterns in normal-children. Epilepsia 1980;21(1):43–55.

[22] Olsson I, Steffenburg S, Gillberg C. Epilepsy in autism and autistic-like conditions—a population-based study. Arch Neurol 1988;45(6):666–8.

[23] Burack JA, Volkmar FR. Development of low-functioning and high-functioning autistic-children. J Child Psychol Psychiatry Allied Discip 1992;33(3):607–16.

[24] Auvin S, Cilio MR, Vezzani A. Current understanding and neurobiology of epileptic encephalopathies. Neurobiol Dis 2016;92:72–89.

[25] Desprairies C, Dozieres-Puyravel B, Ilea A, Bellavoine V, Nasser H, Delanoe C, et al. Early identification of epileptic encephalopathy with continuous spikes-and-waves during sleep: a case-control study. Eur J Paediatr Neurol 2018;22:837–44.

[26] Hrdlicka M, Komarek V, Propper L, Kulisek R, Zumrova A, Faladova L, et al. Not EEG abnormalities but epilepsy is associated with autistic regression and mental functioning in childhood autism. Eur Child Adolesc Psychiatry 2004;13(4):209–13.

[27] Canitano R, Luchetti A, Zappella M. Epilepsy, electroencephalographic abnormalities, and regression in children with autism. J Child Neurol 2005;20(1):27–31.

[28] Rosati A, De Masi S, Guerrini R. Antiepileptic drug treatment in children with epilepsy. CNS Drugs 2015;29(10):847–63.

[29] Rosati A, Ilvento L, Lucenteforte E, Pugi A, Crescioli G, McGreevy KS, et al. Comparative efficacy of antiepileptic drugs in children and adolescents: a network meta-analysis. Epilepsia 2018;59(2):297–314.

[30] Moavero R, Santarone ME, Galasso C, Curatolo P. Cognitive and behavioral effects of new antiepileptic drugs in pediatric epilepsy. Brain Dev 2017;39(6):464–9.

[31] Ulate-Campos A, Fernandez IS. Cognitive and behavioral comorbidities: an unwanted effect of antiepileptic drugs in children. Semin Pediatr Neurol 2017;24(4):320–30.

[32] Halma E, de Louw AJA, Klinkenberg S, Aldenkamp AP, Ijff DM, Majoie M. Behavioral side-effects of levetiracetam in children with epilepsy: a systematic review. Seizure 2014;23(9):685–91.

[33] Andres E, Kerling F, Hamer H, Kasper B, Winterholler M. Behavioural changes in patients with intellectual disability treated with perampanel. Acta Neurol Scand 2017;136(6):645–53.

[34] Juhl S, Rubboli G. Add-on perampanel and aggressive behaviour in severe drug-resistant focal epilepsies. Funct Neurol 2017;32(4):215–20.

[35] Camacho A, Espin JC, Nunez N, Simon R. Levetiracetam-induced reversible autistic regression. Pediatr Neurol 2012;47(1):65–7.

[36] Kossoff EH, Bergey GK, Freeman JM, Vining EPG. Levetiracetam psychosis in children with epilepsy. Epilepsia 2001;42(12):1611–3.

[37] Frye RE, Sreenivasula S, Adams JB. Traditional and non-traditional treatments for autism spectrum disorder with seizures: an online survey. BMC Pediatr 2011;11:37.

[38] Hirota T, Veenstra-VanderWeele J, Hollander E, Kishi T. Antiepileptic medications in autism spectrum disorder: a systematic review and meta-analysis. J Autism Dev Disord 2014;44(4):948–57.

[39] Gonzalez-Heydrich J, Pandina GJ, Fleisher CA, Hsin O, Raches D, Bourgeois BF, et al. No seizure exacerbation from risperidone in youth with comorbid epilepsy and psychiatric disorders: a case series. J Child Adolesc Psychopharmacol 2004;14(2):295–310.

[40] Holzhausen SPF, Guerreiro MM, Baccin CE, Montenegro MA. Use of risperidone in children with epilepsy. Epilepsy Behav 2007;10(3):412–6.

CHAPTER 16

Epilepsy and mood disorders

Marco Mula
Institute of Medical and Biomedical Education, St George's University of London and Atkinson Morley Regional Neuroscience Centre, St George's University Hospitals NHS Foundation Trust, London, United Kingdom

Contents

1. Introduction

Depression is the most frequent psychiatric comorbidity in epilepsy, and the close relationship between these two disorders was first observed, more than 2000 years ago, by the Greek physician Hippocrates who reported that "melancholics ordinarily become epileptics, and epileptics, melancholics: what determines the preference is the direction the malady takes; if it bears upon the body, epilepsy, if upon the intelligence, melancholy" [1]. Since then, the approach to neuropsychiatric problems of epilepsy has changed many times, but the last few decades have seen an increased interest in this subject. This is also captured by the new definition of epilepsy as a disorder of the brain characterized not only by recurrent seizures but also by its neurobiological, cognitive, psychological, and social consequences [2].

The Comorbidities of Epilepsy
https://doi.org/10.1016/B978-0-12-814877-8.00016-7

Many reasons, which are both biological and psychosocial, can explain the close relationship between epilepsy and depression. Epilepsy is still today a highly stigmatized condition, leading to discrimination and/or marginalization; it is a chronic disorder with significant social limitations (e.g., driving license loss); the unpredictable nature of epileptic seizures and the social embarrassment potentially associated with them can lead to poor self-esteem, social withdrawal, isolation, and demoralization [3]. Nevertheless, the relationship between epilepsy and depression also has clear neurobiological underpinnings. In fact, neuroimaging studies of depression outside epilepsy have revealed a brain network of depression involving brain areas that overlap with those involved in temporal lobe epilepsy, namely the amygdala and the hippocampi.

Although depression is a frequently encountered problem, it is still underdiagnosed and undertreated unless it is severe enough to cause major problems or disability. This is due to multiple factors, including the patients' reluctance to volunteer spontaneously mental health issues, a paucity (or total lack) of a specific training of neurologists to recognize and manage psychiatric problems, and a lack of time in very busy outpatient clinics. There are now data clearly suggesting that depression is an important prognostic marker in epilepsy as it is associated not only with poor quality of life [4] but also with antiepileptic drug (AED) resistance [5, 6], increased seizure severity [7], increased side effects of AEDs [8], increased risk of accident and injuries [9], poor outcome after epilepsy surgery [10], and increased mortality [11].

The aim of this chapter is to provide an overview of the epidemiological data about epilepsy and depression and to discuss main clinical problems associated with diagnosis and treatment of mood disorders in the context of epilepsy.

2. Epidemiology
2.1 Studies in adults

Depression is a common condition affecting between 5% and 10% of the general population [12]. Cross-sectional epidemiological studies are showing a uniformly increased prevalence of depression among adult people with epilepsy with rates very similar to those of the general population only among seizure-free patients [13], while the prevalence is definitely higher than that in unselected samples (between 17% and 22%) [14], and it is up to 55% in patients with drug-resistant epilepsy [15]. In general terms, these figures partially reflect the severity of the underlying seizure disorder not only in terms of psychosocial difficulties but also in terms of brain dysfunction. However, cross-sectional studies provide useful public health information about the size of the problem but they have significant limitations, such as the inability to test hypotheses that might explain the co-occurrence of the two conditions. Conversely, studies of incident cohort cases with epilepsy or with depression are able to explore the time order of the relationship. In fact, a number of studies are now suggesting that the relationship between epilepsy and depression is not necessarily unidirectional, but patients with depression per se are at increased risk of developing epilepsy. Data from the UK General Practice Research Database show that the incidence rate ratio of depression is significantly higher in the three years preceding the onset of epilepsy [16]. A population-based study in Sweden shows that the age-adjusted odds ratio for the development of epilepsy is 2.5 for patients with a depressive disorder [17]. Other three population-based studies confirm that patients with a depressive disorder have a three to seven times increased risk to develop epilepsy [18–20]. All these data taken together clearly suggest either that some patients with depression develop epilepsy as part of the "natural course" of the depressive disorder or that depression may represent a premorbid phase of some epileptic syndromes. Further insights are provided by neurobiological studies of depression or epilepsy and are discussed in the following section.

2.2 Studies in children

Epidemiological studies in children with epilepsy are still limited because depression has been historically investigated in the context of adult epilepsies. However, a number of studies are now showing that depression and anxiety disorders are more frequent in children with epilepsy as compared to the general pediatric population. A long-term prospective study in newly diagnosed children with epilepsy followed for up to 9 years reported a 13% prevalence of depression [21]. A large US survey showed depression in 8% of children with current epilepsy, 7% of children with a previous history of seizures, and 2% of controls [22], and similar figures are reported by a UK community-based study of children with epilepsy 5–15 years of age attending schools in Sussex [23]. As already suggested by cross-sectional studies in adults, the prevalence of depression in children seems to reflect the severity of the underlying seizure disorder as mood and anxiety disorders seem to be more common in those with low IQ, language delays, and lower scores on neuropsychological assessment [24–26]. This is further supported by the observation that neurotypical (normal neurologic, cognitive, and imaging examinations) young adults with childhood-onset epilepsy do not present increased rates of psychiatric disorders [27].

But the relationship between depression and epilepsy in children is even more complex than that as many psychological factors are implicated as compared to adults. A US study pointed out that the adolescent attitude toward epilepsy and an external or unknown locus of control correlate strongly with depression [28]. The adverse effect of seizures on the family, limited emotional support, poor communication, inadequate support of child autonomy, and maternal depression are also relevant contributors to anxiety and depression in children with epilepsy [28–30]. It is therefore evident that apart from neurobiological variables, social variables, stigma, and parental attitudes play an important role, and for all these reasons, continuous screening and tailored multidisciplinary approaches including psychotherapy, occupational, and vocational therapy are needed.

Finally, it is important to point out the key role of anxiety disorders in the pediatric population. It is well established outside epilepsy that anxiety disorders are more common in children than in adults [31, 32], but it is also established that an anxiety disorder in childhood is associated with an increased risk of other psychiatric conditions, such as attention-deficit/hyperactivity disorder (ADHD), conduct disorder [33], and further psychiatric problems during adulthood. In fact, 50% of adults with depression have a history of anxiety before the age of 15 [34]. Data on anxiety disorders of children with epilepsy and the potential relationship with depression and ADHD are lacking and further studies are urgently needed, but it seems evident that any screening and prevention program in children with epilepsy should greatly focus on anxiety.

3. Neurobiological basis of the comorbidity between epilepsy and depression

Despite the large number of studies investigating the links between epilepsy and depression, the neurobiological basis of this bidirectional relationship hasn't been entirely clarified. As already pointed out, both depression and temporal lobe epilepsy see a disruption in the same brain networks, but this is obviously not enough to explain the associations and, most importantly, the observed temporal relationship. Results from basic science studies in animal models of epilepsy or depression seem to suggest a few potential hypotheses (Table 1).

Serotonin dysfunction has historically dominated the neurobiology of depression for decades, but it now seems evident that this is also present in epilepsy. In fact, low serotonin levels have been reported in animal models of epilepsy, such as genetically epilepsy-prone rats [35], pilocarpine status epilepticus model in Wistar rats [36], and Rhesus monkeys [37]. A deletion of the 5-HTC2 receptor subunit lowers the threshold for

Table 1 Hypothetical neurobiological contributors to the relationship between epilepsy and depression

Serotonin neurotransmission dysfunction	Reported in animal models of epilepsy, including epilepsy-prone rates, pilocarpine status epilepticus model in Wistar rats and Rhesus monkeys
	Deletion in 5-HTC2
– Low serotonin levels – Dysfunction in serotonin receptors	Downregulation of 5-HT1
Hyperactivation of HPA axis	Acceleration of kindling process
	Reduction of CA3 neuronal cells
Plastic brain changes	Reduction in hippocampal volumes
	Reduction in cortical thickness in frontal lobes, cingulate gyrus, rostral, and caudal orbitofrontal cortex

5-HT, serotonin receptor; CA, cornus ammonis; HPA, hypothalamic-pituitary-adrenal.

audiogenic seizures in mouse models of epilepsy [38] while reduced postsynaptic and increased presynaptic density of 5-HT1 receptors have been documented in animal models of epilepsy and depression [39]. It is, therefore, tempting to speculate that a progressive dysfunction in serotonin neurotransmission is responsible for the occurrence of both conditions. However, in such a case, it would be important to identify a specific threshold in serotonin loss leading to depression or spontaneous seizures and in which serotoninergic pathways are more likely to be responsible for depression or seizures.

Another potential biological explanation for the relationship between epilepsy and depression would be related to the effect of stress on limbic areas. The role of the hypothalamic-pituitary-adrenal (HPA) axis in depression is well established. However, several authors are now supporting a similar role in the neurobiology of epilepsy. In fact, pretreatment with corticosterone accelerates the kindling process in rats [40], and high cortisol levels can promote cortical hyperexcitability through effects on neurotransmitters, including glutamate, serotonin, and GABA. In fact, in animal models of depression, high cortisol levels interfere with neurogenesis of granule cells in the dentate gyrus and lead to a progressive reduction in the total number of CA3 neuronal cells [41]. Still, a number of authors are reporting that patients with depression without epilepsy present with a 10%–20% bilateral decrement in the hippocampal volumes [42], decreased cortical thickness in the frontal lobe, and decreased glial/neuronal cell density in the cingulate gyrus, rostral, and caudal orbitofrontal cortex and dorsal prefrontal cortex [43, 44]. Interestingly, many of these changes have also been reported in patients with chronic temporal lobe epilepsy [45].

Despite the amount of data showing a shared pathophysiology between epilepsy and depression, it is still unknown why only some patients develop the two disorders. One possibility is that the complex reorganization of brain circuits leading to the two conditions occur in predisposed individuals and such a predisposition is due to a combination of genetic background and environmental stressors [45]. The diathesis-stress model represents a potential explanation for the interaction between psychiatric disorders and epilepsy. According to this model, if the combination of the background predisposition and stress exceeds a threshold, the subject will develop specific disorders [46]. The diathesis-stress model has been historically used to explain schizophrenia or mood disorders [47], but it can easily be applied to this context as well, explaining why some patients develop only epilepsy or only depression or both depending on the individual combinations of predisposing factors and environmental contributors/stressors.

4. Clinical aspects

The first step in the management of depression in epilepsy is to dissect out the various potential contributors, such as psychosocial issues, treatment-emergent adverse effects of the AEDs or neurobiological factors directly related to the seizures or the epileptic disorder. In fact, different contributing factors may need different approaches, including psychotherapy, counseling, antidepressant drugs, and changes in AEDs. The practicality of classifying psychiatric symptoms according to their temporal relation to seizure occurrence (peri-ictal/para-ictal symptoms vs. interictal symptoms) is well established, and it can help clinicians in identifying concomitant contributors (Table 2).

Peri-ictal phenomena have been well described by many authors [48, 49] and distinguishing between peri-ictal and interictal psychiatric symptoms has relevant implications in terms of management.

4.1 Peri-ictal mood symptoms

Historically, it has been reported that some patients may present mood swings or irritability lasting hours to days before a convulsion [50]. More systematic studies showed that up to 30% of patients with focal epilepsies can report a variety of premonitory symptoms [51]. However, pre-ictal psychiatric symptoms are still a matter of debate and their neurobiology is still unclear.

Ictal depression has been occasionally reported and, according to some authors, can be seen in 1% of patients with temporal lobe epilepsy [52]. It is characterized by an extremely intense anhedonia, feelings of guilt and/or suicidal ideation, completely out of context and lasting for a few seconds or minutes with preserved awareness. No lateralizing or localizing value identified. Ictal fear or ictal panic is definitely more frequent than ictal depression, and it has a strong localizing and lateralizing value [53], being associated with

Table 2 Mood symptoms in relationship to seizures

Peri-ictal depression	Pre-ictal	Dysphoric moods or insomnia up to 24 h before a convulsion (reported by up to 30% of patients with TLE but still controversial)
	Ictal	Rare (less than 1% of patients with focal seizures). No lateralizing or localizing value identified
	Postictal	Up to 18% of patients (data from monitoring unit)
		Consider also postictal mood worsening in patients with interictal depression
Para-ictal depression	Forced normalization	Rare but reported (prevalence unknown)
Interictal depression	Comorbid DSM-5 mood disorders	Major depressive disorder
		Persistent depressive disorder
	Other clinical entities	Interictal dysphoric disorder

DMS, Diagnostic and Statistical Manual of Mental Disorders; *TLE*, temporal lobe epilepsy.

the right mesial temporal lobe structures [54], and some authors suggested a possible association with a poor seizure outcome after epilepsy surgery [55].

Postictal depressed mood and postictal worsening of depression are also reported. A case series in a monitoring unit show that up to 18% of patients can report depressive symptoms lasting more than 24 h [56]. Interestingly, contropolar mood changes such as manic/hypomanic symptoms are reported postictally by a similar proportion of patients (i.e., 22%) but are often associated with psychotic symptoms [56]. Postictal mania has a stronger localizing value than postictal depression, and it seems to be associated with frontal electroencephalogram (EEG) discharges and nondominant hemisphere involvement [57].

Postictal anxiety is reported by 45% of patients and can last variably from 6 h to more than 24 h but in one third of cases is reported by people with a preexisting anxiety disorder and, in this specific subgroup, should be considered a postictal worsening or exacerbation rather than postictal manifestations.

4.2 Phenomenology of interictal depression

The phenomenology of interictal depression has been a matter of debate for many years. Although it is established that patients with epilepsy can develop mood disorders that are clinically identical to those of patients without epilepsy [58], several authors have pointed out that mood disorders in epilepsy can be characterized by atypical features that are poorly reflected by conventional classificatory systems, such as the Diagnostic and Statistical Manual of Mental Disorders (DSM) and International Classification of Diseases [59, 60]. Historically, both Kraepelin and Bleuler have reported that patients with epilepsy can develop a pleomorphic pattern of depressive symptoms intermixed with euphoric moods, irritability, fear, and anxiety as well as anergia, pain, and insomnia [61]. This formulation has been subsequently rejuvenated by Blumer who coined the term "interictal dysphoric disorder" (IDD) to refer to a peculiar somatoform-depressive disorder claimed as typical of patients with epilepsy [62]. Modern studies pointed out that such a condition can be diagnosed in up to 12% of patients, but it is not specific of epilepsy per se, as it can also be diagnosed in other neurological disorders [60]. As pointed out by Blumer, it is indeed characterized by mood instability and a significant component of comorbid anxiety (social phobia and/or generalized anxiety disorder) [60], but peri-ictal mood symptoms are probably responsible for some of the atypical and pleomorphic features of this condition [63].

In conclusion, it seems evident that interictal depression in epilepsy is characterized by a large spectrum of manifestations due to a number of factors, namely the high rates of comorbidities with anxiety disorders, the presence of peri-ictal symptoms, the presence of cognitive problems due to the underlying neurologic condition, and the psychotropic effect of AEDs. All these elements have to be taken into account when diagnosing mood disorders in epilepsy.

4.3 Diagnosing depression in epilepsy

The complex phenomenology of interictal depression clearly suggests the use of clinical instruments validated in the epilepsy population. A number of well-known rating scales for depression have now been validated in people with epilepsy including the Beck Depression Inventory, the Hamilton Rating Scale for Depression (HRSD), and the Hospital Anxiety and Depression Scale [64]. For example, the Beck Depression Inventory has been validated in the epilepsy setting against the Structured Clinical Interview for Axis I DSM disorders (SCID-I), showing good sensitivity (93%), acceptable specificity (81%), an excellent negative predictive value (98%), and a low positive predictive value (47%) [65]. The issue of a low positive predictive value seems to be a common problem for clinical instruments for depression as shown for the HRSD. The HRSD was validated against the Mini-International Neuropsychiatry Interview (MINI) Plus, showing a sensitivity of 94%, a specificity of 80%, a negative predictive value of 99%, and a positive predictive value of 46% [66]. The Neurological Disorder Depression Inventory for Epilepsy (NDDIE) is the only clinical instrument specifically developed for patients with epilepsy [67]. It is currently one of the most popular screening instruments because it is short and easy to use. In addition, it has the advantage of being constructed specifically to minimize confounding factors, such as adverse events related to AEDs or cognitive problems associated with epilepsy. The NDDIE showed a specificity of 90% and a sensitivity of 81% [67]. In addition, the NDDIE has been also validated as a suicidality screening tool showing a sensitivity of 84% and a specificity of 91% [68].

In general terms, it is evident that all clinical instruments used outside epilepsy show a low positive predictive value. This is partially due to the small sample size of validation studies, but it is also related to the pleomorphic and atypical phenomenology of interictal depression. For this reason, a number of authors tried to develop clinical instruments tailored on these atypical manifestations. Among structured interviews, an adapted version of the SCID-I, named SCID-E, has been suggested [69], and a specific epilepsy questionnaire to be used with the MINI, called the Epilepsy Addendum for Psychiatric Assessment, has been also developed [70]. However, the relative benefits of these various instruments, in the assessment of generic psychopathology in community-based studies, are the subject of considerable debate.

There are a couple of questionnaires for the assessment of the IDD. The Seizure Questionnaire [71] contains an inquiry for the eight key symptoms of the IDD. Patient and next of kin answer them jointly and the examiner, for completeness and accuracy, then reviews all answers. Another questionnaire, developed mainly for research purposes, named Interictal Dysphoric Disorder Inventory, has been also developed [60]. The reliability of these questionnaires has been debated. The pleomorphic nature of the IDD itself along with the issue of peri-ictal symptoms make the development of an epilepsy-specific clinical instrument quite challenging.

5. Depression as a treatment-emergent adverse event

5.1 Depression and antiepileptic drugs

Historically, the emergence of depressive symptoms during AED treatment has been linked mainly with GABAergic drugs. Subsequently, it became evident that several AEDs can be responsible for treatment-emergent depressive symptoms [72], and within this literature the concept of forced normalization has been revived. The forced normalization phenomenon is the sudden improvement or even normalization of EEGs in people with intractable epilepsy who then develop psychiatric symptoms, very often a psychotic episode, but depressed mood has also been reported [73].

It is now established that the effect of AEDs is not only restricted to the modulation of cortical excitability but they also modulate systems that regulate mood and behavior [74]. It is also established that AEDs are associated with treatment-emergent behavioral problems that are reported not as frequently as in epilepsy, when AEDs are used in other conditions, such as pain, migraine, or movement disorders [75]. As already suggested, the AEDs most frequently associated with depression are those modulating GABAergic neurotransmission like tiagabine, topiramate, and vigabatrin, but other drugs with a completely different mechanism of action, like levetiracetam, have shown similar effects [72]. It has been reported that about 8% of patients with drug-resistant epilepsy develop treatment-emergent psychiatric adverse events regardless of the mechanism of action of the individual AED, and this is apparently driven by an underlying individual predisposition [76]. In patients with epilepsy, a dysfunction in the temporolimbic structures and the presence of a psychiatric comorbidity represent the fertile ground on which these paradoxical reactions develop [72], further reinforcing the importance of periodic screening for psychiatric disorders in order to identify patients at risk.

The rapidity of the titration rate of an AED is another relevant variable. In fact, even if it is true that some compounds seem to be more frequently associated with behavioral problems than others [72, 74, 77], it is also established that the rapidity of the titration can significantly increase the likelihood to develop treatment-emergent psychiatric problems [78, 79]. A retrospective study in a large cohort of consecutive patients treated with topiramate shows that while a previous history of depression is associated with a 3.5-times increased risk of developing depression as a treatment-emergent adverse event, the use of a rapid titration schedule on top of a previous history of depression is associated with a 23-fold increased risk [80]. For this reason, individualized titration schedules should be adopted in different patients in order to minimize the risk of treatment-emergent psychiatric adverse events.

5.2 Depression after epilepsy surgery

Despite the amount of published case series of postsurgical psychiatric complications, our understanding of these conditions is still limited. The majority of studies agree that depressive symptoms can be identified in about 10%–30% of patients at three months after epilepsy surgery [81, 82]. The phenomenology of postsurgical depression seems to be quite variable. While interictal depression often appears more with dysthymic or dysphoric features, postoperative depression seems to be more persistent, more severe, and more frequently associated with clear anhedonic features as compared to interictal depression [82]. Other patients may present with physical and mental asthenia with avoidance behavior and social withdrawal but no typical anhedonic features [83]. For all these reasons careful clinical monitoring after surgery is usually recommended. The majority of studies suggest that patients with a preexisting depressive disorder are at increased risk developing psychiatric complications, but further data are needed in order to identify patients at risk, especially regarding de novo psychiatric complications.

6. Suicide in epilepsy

In Western countries, suicide represents the 11th cause of death and the 2nd in the group aged 25–34 years, but in patients with epilepsy, the overall risk of committing suicide is almost three times higher than that of the general population. Several studies tried to understand why people with epilepsy are at high risk as the presence of depression does not seem to account entirely for such an increased risk [84]. As already discussed at the beginning of this chapter, the relationship between psychiatric disorders and epilepsy is quite complex and also for suicide, epidemiological studies have pointed out a clear bidirectional relationship with an already increased risk before the onset of the epilepsy [20]. Some authors have suggested a link with temporal lobe epilepsy [85], but others found no association with epilepsy-related variables [86].

During the last 10 years, the issue of suicide in epilepsy has been linked with AEDs as potentially responsible for such an increased risk [87]. It seems now evident that there are no robust data supporting a causal role for AEDs, although clinicians should always consider treatment-emergent psychiatric adverse events during AED treatment [88]. Suicide prevention strategies are increasingly recognized in tertiary epilepsy clinics, and possible screening instruments have been suggested [68].

7. Treatment issues

Evidence based data on treatment of depression in epilepsy is still limited and relies heavily on clinical experience. The only double-blind trial on antidepressants in epilepsy was published 30 years ago and compared nomifensine, amitriptyline, and placebo [89]. Since then, a number of open studies in small samples of unselected patients with different epilepsy types have been published (i.e., sertraline, citalopram, reboxetine, mirtazapine, and fluoxetine) [90]. One study is of particular interest because it is the only published study in children and adolescents with epilepsy and depression [91]. All these antidepressants seem to be effective and well tolerated, but due to the lack of controlled data, the Epilepsy Foundation [92] and the International League Against Epilepsy [93, 94] published a number of recommendations to guide clinicians. In general terms, it is reasonable to follow internationally accepted guidelines for the treatment of mood disorders outside epilepsy, applying individual adjustments, in the individual patient, according to the epilepsy type and the potential for interactions with concomitant AEDs.

7.1 Interactions between antidepressants and antiepileptic drugs

Antidepressants are usually classified into older or classic agents, such as tricyclic antidepressants and monoamine oxidase inhibitors, and newer antidepressants, such as selective serotonin reuptake inhibitors (SSRIs), serotonin and noradrenaline reuptake inhibitors, and other antidepressants with varying mechanisms of actions.

Among first generation of AEDs, carbamazepine (CBZ), phenytoin (PHT), and barbiturates are powerful inducers of several drug-metabolizing enzymes including the CYP and the UGT systems. Valproate (VPA) has been traditionally considered a broad spectrum enzyme inhibitor on the CYPs and UGTs [90, 95]. As all these enzymes contribute to the metabolism of the majority of antidepressants, these AEDs may present pharmacokinetic interactions with antidepressants. Regarding SSRIs, first generation inducers (i.e., CBZ, PHT, and phenobarbial) seem to reduce the plasma levels of the majority of them by at least 25%, but whether this is clinically relevant depends on the individual patient. Studies on VPA are limited, but it seems that there are no clinically relevant pharmacokinetic interactions. As far as other antidepressants are concerned, inducers like CBZ, PHT, or barbiturates obviously reduce the plasma levels of mirtazapine, venlafaxine, and bupropion. This seems to be particularly evident for bupropion with up to 90% reduction in AUC when CBZ is added to a stable bupropion regime of 150 mg [90].

Compared to first-generation AEDs, new compounds have a better pharmacokinetic profile with a low risk of interactions. Oxcarbazepine and topiramate may have weak inducing properties, especially at high doses, but systematic studies are lacking. Newest drugs like levetiracetam and lacosamide have clean pharmacokinetics with very low potential for interactions.

7.2 Seizure worsening

Neurologists are often concerned by the potential risk of seizures with antidepressants. However, this was based on an a priori assumption rather than on clinical evidence [90]. The issue of drug-related seizures is quite complex, and it is not only confined to psychotropic medications as it has been described with a number of other drugs. In general terms, multiple factors have to be taken into account, and studies in animal models suggest that serotonin potentiation may even be anticonvulsant [35]. Among all antidepressants, a clear association with seizures has been established only for maprotiline, high doses of clomipramine and amitriptyline (>200 mg), and high doses of bupropion in the immediate release formulation (>450 mg) [90]. For all other antidepressant drugs, there is no clear evidence of an increased risk of seizures. If we take into account the increased risk of seizures given by the bidirectional relationship, the reported prevalence of epileptic seizures during treatment with antidepressants in patients with mood disorders [96] is even lower than the expected one, suggesting, in conclusion, that antidepressant drugs reduce the risk of seizures [90]. In this regard, it is important to bear in mind that current knowledge on seizure prevalence during antidepressant drug treatment is based on psychiatric populations, and it is still unknown whether these data can be transferred to patients with epilepsy and whether some epileptic syndromes are more at risk than others.

8. Conclusions

There no doubt that depression in epilepsy is a relevant clinical problem and that the two conditions share a complex relationship. The phenomenology of depression can be different from that seen outside epilepsy, but robust data about treatment and prognosis are still limited. Further studies are needed in order to develop specific guidelines of treatment for patients with epilepsy. Furthermore, studies on the neurobiology of this comorbidity will probably shed light on the neurobiology of epilepsy itself and may potentially lead to the development of new treatments.

References

[1] Temkin O. The falling sickness: a history of epilepsy from the Greeks to the beginnings of modern neurology. JHU Press; 1994. p.492.

[2] Fisher RS, Acevedo C, Arzimanoglou A, Bogacz A, Cross JH, Elger CE, et al. ILAE official report: a practical clinical definition of epilepsy. Epilepsia 2014;55(4):475–82.

[3] Mula M, Sander JW. Psychosocial aspects of epilepsy: a wider approach. BJPsych Open 2016;2 (4):270–4.

[4] Boylan LS, Flint LA, Labovitz DL, Jackson SC, Starner K, Devinsky O. Depression but not seizure frequency predicts quality of life in treatment-resistant epilepsy. Neurology 2004;62:258–61.

[5] Hitiris N, Mohanraj R, Norrie J, Sills GJ, Brodie MJ. Predictors of pharmacoresistant epilepsy. Epilepsy Res 2007;75(2-3):192–6.

[6] Nogueira MH, Yasuda CL, Coan AC, Kanner AM, Cendes F. Concurrent mood and anxiety disorders are associated with pharmacoresistant seizures in patients with MTLE. Epilepsia 2017;58(7):1268–76.

[7] Cramer JA, Blum D, Reed M, Fanning K. The influence of comorbid depression on seizure severity. Epilepsia 2003;44:1578–84.

[8] Mula M, von Oertzen TJ, Cock HR, Lozsadi DA, Agrawal N. Clinical correlates of memory complaints during AED treatment. Acta Neurol Scand 2016;134(5):368–73.

[9] Gur-Ozmen S, Mula M, Agrawal N, Cock HR, Lozsadi D, von Oertzen TJ. The effect of depression and side effects of antiepileptic drugs on injuries in patients with epilepsy. Eur J Neurol 2017;24 (9):1135–9.

[10] Kanner AM, Byrne R, Chicharro A, Wuu J, Frey M. A lifetime psychiatric history predicts a worse seizure outcome following temporal lobectomy. Neurology 2009;72(9):793–9.

[11] Fazel S, Wolf A, Långström N, Newton CR, Lichtenstein P. Premature mortality in epilepsy and the role of psychiatric comorbidity: a total population study. Lancet 2013;382(9905):1646–54.

[12] World Health Organization. Depression and other common mental disorders: global health estimates; 2017.

[13] Jacoby A, Baker GA, Steen N, Potts P, Chadwick DW. The clinical course of epilepsy and its psychosocial correlates: findings from a U.K. community study. Epilepsia 1996;37(2):148–61.

[14] Tellez-Zenteno JF, Patten SB, Jetté N, Williams J, Wiebe S. Psychiatric comorbidity in epilepsy: a population-based analysis. Epilepsia 2007;48(12):2336–44.

[15] Gilliam FG, Santos J, Vahle V, Carter J, Brown K, Hecimovic H. Depression in epilepsy: ignoring clinical expression of neuronal network dysfunction? Epilepsia 2004;45(Suppl. 2):28–33.

[16] Hesdorffer DC, Ishihara L, Mynepalli L, Webb DJ, Weil J, Hauser WA. Epilepsy, suicidality, and psychiatric disorders: a bidirectional association. Ann Neurol 2012;72(2):184–91.

[17] Adelow C, Andersson T, Ahlbom A, Tomson T. Hospitalization for psychiatric disorders before and after onset of unprovoked seizures/epilepsy. Neurology 2012;78(6):396–401.

[18] Forsgren L, Nystrom L. An incident case-referent study of epileptic seizures in adults. Epilepsy Res 1990;6(1):66–81.

[19] Hesdorffer DC, Hauser WA, Annegers JF, Cascino G. Major depression is a risk factor for seizures in older adults. Ann Neurol 2000;47(2):246–9.

[20] Hesdorffer DC, Allen Hauser W, Olafsson E, Ludvigsson P, Kjartansson O. Depression and suicide attempt as risk factors for incident unprovoked seizures. Ann Neurol 2006;59(1):35–41.

[21] Berg AT, Caplan R, Hesdorffer DC. Psychiatric and neurodevelopmental disorders in childhood-onset epilepsy. Epilepsy Behav 2011;20(3):550–5.

[22] Russ SA, Larson K, Halfon N. A national profile of childhood epilepsy and seizure disorder. Pediatrics 2012;129(2):256–64.

[23] Reilly C, Atkinson P, Das K, Chin R. Neurobehavioral comorbidities in children with active epilepsy: a population-based study. Pediatrics 2014;133(6):1586–603.

[24] Buelow JM, Austin JK, Perkins SM, Shen J, Dunn DW, Fastenau PS. Behavior and mental health problems in children with epilepsy and low IQ. Dev Med Child Neurol 2003;45(10):683–92.

[25] Caplan R, Siddarth P, Gurbani S, Hanson R, Sankar R, Shields WD. Depression and anxiety disorders in pediatric epilepsy. Epilepsia 2005;46(5):720–30.

[26] Austin JK, Perkins SM, Johnson CS, Fastenau PS, Byars AW, deGrauw TJ, et al. Self-esteem and symptoms of depression in children with seizures: relationships with neuropsychological functioning and family variables over time. Epilepsia 2010;51(10):2074–83.

[27] Baldin E, Hesdorffer DC, Caplan R, Berg AT. Psychiatric disorders and suicidal behavior in neurotypical young adults with childhood-onset epilepsy. Epilepsia 2015;56(10):1623–8.

[28] Dunn DW, Austin JK, Huster GA. Symptoms of depression in adolescents with epilepsy. J Am Acad Child Adolesc Psychiatry 1999;38(9):1132–8.

[29] Rodenburg R, Marie Meijer A, Dekovic M, Aldenkamp AP. Family predictors of psychopathology in children with epilepsy. Epilepsia 2006;47(3):601–14.

[30] Ferro MA, Speechley KN. Depressive symptoms among mothers of children with epilepsy: a review of prevalence, associated factors, and impact on children. Epilepsia 2009;50(11):2344–54.

[31] Franz L, Angold A, Copeland W, Costello EJ, Towe-Goodman N, Egger H. Preschool anxiety disorders in pediatric primary care: prevalence and comorbidity. J Am Acad Child Adolesc Psychiatry 2013;52(12):1294–303.

[32] Costello EJ, Egger HL, Angold A. The developmental epidemiology of anxiety disorders: phenomenology, prevalence, and comorbidity. Child Adolesc Psychiatr Clin N Am 2005;14(4):631–48.

[33] Kendall PC, Compton SN, Walkup JT, Birmaher B, Albano AM, Sherrill J, et al. Clinical characteristics of anxiety disordered youth. J Anxiety Disord 2010;24(3):360–5.

[34] Kim-Cohen J, Caspi A, Moffitt TE, Harrington H, Milne BJ, Poulton R. Prior juvenile diagnoses in adults with mental disorder: developmental follow-back of a prospective-longitudinal cohort. Arch Gen Psychiatry 2003;60(7):709–17.

[35] Kanner AM. Can neurobiological pathogenic mechanisms of depression facilitate the development of seizure disorders? Lancet Neurol 2012;11(12):1093–102.

[36] Mazarati A, Siddarth P, Baldwin RA, Shin D, Caplan R, Sankar R. Depression after status epilepticus: behavioural and biochemical deficits and effects of fluoxetine. Brain 2008;131(8):2071–83.

[37] Jobe PC. Common pathogenic mechanisms between depression and epilepsy: an experimental perspective. Epilepsy Behav 2003;4(Suppl. 3):S14–24.

[38] Brennan TJ, Seeley WW, Kilgard M, Schreiner CE, Tecott LH. Sound-induced seizures in serotonin 5-HT2c receptor mutant mice. Nat Genet 1997;16(4):387–90.

[39] Ravizza T, Onat FY, Brooks-Kayal AR, Depaulis A, Galanopoulou AS, Mazarati A, et al. WONOEP appraisal: biomarkers of epilepsy-associated comorbidities. Epilepsia 2017;58(3):331–42.

[40] Kumar G, Couper A, O'Brien TJ, Salzberg MR, Jones NC, Rees SM, et al. The acceleration of amygdala kindling epileptogenesis by chronic low-dose corticosterone involves both mineralocorticoid and glucocorticoid receptors. Psychoneuroendocrinology 2007;32(7):834–42.

[41] Rajkowska G, Miguel-Hidalgo JJ, Wei J, Dilley G, Pittman SD, Meltzer HY, et al. Morphometric evidence for neuronal and glial prefrontal cell pathology in major depression. Biol Psychiatry 1999;45(9):1085–98.

[42] Sheline YI, Gado MH, Kraemer HC. Untreated depression and hippocampal volume loss. Am J Psychiatry 2003;160(8):1516–8.

[43] Cotter DR, Pariante CM, Everall IP. Glial cell abnormalities in major psychiatric disorders: the evidence and implications. Brain Res Bull 2001;55(5):585–95.

[44] Cotter D, Mackay D, Chana G, Beasley C, Landau S, Everall IP. Reduced neuronal size and glial cell density in area 9 of the dorsolateral prefrontal cortex in subjects with major depressive disorder. Cereb Cortex 2002;12(4):386–94.

[45] Kanner AM, Scharfman H, Jette N, Anagnostou E, Bernard C, Camfield C, et al. Epilepsy as a network disorder (1): what can we learn from other network disorders such as autistic spectrum disorder and mood disorders? Epilepsy Behav 2017;77:106–13.

[46] Belsky J, Pluess M. Beyond diathesis stress: differential susceptibility to environmental influences. Psychol Bull 2009;135(6):885–908.

[47] Walker EF, Diforio D. Schizophrenia: a neural diathesis-stress model. Psychol Rev 1997;104 (4):667–85.

[48] Boylan LS. Peri-ictal behavioral and cognitive changes. Epilepsy Behav 2002;3:16–26.

[49] Mula M, Monaco F. Ictal and peri-ictal psychopathology. Behav Neurol 2011;24(1):21–5.

[50] Blanchet P, Frommer GP. Mood change preceding epileptic seizures. J Nerv Ment Dis 1986;174:471–6.

[51] Scaramelli A, Braga P, Avellanal A, Bogacz A, Camejo C, Rega I, et al. Prodromal symptoms in epileptic patients: clinical characterization of the pre-ictal phase. Seizure 2009;18(4):246–50.

[52] Gaitatzis A, Trimble MR, Sander JW. The psychiatric comorbidity of epilepsy. Acta Neurol Scand 2004;110(4):207–20.

[53] Mula M. Epilepsy-induced behavioral changes during the ictal phase. Epilepsy Behav 2014;30:14–6.

[54] Guimond A, Braun CMJ, Bélanger E, Rouleau I. Ictal fear depends on the cerebral laterality of the epileptic activity. Epileptic Disord: Int Epilepsy J Videotape 2008;10(2):101–12.

[55] Feichtinger M, Pauli E, Schäfer I, Eberhardt KW, Tomandl B, Huk J, et al. Ictal fear in temporal lobe epilepsy: surgical outcome and focal hippocampal changes revealed by proton magnetic resonance spectroscopy imaging. Arch Neurol 2001;58(5):771–7.

[56] Kanner AM, Soto A, Gross-Kanner H. Prevalence and clinical characteristics of postictal psychiatric symptoms in partial epilepsy. Neurology 2004;62(5):708–13.

[57] Nishida T, Kudo T, Inoue Y, Nakamura F, Yoshimura M, Matsuda K, et al. Postictal mania versus postictal psychosis: differences in clinical features, epileptogenic zone, and brain functional changes during postictal period. Epilepsia 2006;47(12):2104–14.

[58] Jones JE, Hermann BP, Barry JJ, Gilliam F, Kanner AM, Meador KJ. Clinical assessment of Axis I psychiatric morbidity in chronic epilepsy: a multicenter investigation. J Neuropsychiatr Clin Neurosci 2005;17(2):172–9.

[59] Kanner AM, Kozak AM, Frey M. The use of sertraline in patients with epilepsy: is it safe? Epilepsy Behav 2000;1(2):100–5.

[60] Mula M, Jauch R, Cavanna A, Collimedaglia L, Barbagli D, Gaus V, et al. Clinical and psychopathological definition of the interictal dysphoric disorder of epilepsy. Epilepsia 2008;49(4):650–6.

[61] Bleuler E. Textbook of psychiatry. New York: The Macmillan Co.; 1924.

[62] Blumer D. Dysphoric disorders and paroxysmal affects: recognition and treatment of epilepsy-related psychiatric disorders. Harv Rev Psychiatry 2000;8:8–17.

[63] Mula M, Jauch R, Cavanna A, Gaus V, Kretz R, Collimedaglia L, et al. Interictal dysphoric disorder and periictal dysphoric symptoms in patients with epilepsy. Epilepsia 2010;51(7):1139–45.

[64] Gill SJ, Lukmanji S, Fiest KM, Patten SB, Wiebe S, Jetté N. Depression screening tools in persons with epilepsy: a systematic review of validated tools. Epilepsia 2017;58(5):695–705.

[65] Jones JE, Hermann BP, Woodard JL, Barry JJ, Gilliam F, Kanner AM, et al. Screening for major depression in epilepsy with common self-report depression inventories. Epilepsia 2005;46(5):731–5.

[66] Mula M, Iudice A, La Neve A, Mazza M, Mazza S, Cantello R, et al. Validation of the hamilton rating scale for depression in adults with epilepsy. Epilepsy Behav 2014;41:122–5.

[67] Gilliam FG, Barry JJ, Hermann BP, Meador KJ, Vahle V, Kanner AM. Rapid detection of major depression in epilepsy: a multicentre study. Lancet Neurol 2006;5(5):399–405.

[68] Mula M, McGonigal A, Micoulaud-Franchi J-A, May TW, Labudda K, Brandt C. Validation of rapid suicidality screening in epilepsy using the NDDIE. Epilepsia 2016;57(6):949–55.

[69] Krishnamoorthy ES. The evaluation of behavioral disturbances in epilepsy. Epilepsia 2006;47(Suppl. 2):3–8.

[70] Mintzer S, Lopez F. Comorbidity of ictal fear and panic disorder. Epilepsy Behav 2002;3(4):330–7.

[71] Blumer D. Psychiatric aspects of intractable epilepsy. Adv Exp Med Biol 2002;497:133–47.

[72] Mula M, Sander JW. Negative effects of antiepileptic drugs on mood in patients with epilepsy. Drug Saf Int J Med Toxicol Drug Exp 2007;30(7):555–67.

[73] Trimble MR, Schmitz B. Forced normalization and alternative psychoses of epilepsy. Wrightson Biomedical Pub.; 1998. 235 p.

[74] Perucca P, Mula M. Antiepileptic drug effects on mood and behavior: molecular targets. Epilepsy Behav 2013;26(3):440–9.

[75] Mula M. Topiramate and cognitive impairment: evidence and clinical implications. Ther Adv Drug Saf 2012;3(6):279–89.

[76] Mula M, Trimble MR, Sander JW. Are psychiatric adverse events of antiepileptic drugs a unique entity? A study on topiramate and levetiracetam. Epilepsia 2007;48(12):2322–6.

[77] Stephen LJ, Wishart A, Brodie MJ. Psychiatric side effects and antiepileptic drugs: observations from prospective audits. Epilepsy Behav 2017;71(Pt A):73–8.

[78] Mula M, Trimble MR, Lhatoo SD, Sander JWAS. Topiramate and psychiatric adverse events in patients with epilepsy. Epilepsia 2003;44(5):659–63.

[79] White JR, Walczak TS, Leppik IE, Rarick J, Tran T, Beniak TE, et al. Discontinuation of levetiracetam because of behavioral side effects: a case-control study. Neurology 2003;61(9):1218–21.

[80] Mula M, Hesdorffer DC, Trimble M, Sander JW. The role of titration schedule of topiramate for the development of depression in patients with epilepsy. Epilepsia 2009;50(5):1072–6.

[81] Macrodimitris S, Sherman EMS, Forde S, Tellez-Zenteno JF, Metcalfe A, Hernandez-Ronquillo L, et al. Psychiatric outcomes of epilepsy surgery: a systematic review. Epilepsia 2011;52(5):880–90.

[82] Koch-Stoecker S, Schmitz B, Kanner AM. Treatment of postsurgical psychiatric complications. Epilepsia 2013;54(Suppl. 1):46–52.

[83] Malmgren K, Starmark JE, Ekstedt G, Rosén H, Sjöberg-Larsson C. Nonorganic and organic psychiatric disorders in patients after epilepsy surgery. Epilepsy Behav 2002;3(1):67–75.

[84] Christensen J, Vestergaard M, Mortensen PB, Sidenius P, Agerbo E. Epilepsy and risk of suicide: a population-based case-control study. Lancet Neurol 2007;6:693–8.

[85] Park S-J, Lee HB, Ahn MH, Park S, Choi EJ, Lee H-J, et al. Identifying clinical correlates for suicide among epilepsy patients in South Korea: a case-control study. Epilepsia 2015;56(12):1966–72.

[86] Hecimovic H, Santos JM, Carter J, Attarian HP, Fessler AJ, Vahle V, et al. Depression but not seizure factors or quality of life predicts suicidality in epilepsy. Epilepsy Behav 2012;24(4):426–9.

[87] Mula M, Sander JW. Suicide and epilepsy: do antiepileptic drugs increase the risk? Expert Opin Drug Saf 2015;14(4):553–8.

[88] Mula M, Kanner AM, Schmitz B, Schachter S. Antiepileptic drugs and suicidality: an expert consensus statement from the task force on therapeutic strategies of the ilae commission on neuropsychobiology. Epilepsia 2013;54(1):199–203.

[89] Robertson MM, Trimble MR. The treatment of depression in patients with epilepsy. A double-blind trial. J Affect Disord 1985;9(2):127–36.

[90] Mula M. The pharmacological management of psychiatric comorbidities in patients with epilepsy. Pharmacol Res 2016;107:147–53.

[91] Thomé-Souza MS, Kuczynski E, Valente KD. Sertraline and fluoxetine: safe treatments for children and adolescents with epilepsy and depression. Epilepsy Behav 2007;10(3):417–25.

[92] Barry JJ, Ettinger AB, Friel P, Gilliam FG, Harden CL, Hermann B, et al. Consensus statement: the evaluation and treatment of people with epilepsy and affective disorders. Epilepsy Behav 2008;13 (Suppl. 1):S1–29.

[93] Kerr MP, Mensah S, Besag F, de Toffol B, Ettinger A, Kanemoto K, et al. International consensus clinical practice statements for the treatment of neuropsychiatric conditions associated with epilepsy. Epilepsia 2011;52(11):2133–8.

[94] Mula M, Kanner AM. Introduction—treatment of psychiatric disorders in adults with epilepsy: what every epileptologist should know. Epilepsia 2013;54(Suppl. 1):1–2.

[95] Mula M. Anticonvulsants—antidepressants pharmacokinetic drug interactions: the role of the CYP450 system in psychopharmacology. Curr Drug Metab 2008;9(8):730–7.

[96] Alper K, Schwartz KA, Kolts RL, Khan A. Seizure incidence in psychopharmacological clinical trials: an analysis of Food and Drug Administration (FDA) summary basis of approval reports. Biol Psychiatry 2007;62:345–54.

CHAPTER 17

Epilepsy and psychosis

Joanna Whitson, Niruj Agrawal
Department of Neuropsychiatry, St George's Hospital, London, United Kingdom

Contents

Abbreviations

AED	antiepileptic drug
APD	antipsychotic drug
AIPD	antiepileptic drug-induced psychotic disorder
BIP	brief interictal psychosis
CIP	chronic interictal psychosis
CPS	complex partial seizures
CT	computed tomography
ECT	electroconvulsive therapy
EEG	electroencephalogram
GABA	gamma-Aminobutyric acid
HV	healthy volunteer
HMPAO-SPECT	hexamethylpropyleneamine-oxime single-photon emission computed tomography
MRI	magnetic resonance imaging
MTR	magnetization transfer
NCSE	nonconvulsive status epilepticus
NMDA	N-methyl-D-aspartate
PLA2	phospholipase A2
PIP	postictal psychosis

The Comorbidities of Epilepsy
https://doi.org/10.1016/B978-0-12-814877-8.00017-9

POE	psychosis of epilepsy
SPECT	single-photon emission computed tomography
TLE	temporal lobe epilepsy

1. Introduction

Psychosis ("losing touch with reality") is a disorder of the mind that affects thoughts, feelings, and behavior. Psychosis can be the result of a psychogenic cause, such as a mental illness (e.g., depression, bipolar affective disorder, schizophrenia, schizoaffective disorder, etc.), or it can be organic in nature triggered by a physical condition as is the case in psychosis with epilepsy. Schizophrenia commonly presents with positive (psychosis) symptoms, such as delusions, hallucinations (in any sensory modality), thought disorder (insertion, withdrawal, and broadcast, resulting in disorganized speech), and feelings of being controlled (presenting as disorganized behavior), or negative symptoms (similar to depression), such as diminished emotional expression, avolition, anhedonia, and alogia. Psychosis can be a very frightening experience and can affect relationships, judgment, activities of daily living, and insight, with associated risks.

Psychosis and epilepsy have similar point prevalence rates in the general population of around 1%, and psychosis has a higher prevalence in epileptic patients, making epilepsy a risk factor for psychosis and vice versa [1]. There is a lack of consistency in findings on the actual prevalence of psychosis in epilepsy; estimates vary from 3.8% to 35.7%, reflected by different methodological differences and changing diagnostic classifications within neurology and psychiatry [2]. A systematic review carried out by Clancy et al. [1] found the pooled prevalence of psychosis in epilepsy was 5.2% (95% CI: 3.3–7.2). The psychosis prevalence was 13% higher in complex partial seizures (CPS) and 7%–12% higher in temporal lobe epilepsy (TLE), supported by many studies [1–5]. Psychosis is seen with greater prevalence in lesions in the temporal lobe/limbic system, hippocampal sclerosis, "alien tissue" (e.g., small tumors, gangliogliomas, and hamartomas), lesions in frontal areas [6], and left-hemisphere abnormalities [7]. Understanding psychosis of epilepsy (POE) has the potential to improve our recognition of both disorders and the underlying neuropathophysiology, leading to advances in overall management, reducing the enormous burden of morbidity psychosis and epilepsy cause. Life expectancy is reported to be reduced in both psychosis (around 10 years) and epilepsy (approximately 20 years). In mental health patients the causes of death is frequently related to respiratory diseases. In epilepsy patients, the seizures and their accidents and risk of sudden death constitute the main causes of a lower life expectancy [8].

2. History and etiopathogenesis of POE

Most work on epilepsy and psychosis began in the 19th century. However, associations have been made between epilepsy and mental illness since Hippocrates in the

4th century BCE [9]. Today epilepsy is treated as any other illness, but in the past epilepsy was met with terror and dismay because of its striking manifestations [9]. In the mid–18th century spontaneous fits of epilepsy were thought to be antagonistic to psychosis. This inspired Auenbrugger, who invented percussion used today in medical examinations, to explore the idea that fits might protect from mental illness including psychosis [10]. He used camphor, which has epileptogenic properties to treat psychotic patients. This was first attempted in the 16th century by Paracelsu, in 1751 by Whytt, and in 1785 by Oliver [10]. Auenbrugger gave increasing doses to his patients until severe convulsions were induced. In the 1930s camphor was introduced as a treatment of schizophrenia on the presumption of supposed biological antagonism that epilepsy and schizophrenia never occur together. In the 1930s camphor was replaced by pentylenetetrazole (metrazole). Belgrave wrote in 1868 on bromide's antiepileptic effect and concomitant insanity [11]. In 1868 Holm observed that bromide reduced frequency of seizures at the same time as psychotic symptoms appeared. This antagonistic theory led to the subsequent development of the electroconvulsive therapy (ECT) still practiced today and first used in the United Kingdom in 1939 [10]. Landolt coined the term "forced normalization" in the 1950s to describe psychotic episodes associated with the remission of seizures and disappearance of epileptiform activity on electroencephalograms (EEGs) in individuals with epilepsy [12]. Despite extensive research, the mechanism of forced normalization remained unclear [12]. Landolt pointed out the reciprocal relationship between abnormal mental states and seizures. This reciprocal nature led to the term "alternative psychosis" used as a clinical expression, which does not automatically imply cessation of the interictal epileptiform discharge [13]. Kawakami et al. in 2017 discussed the role of dopamine (DA), which appears to be a key factor in the mechanism of forced normalization [12].

In the 19th century, Lombroso tried to demonstrate the common origin of epilepsy, criminality, madness, and genius [9]. Lombroso described developmental frontal cortex lesions in epileptic patients (today Taylor's dysplasia), and these observations supported the erroneous conviction of a relationship between criminality and epilepsy. He seized on the opportunity to meet author Leo Tolstoy in 1897 and thought he had the chance to put his theories to the test by meeting a "man of genius" whom he suspected to be nothing but a madman. Their encounter was not a huge success; both had different opinions, which they did not share with each other. But Tolstoy allegedly revealed his in his novel *Resurrection* [9].

In 1923 Freud [13a] commented on a 17th century painter's account of his epileptic seizures, trances, and visions as "demonological neurosis" without discussing the seizures. Attention was drawn to the concurrence of POE in this early autobiographical source [14]. It was only after the first experimental research by Gall, Hitzig, Reynolds, Gowers, Wenzel, Burdach, Brown-Séquard, among others that decisive advancements of epilepsy research were made. The studies demonstrated that an epileptic crisis is due to a sudden, excessive, uncontrolled electrical discharge of nervous cells, which can involve the whole or only a part of the brain [9]. For some authors the stigma remained. Charcot himself defined the conditions of hysteria epilepsy, proposing to extend the clinical conception of epilepsy to disorders characterized by psychogenic seizures [9]. It was neurologist Jackson in 1873 [14a] who formulated his own evolutionistic theory of the nervous system, separated on three levels: low (spinal cord and extended spine), medium (basal ganglia), and high (brain cortex), explaining epilepsy as a loss of control perpetuated from the superior to the inferior level [5]. Jackson's theory had an extraordinary positive influence on neurology. Thanks to Jackson's studies it became possible to demonstrate that cerebral crises, which characterize epilepsy, are due to a sudden, excessive, and uncontrolled electric discharge of nervous cells affecting part or the whole brain. In the same years, Maudsley delineated strict correlation between insanity and epilepsy [9]: "As far as this is concerned, the two most intimately bound diseases are madness and epilepsy; anyone who descends from epileptics has equal probabilities to become both epileptic and mad; and it is not rare to notice epileptics among the descendants of a madman" [9] (Fig. 1).

Neuropathologist and psychiatrist Corsellis and Taylor in 1971 are linked to the recognition of focal cortical dysplasia as an entity of seizure etiology, TLE, and epilepsy surgery in general. Corsellis and Burton in 1983 provided the first systematic studies on the pathology of status epilepticus [15]. Corsellis contributed studies focusing on important aspects of epileptology, tissue changes after ECT, and ECT being safe and not causing brain damage [15].

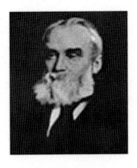

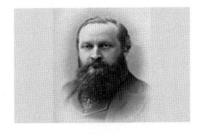

John Hughlings Jackson
Neurologist
(1835–1911)

Henry Maudsley
Psychiatrist
(1835–1918)

Fig. 1 Photographs of two high-profile figures, Jackson and Maudsley.

Hill et al. [15a] suggested an overrepresentation of psychotic patients in TLE. One of the strongest biological findings in schizophrenia is volume loss of temporal lobe structures and the hippocampus in particular. The temporal lobe hypothesis of schizophrenia was put forward by Slater et al. [15b] in 1963 that episodes with paranoid psychoses are more prevalent in TLE [16]. POE has been found to be associated with tumors involving mesial temporal lobe structures [17]. Mendez et al. [17a] reported a higher rate of CPS, but not temporal lobe foci, in their POE group than in their nonpsychotic epilepsy subjects [18]. Crow et al. [18a] investigations support the two-process view that disruptions of the temporolimbic dopaminergic system correlate with positive schizophrenic symptomatology. Jibiki et al. (1993) demonstrated that temporolimbic dysfunction, in particular hyperfunction in the temporolimbic system in the left dominant hemisphere, arises at the time of the psychotic state in epileptic psychosis using regional cerebral blood flow patterns with single-photon emission computed tomography (SPECT) [19, 20]. A retrospective study by Tebartz Van Elst et al. (2002) comparing TLE ± psychosis and healthy volunteers (HVs) using magnetic resonance imaging (MRI) found there no difference in hippocampal volumes between the three groups but there was a significant 16%–18% enlargement of the amygdala in patients with POE [16]. Bruton et al. in 1994 compared clinical, EEG, and neuropathological data from a group of subjects who had both POE and epilepsy without psychosis. Psychotic epileptic patients had larger cerebral ventricles, excess periventricular gliosis, and more focal cerebral damage compared with epileptic patients who had no psychotic illness [21]. Kendrick and Gibbs in 1957 [21a] first used implanted electrodes to study the electrophysiology disturbance in schizophrenia and psychosis of psychomotor epilepsy, spike discharges were noted in medial, frontal, and temporal structures in both patient groups [18]. Heath [21b] noted similar abnormal discharges that did not spread across the amygdala, hippocampus, and septal regions, again in both groups [18]. This led Kendrick and Gibb to report that surgery on medial temporal structures was beneficial for schizophrenia [18]. Due to ethical reasons their research could not continue.

Sato et al. in 1976 considered kindling effect neurochemical disorders caused by repeated electrical disorders, which was discovered by Goddard in 1969, as a good model of epilepsy, psychosis, and memory loss [22]. He first carried out amygdala kindling effect then continued to study hippocampus kindling and temporal lobe cortex kindling and their transference phenomenon. He later studied so-called DA kindling but pointed out the necessity to differentiate this phenomenon from kindling and called this "reverse tolerance phenomenon" [23]. Professor Sato found that repeated use of central stimulants generates psychosis similar to schizophrenia and reported that chronic intake of catecholaminergic agents can cause long-term changes of the brain with cross sensitization and clarified that reverse tolerance phenomenon can be triggered by other kinds of catecholaminergic agents and that DA receptor blockers can suppress this phenomenon [22]. Furthermore, these results, suggesting an antagonistic relationship between experimental epilepsy and schizophrenia, may provide a theoretical basis for the concept of "forced normalization," that is, an antagonism between schizophrenic symptoms and epileptic seizures [22].

Using magnetoencephalography Canuet et al. 2011 found increased theta oscillations in regions, namely the medial and lateral parietal cortex bilaterally in the POE patients relative to their nonpsychotic counterparts. In addition, patients with psychosis had increased beta temporo-prefrontal connectivity in the hemisphere with predominant seizure focus. This functional connectivity in temporo-prefrontal circuits correlated with positive symptoms [24]. Adachi et al. [24a] concluded POE with religious delusion was related to control mechanisms in the prefrontal lobe-related processes rather than medial temporal lobe-related processes [25]. TLE with psychosis has also been postulated to arise from abnormalities in fetal brain development and to represent a model or mock up of schizophrenia. It is recognized that these conditions share common genetic or environmental causes [24]. Slater and Moran [25a] established the modern concept of POE in which paranoid psychosis came on years after epileptic fits [26]. In recent literature, POE is likely associated with epilepsy-related processes [26a, 26b], but other types of POE exist; rather than organic psychosis, POE can be a consequence of iatrogenic factors such as side effects from antiepileptic drugs (AEDs). There are descriptions of psychosis preexisting before epilepsy as a variant epilepsy-related psychosis [18, 27]. Recent studies have illustrated that not only epileptic factors but also nonepileptic factors are associated with POE [26, 27a].

3. Clinical presentations of POE

POE can be subdivided into the five following groups depending upon when the psychosis occurs in relation to an epileptic seizure:

1. Preictal: occurring immediately before a seizure.
2. Ictal: those directly related to the seizures; namely, the epileptic clouded or twilight states; petit mal status, psychomotor status.
3. Postictal: clouded psychotic states due to direct and widespread interference of cortical function by the ictal discharge.
4. Interictal psychoses: not directly related to the ictal discharge, but where involvement of the limbic system structures by abnormal electrical activity and/or the lesion causing the fits.
5. Psychosis brought on by treatment of epilepsy: such as medication or surgery, following the forced normalization theory [28, 29]. These groups will be discussed individually in the following sections.

3.1 Preictal psychosis

There is little literature on preictal psychosis. Patients may experience a variety of vague symptoms during the days and hours leading up to seizure as prodromal symptoms. An aura may occur immediately prior to seizure onset. This is most common in CPS, TLE, or extra-temporal epilepsy (e.g., frontal CPS). Auras are typically stereotyped, for example, autonomic or visceral aura, derealization and depersonalization experiences, cognitive symptoms (dysphasia, forced thinking, ideomotor aura, déjà vu, jamais vu, fugue, and twilight states), affective symptoms (anxiety, euphoria), and perceptual experiences (hallucinations or illusions) [30, 31].

A 49-year-old patient with a history of TLE for >20 years with two distinct types of psychoses, preictal and interictal psychosis, was observed; during preictal psychoses presented as forced thinking and auditory hallucinations, EEG tracing showed emerging seizure activity while a relatively normal EEG tracing was present during interictal psychosis [31]. This case study highlights the importance of a good clinical assessment to differentiate between these two conditions [31]. If the psychosis develops gradually before and in parallel with increasing seizure frequency, it is likely to be preictal [18]. Normally optimized control of the seizures helps control preictal psychosis; specific antipsychotic drugs (APDs) are not indicated.

3.2 Ictal

Ictal psychosis is most commonly linked with CPS (or psychomotor status) [18]. Epilepsy partialis continua is a condition of prolonged CPS, for example, temporal, frontal, or cingulate seizures lasting hours to days, which may be confused with delirium or psychosis [30, 31]. Simple partial status may produce autonomic, affective, and psychotic symptoms (including hallucinations and thought disorder) in clear consciousness. In such cases, insight is usually retained, but symptoms can be embellished resulting in behavioral disturbances [18]. By definition, ictal psychosis is concurrently associated with epileptic discharges in the brain, except for some patients with simple partial status [18]. The majority of EEG discharges have a focus in the limbic system and isocortical components of the temporal lobe. In 30% of patients the focus is extra temporal, usually frontal or cingulate cortex [18]. The psychosis is brief, usually hours to days. When prolonged into days it is likely to be ictal behavior that extends postictally [18]. Patients present with a wide range of perceptual, behavioral, cognitive, and affective symptoms often in connection with automatisms. Automatisms (involving oral activity, eyelid fluttering, picking at clothes, mutism, simple or complex stereotyped movements that tend to be disorganized and purposeless), which occur during a seizure suggest focal origin such as medial temporal lobe. There are alterations in consciousness during ictus and amnesia for the automatism, which usually lasts <5 min. Automatisms may be the basis of twilight and fugue states (EEG may aid differential diagnosis) [18].

Ictal psychosis, some theories suggest, is caused by the positive effect of the seizure, the epileptic discharges activating behavioral mechanisms. Automatisms are thought to be due to positive effects but also negative effects of epileptic discharge when the individual is unable to engage in a particular behavior due to paralysis of the anatomical substrate for that behavior [18, 31]. Normally ictal psychosis resolves with effective management of epilepsy, without having to treat the psychosis directly [32]. Specific APDs are not indicated.

Nonconvulsive status epilepticus (NCSE) may present in association with a variety of underlying disorders and can be mistaken for idiopathic forms of chronic psychosis. Fluctuating attention and concentration, signs and symptoms of encephalopathy, and refractoriness to treatment with APDs can be clues to its presence [33]. Prompt recognition and treatment are important to prevent continuing seizure activity. A case report of NCSE in a 46-year-old female with longstanding schizoaffective disorder and hearing loss treated with clozapine and levetiracetam, presented with confusion, hallucinations (noise and voice), and normal affect and was observed to have myoclonic movements and fluctuating attention [33]. She had a history of generalized seizures but also partial seizures at times. NCSE was suspected and an EEG demonstrated epileptiform activity. Oral phenytoin was administered and all symptoms improved [33]. The clinical challenges of NCSE include recognition with attention to medication interaction and toxicity as well as underlying causes [33]. The importance of video-EEG recordings was again highlighted in a case study of a 16-year-old girl with psychotic symptoms, including auditory hallucinations and paranoia especially at night [34], which lasted 2–3 min and up to 30 min. During episodes she retained consciousness. Increased dosages of APDs had no effect. MRI was normal. A routine and later a sleep-deprived EEG revealed intermittent polymorphic theta slowing over the left temporal region. Clobazam was added for her nighttime symptoms and a slight improvement was noted. A video EEG revealed very frequent spikes and slowing over the left temporal region. APDs were withdrawn and carbamazepine was commenced at 400 mg daily; she then became free of hallucinations [34]. A 55-year-old lady was admitted due to a change in behavior in terms of declining mood, paranoia, and olfactory hallucinations. She had a prior diagnosis of bipolar affective disorder and was being treated with lithium but was noncompliant. Upon admission her computed tomography (CT) was normal but EEG was grossly abnormal [35]. Carbamazepine was commenced in view of the change in diagnosis to TLE [35]. The patient responded very well to carbamazepine in all spheres [35].

3.3 Postictal

Postictal delirium is a very common confusional state following a seizure. Postictal psychosis (PIP) is a well-known complication, occurring in 7%–10% of TLE [36, 37] or extra temporal localization and encephalitis [38]. It usually follows seizure clusters or a recent exacerbation in seizure frequency that may be related to withdrawal of anticonvulsants [18, 27]. The psychosis commonly appears following a lucid interval, 12–72 h in the Kanner [38a] study and up to 1 week according to Refs. [18, 30, 38b, 39]. Thereafter the individual will develop a brief psychotic episode with variable psychotic symptoms including delusions (persecutory, grandiose, referential, somatic, and religious), hallucinations, catatonia, and affective symptoms; clouding of consciousness is sometimes present before or during PIP [18]. Aggressive behavior has also been reported during PIP, 22.9% in one study [27]. Kanemoto et al. carried out a study illustrating aggression, and self-harm is linked with PIP but not other forms of POE [40]. Since PIP is brief, lasting a few days to 1 month, mean duration 70 h, and occurs in close proximity with seizures, this is ideal for investigating some pathogenetic mechanisms. It may recur two or three times in a year, and it becomes chronic in 15% [18, 30]. The majority of patients suffer from secondarily generalized CPS, with epilepsy predating the psychosis for about 10 years [18, 30]. PIP is well known in adults but only sparsely reported in the pediatric population [39].

Predisposing factors are not fully understood; a positive family history of psychosis [38, 41], longer duration of epilepsy, impaired intellectual function, bilateral ictal discharges, interictal epileptiform activity [27, 37, 38], high rate of ictal fear, and gross structural lesions have been associated with PIP [18]. EEG shows marked changes during psychotic episodes [30]. Some patients have demonstrated frequent bitemporal independent epileptiform discharges, greatest in the mesial temporal regions [18]. Falip et al. investigated TLE with video EEG, observed PIP, and noted that most PIP often develops in patients with bitemporal lobe dysfunction [27]. Logsdail and Toone observed CT abnormalities in the temporal lobe in patients with PIP [42]. MRI studies by Kanemoto et al. showed a high incidence of PIP in resistant temporal sclerosis, especially on the left side, and this group was likely to have atrophy of the temporal neocortex [18]. Other studies illustrated bilateral or widespread functional central nervous system disturbances rather than distinct structural brain alterations as predisposing etiologies [37]. This was further supported by a case study that PIP is more likely to be pathophysiological than structural [43]. There has been a recent interest in the relationship between autoimmunity and the pathogenesis of both epilepsy and psychosis. Studies have demonstrated the presence of antibodies directed against synaptic autoantigens (such as the N-methyl-D-aspartate [NMDA] receptor or the voltage-gated potassium channel complex) in approximately 10% of cases of sporadic epilepsy [44]. These same autoantibodies are known to cause encephalopathy syndromes that feature psychiatric symptoms [44]. It was hypothesized that PIP may be an autoimmune phenomenon mediated by autoantibodies against synaptic antigens. In essence, it was proposed that PIP is a time-limited, seizure-dependent, autoantibody-mediated encephalopathy syndrome. There are a number of features of PIP that are explained by this mechanism, such as the lucid interval between seizures and onset of psychosis and the progression in some cases to a chronic PIP [44].

Leutmezer et al. studied five patients with TLE in whom PIP developed during the course of video-EEG [36]; they were studied with hexamethylpropyleneamine-oxime SPECT (HMPAO-SPECT). The results showed in comparison to the interictal state, all SPECT scans obtained during PIP were remarkable for bifrontal and bitemporal hyperperfusion patterns. Some studies also demonstrated unilateral left lateral frontal hyperperfusion. Conclusions drawn indicated that PIP in TLE patients is associated with hyperactivation of both temporal and frontal lobe structures. This hyperperfusion may reflect ongoing (subcortical) discharges, active inhibitory mechanisms that terminate the seizure, or simply a dysregulation of cerebral blood flow [36]. A case study illustrated after repeated EEGs during the period of psychosis that their habitual focal epileptiform abnormalities had disappeared. Their psychotic symptoms alleviated after their epileptiform abnormalities reappeared. These observations may suggest possible overlapping mechanisms between a prolongation of psychosis and suppression of epileptiform discharges on a scalp EEG [45].

PIP usually runs a benign course [40], but resolution can be aided by low doses of APDs, such as risperidone or quetiapine [32]. A further seizure may exacerbate the psychosis, and anticonvulsant treatment is normally required [18]. Using quetiapine 400 mgOD to treat the psychotic symptoms was found to have an added effect of reducing suicidal ideation/intent [46]. A case presentation of a 14-year-old boy with borderline IQ 75 and PIP presenting with symptoms of irritability, auditory, and visual hallucinations and persecutory delusions [47] had been receiving treatment for epilepsy since he was 7 years old. The patient was using carbamazepine, levetiracetam, and primidone. Epileptiform activity at the left frontal-temporal-central area was observed with EEG while quetiapine 25 mgOD was started. The dose was titrated gradually to 200 mgOD and successfully controlled his psychotic symptoms [47]. Another epileptic patient who developed PIP presented with delusions and acoustic hallucinations two days after a prolonged CPS; upon treatment with diazepam and haloperidol, the psychosis subsided within 3 days [48]. Brown et al. demonstrated the efficacy of lithium in the treatment of PIP [49]. Some case studies with rare pediatric patients have shown psychosis improving on AEDs (e.g., levetiracetam) alone [39]. These cases illustrate the importance of close collaboration between neurologists and psychiatrists for the optimal success of therapy [47].

Neuronal antibody encephalitis, such as anti-NMDA receptor encephalitis can present with seizures and psychosis, both of which can resolve with prompt, appropriate immunotherapy. The management of epilepsy-related psychosis in young people is similar to that in adults. APDs should not be withheld if it is needed on clinical grounds. If the psychosis has been induced by AEDs, a medication review is necessary [50].

There are many controversies in the literature; while some PIP patients get better from their psychiatric condition after epileptic surgery, others develop de novo depression or psychosis [51]. Patients with recurrent PIP episodes who undergo TLE surgery are at increased risk of developing de novo psychiatric disorders, particularly mood disorders. This has implications for preoperative counseling and highlights a need for postsurgical psychiatric monitoring for these patients [41]. In a case base study on TLE undergoing surgery, D'Alessio et al. found that while some patients with a history of psychotic disorders get better from psychoses after epilepsy surgery, others continue having psychotic symptoms or developed other psychiatric conditions such as depression [41].

3.4 Interictal psychosis
3.4.1 Brief interictal psychosis
Brief interictal psychosis (BIP) occurs unrelated to a seizure when there is good control of epilepsy [30]. The psychosis lasts from days to weeks and is normally self-limiting [18]. There may be premonitory symptoms such as anxiety and insomnia, hence why treatment with anxiolytics at this stage has been found to prevent BIP [18]. The psychosis is characterized by paranoid delusions, and auditory hallucinations, affective symptoms, and behavioral symptoms may occur [18]. Patients with brief BIP have been reported to have either CPS or primary generalized epilepsy, while temporal lobe onset is uncommon. In a study by Wolf [51a], all patients had generalized seizures [18].

3.4.2 Chronic interictal psychosis
Chronic interictal psychosis (CIP) is more common in chronic epilepsy cases with a history of febrile convulsions, status epilepticus, and lateralization of epileptiform discharges, epileptic women and those with cognitive impairment [52–54]. There is often a period of 10–15 years that elapses between epilepsy and the onset of psychoses; Slater reported a mean onset at age 30 years old [13, 30]. Clinically the illness is very similar to idiopathic schizophrenia, although there tends to be a prominent affective component and autonomic auras [13, 30]; there is also a preserved premorbid personality and fewer negative symptoms. The psychotic symptoms are largely paranoid delusions, hallucinations (including visual), catatonia, affective blunting, and volitional symptoms [18]. CIP is suggested to conform to current DSM-IV classification of schizophrenia; therefore, it is often named "Schizophrenia-like psychosis" [55].

CIP is particularly associated with CPS (including TLE and hippocampal sclerosis) [54, 55] or generalized tonic-clonic seizures [53]. Studies looking at unilateral TLE without psychosis, schizophrenia, and HVs performed coronal spin-echo MRI and found relative to controls all patient groups had ventricular enlargement and smaller temporal lobe, frontal-parietal, and superior temporal gyrus gray matter volumes, with the extent of these abnormalities greater in CIP [56].

A positron emission tomography (PET) study using (15O) H$_2$O demonstrated lower oxygen extraction ratios in the frontal, temporal, and basal ganglia regions in CIP patients but not nonpsychotic epileptic patients [18], and a small study using SPECT illustrated lower left medial temporal blood flow in CIP but not nonpsychotic epileptic patients [18]. Another PET study showed higher than normal levels of DOPA decarboxylase activity in CIP and schizophrenia patients. Reith et al. [56a] suggested this was due to suppressed tonic release of DA in striatum because of low corticostriatal glutamatergic input [18]. CIP had a substantial preponderance of temporal mediobasal spike foci, recorded on sphenoidal electrodes and an excess of epigastric auras [18]. The majority of the evidence points to a mediobasal rather than neocortical temporal lobe abnormality underpinning psychosis [18], and psychosis is thought to involve dysfunction of frontal and medial temporal limbic brain regions, which are key areas in emotional regulation.

Discussions about pathophysiology have centered broadly on mechanisms that psychosis is due to repeated electrical discharges, either directly or through the development of neurophysiology or neurochemical abnormalities. Kindling has been proposed as one possible mechanism for CIP by Sato [22]. Cifelli and Grace demonstrated in a TLE study using rats that pathologically increased drive from ventral hippocampus can induce aberrant DA signaling. Their data provide support of a direct link between increased hippocampal activity due to TLE and the hyperresponsivity of the DA system that is believed to underlie the psychotic behavior in CIP [57]. Another mechanism is frequent seizures causing the production of plastic regenerative changes, especially affecting the medial temporal lobe. It has been demonstrated that stimulation of the hippocampus leads to anomalous axonal sprouting from dentate granule cells before the development of seizures. This is supported by expansion of glutamatergic presynaptic mossy fibers and an increase in postsynaptic densities on granule cells in temporal lobectomy specimens, changes possibly triggered by increased expression of messenger RNA for c-fos and NGF by recurrent limbic seizures, the resultant miswiring could be the basis for CIP [18].

Work was carried out to investigate whether increased activity of the enzyme phospholipase A2 (PLA2) in the brain, as frequently reported in schizophrenia, is also related to CIP, and it was found that an increment in brain PLA2 is also associated with POE [58]. Suckling et al. [58a] investigated relationships between hippocampal/temporal lobe neuropathology and psychosis in subjects with TLE, paying particular attention to possible differences in density of hippocampal neurons immunoreactive for calcium-binding proteins. Psychotic cases differed from nonpsychotic ones in having more focal lesions outside the hippocampus, and cases of TLE with psychosis were distinguishable on the basis of a higher density of calbindin-reactive neurons in CA4 as well as on more general aspects of their pathology [58]. Calcium-binding protein (S100B) is a 21 kDa protein expressed primarily in astrocytes and has been related with brain dysfunction. There is evidence for increased S100B in schizophrenia, including first-episode psychosis, and in POE, especially after seizures. Pico and nanomolar levels of S100B are neurotrophic, and micromolar levels are toxic and apoptotic [59]. Compared to healthy subjects, levels were ten times higher in epilepsy (without psychosis), a hundred times higher with psychosis, and thousands of times higher in CIP. Barrau et al. (2012) interpreted these results as an intense activation of astrocytes by a double brain insult of epilepsy and psychosis [59].

Monji et al. [59a] investigated whether a functional folate deficiency and/or elevated levels of plasma homocysteine may be related to CIP. The epileptic patients with CIP had significantly lower folate levels and higher homocysteine levels than those without psychosis. There were no significant differences in the vitamin B12 levels between the two groups [57]. This study suggests that low plasma folate and high plasma homocysteine levels may be related to the CIP pathophysiology [57]. Scherer et al. (2011) investigated noradrenaline, DA, serotonin (5-HT), and substance P (NK1) receptors' role in hippocampi removed from people with TLE with or without psychiatric comorbidity [60]. He did this in order to assess whether there are differences in different neurotransmitters' roles in TLE with or without psychiatric comorbidity, using PCR. Results illustrated DA receptors AD2A and AD2C showed differences and more expression in the epilepsy group when compared with controls. In the psychosis group AD2A showed significance in the antiepileptic variable, a substance that activates AD2A in the hippocampus. The differences in AD2A and AD2C receptor expression between epilepsy and in the psychosis group suggest different adrenergic mechanisms connected with psychosis and epilepsy. The role of 5-HT2A in TLE is indicated by its greater expression in the epilepsy group when compared with the control, with significance for the epileptic seizures frequency. No significant results were found for D4, 5-HT1A, 5-HT2C, and NK1 between the three groups [60].

Theories imply that, rather than psychosis being a consequence of epileptiform activity, both psychosis and epilepsy are symptomatic of an underlying neuropathological or physiological dysfunction with two major possibilities: [18] neurodevelopmental disorders leading to cortical dysgenesis; and [1] diffusion of brain damage causing both epilepsy and psychosis [18]. With cortical dysgenesis hypothesis TLE have found a high majority of patients to have hippocampal cell loss and sclerosis particularly in the presubiculum and CA1 regions, and other TLE patients have gliomas, hamartomas, and heterotopias, and the presence of this alien tissue suggests defective neuroembryogenesis [18].

Patients with mesial sclerosis commonly have heterotopias, hippocampal neuronal loss, and synaptic reorganization [18]. Cryptic insults, such as childhood viruses, fever, or hypoxia, may lead to synaptic reorganization in vulnerable brains [18]. It is of interest that there is significant evidence emerging that schizophrenia is associated with cortical maldevelopment [18]. More than a decade ago it was illustrated that patients with schizophrenia had disorganization of the pyramidal cell layer, thought to migrate in to the hippocampal area. Heterotopias and synaptic reorganizations have also been demonstrated in schizophrenia patients [18]. These disturbances could be genetic or early insults on neurodevelopment, and perhaps epilepsy activity may, in addition, exacerbate an underlying dysgenesis for psychosis, explaining the delay in onset [18].

Bringing these entire hypotheses together it could be possible that epileptic patients with CIP have a brain lesion that makes them vulnerable to psychosis as well as epilepsy. This lesion could be neurodevelopmental, leading to cortical dysgenesis or acquired (e.g., by trauma, infection, or hypoxia). The abnormality may be widespread but probably involves the limbic structures. The abnormality is likely to cause electrical storms in the limbic cortex, resulting in seizures at an early age. This could trigger kindling mechanisms, regenerative changes involving axonal sprouting, and synaptic reorganization leading to CIP [18]. Either by the presence of continuous subictal activity or by modulation of catecholamine, glutamatergic, and GABAergic pathways modulating psychosis either triggering or inhibiting psychosis, the latter explains the impression of antagonism ("forced normalization") [18]. This is further complicated by long-term medication use for epilepsy and the psychosocial factors of epilepsy [18] (Fig. 2).

Magnetization transfer (MTR) imaging with TLE patients with CIP demonstrated that these patients were significantly more cognitively impaired on executive and semantic memory tasks than the nonpsychotic TLE group. This was illustrated by vocabulary test scores in the psychotic but not the nonpsychotic group correlating significantly with MTR reduction in the left fusiform gyrus (occipitotemporal gyrus) part of the temporal lobe, involved in cognitive function/memory and is particularly linked to dyslexia, synesthesia, dyslexia, and prosopagnosia [54]. These findings suggest that the cognitive deterioration in these patients may occur as the illness progresses and the causes are multifactorial [54]. In CIP patients, cortical thickness was reduced in the inferior frontal gyrus, and their current IQ was associated with decreases in area, but not thickness, in regions of the frontotemporal cortex [54]. This likely reflects the interplay of psychosis-related genetic factors and the cumulative effects of seizure activity on the brain [54]. Cortical thinning in the inferior frontal gyrus, a region implicated in schizophrenia, is likely to be related to seizure activity, whereas changes in IQ, associated with reductions in area of the frontotemporal cortex, may be related to the presence of psychosis [54].

4. Treatment issues

The treatment of all forms of POE, with the exception of ictal psychotic episodes, may require the use of APDs, despite theories of APDs lowering seizure threshold; preferably atypical APDs that have low or negligible potential to lower seizure threshold (e.g., risperidone, aripiprazole, or quetiapine), starting at a low dose with stepwise increments [61]. All APDs have the propensity to reduce seizure threshold related to drug type and dose, and clozapine is thought to be the most epileptogenic of the APDs [19, 62]. However cases have illustrated that control of psychosis with APDs has also improved patients' epilepsy, even with clozapine. In a case study with an 8-year-old male with vivid visual and auditory hallucinations and loss of consciousness, MRI revealed cortical dysgenesis in

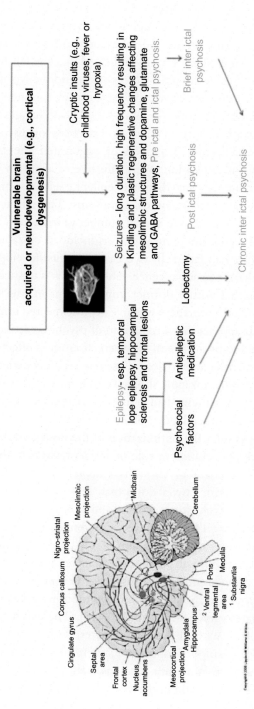

Fig. 2 Pathophysiology of chronic interictal psychosis [18].

the left inferior frontal cortex and adjacent subcortical structures [63]. SPECT imaging revealed left temporal hypoperfusion. Risperidone therapy was initiated because there was no remission after carbamazepine and valproate treatment. After risperidone treatment, symptoms remitted. A SPECT study indicated that the left temporal hypoperfusion was normalized [63]. After discontinuation of risperidone, symptoms returned, and EEG revealed generalized slow-wave activity particularly prominent in the left temporal region. This is one of the first reports of cerebral blood flow changes in a pediatric patient with psychosis after treatment [63]. In 11 cases, a decrease or discontinuation of APDs (mostly haloperidol) significantly provoked or aggravated the psychotic symptoms [64]. While olanzapine and risperidone were effective to a certain extent, two patients treated with olanzapine showed exacerbation of epileptic seizures, and one patient treated with risperidone developed extrapyramidal symptoms. The efficacy of quetiapine and aripiprazole is difficult to judge due to a small number of trials [65]. Treatment strategies in adolescents with CPS and emerging psychosis included clozapine, which was only considered if other APDs had failed. In two cases patients developed epilepsy in early childhood and schizophrenia in adolescence. Their CPS was unsuccessfully treated with AEDs. Clozapine was tried with a distinct improvement in psychotic symptoms and functional level [65]. In both cases there was an early unexpected improvement in seizure control on clozapine. It appears that a reduction of psychotic activity improved seizure control. There appeared to be a tradeoff between clozapine's effect on psychotic symptoms and recurrence of seizure activity [65]. Case reports of six patients with epilepsy and severe psychosis treated with clozapine showed that none of the patients had an increase in seizure frequency; three patients had a substantial reduction in seizures, while one patient had a reduction in nonepileptic seizures as well [66].

Treatment should consider the optimization of the dosage of AEDs in combination with APDs [55]. There is a prominent role of antidepressants with CIP [55], as a high number of patients with interictal psychosis have depression [67]. Treatment with APDs usually needs to be long term. Lower doses than those used in primary schizophrenia seem to be effective [19]. Psychosocial support and family education are also important.

CIP is found in refractory TLE. However, CIP refractory epilepsy patients are often rejected from many epilepsy surgery programs purely on psychiatric grounds. It is often assumed that disturbed behavior will prevent adequate preoperative evaluation or that the patients are unable to provide informed consent for preoperative investigations and for surgery [68], and de novo psychosis may develop months or years after temporal lobe lobectomy; reported rates vary from 3% to 28% [18]. The psychosis is usually paranoia with hallucinations often with depressive features. However, there are reports of improvement of CIP with temporal lobectomy, interestingly, in cases associated with left sided surgery [18]. Marchetti et al., in a case-based study involving patients with medically intractable TLE and CIP who underwent temporal lobe resection [69], illustrated that with appropriate psychiatric intervention, patients with refractory epilepsy and CIP may undergo surgery successfully [69]. This is supported by a case study of five patients with the dual diagnoses of medically intractable TLE and CIP who underwent temporal lobe resection. The patients were able to provide informed consent and were easily managed during preoperative investigations. Seizure outcome has been excellent in all. Neither temporal lobe resection nor remission of seizures influenced the nature or evolution of the psychosis. Subjectively the patients functioned better in activities of daily living and freedom from seizures improved quality of life. With appropriate psychiatric intervention, patients with chronic psychosis and refractory epilepsy can undergo surgery successfully [68].

In a case report of a 49-year-old man with a hypothalamic hamartoma and a history of both gelastic and temporal lobe seizures, the patient was rendered seizure-free after three neurosurgical procedures but developed a drug-resistant paranoid psychosis. He was treated with ECT. After 2 weeks with six stimulations that resulted in seizures, the psychiatric phenomena disappeared completely. There was no relapse of either the psychiatric symptoms or the seizures during the 42 months of follow-up. This case report illustrates the therapeutic properties of ECT in POE [69]. Psychiatric disorders that indicate the use of ECT also occur in epileptic patients, but there is a lack of medical authority concerning the use of ECT in epileptic patients. There is emerging evidence that ECT has an anticonvulsive effect [69]. Another case study of an epileptic patient resistant to AEDs at the same time had schizophreniform psychosis [69]. ECT resulted in the longest symptom-free balanced period in the patient [69]. In view of the epileptogenic risk factors of classical APDs and the anticonvulsive potential of ECT in cases of severe POE, ECT is an attractive potential therapeutic option for CIP [69].

5. POE induced by treatment for epilepsy
5.1 Psychosis induced by AEDs

There are no agreed definitions or diagnosis criteria for AED-induced psychotic disorder (AIPD) in the classification systems [70]. Disorganized behaviors and abnormal thinking are predominant symptoms of AIPD, but AIPD differed from nondrug-induced psychotic disorders in having a much better outcome [70]. A study investigated the clinical spectrum of AIPD; they evaluated 2630 patients with epilepsy and psychotic disorders. Results revealed four factors associated with AIPD: female gender, TLE and use of levetiracetam, topiramate, and a negative association with carbamazepine [70]. The antagonistic relationship between seizures and psychosis is highlighted when anticonvulsants (AEDs) trigger an onset of psychosis, and APDs have a proconvulsive effect in a few patients, but literature is confounded by the inclusion of affective and confusion disorders [30, 62]. Studies have associated several AEDs, for example, carbamazepine, barbiturates, benzodiazepines (e.g., clobazam), ethosuximide, gabapentin, lamotrigine, levetiracetam, piracetam, pregabalin, primidone tiagabine, topiramate, valproate, vigabatrin, and zonisamide [62], with triggering psychosis, but other studies have found the opposite or that this is a rare adverse effect [18, 62]. Patients with drug-resistant epilepsy have a higher incidence of psychiatric problems. Concern has been raised that gamma–Aminobutyric acid (GABA) drugs may be associated with treatment-emergent psychosis [69]. Three adolescents with epilepsy had historical findings consistent with mild behavioral problems and cognitive deficits before initiating levetiracetam; following treatment with levetiracetam, emergent psychosis was observed in all three cases, which was reversible. Whether rapid initiation or prior neurobehavioral problems predispose to this side effect is not clear [70]. Other studies have shown topiramate may induce psychotic symptoms, possibly by the inhibition of frontal and prefrontal areas. The clinical history of a 34-year-old man with epilepsy associated to tuberous sclerosis complex and without a previous history of mental illness presented acutely with florid psychotic symptoms. These symptoms appeared 1 month after the introduction of topiramate, added to leve-tiracetam and carbamazepine, when topiramate reached the dose of 200 mgOD. Once topiramate was discontinued, the psychotic symptoms disappeared. It was hypothesized that psychotic symptoms appeared 1 month after the topiramate introduction because of the slow topiramate titration and protective effect of carbamazepine [71]. Eight patients with difficult-to-control epilepsy and an active or a history of psychosis were treated with vigabatrin, and the results of this clinical intervention are five cases that had no untoward deterioration of mental state. Three cases developed psychosis, which was reversed by judicious adjustment of both the anticonvulsant and APDs [72].

Lamotrigine is a generally well-tolerated AED with broad-spectrum efficacy in several forms of partial and generalized epilepsy and is also licensed for use in bipolar disorder. Six patients out of 1400 patients studied developed psychosis under treatment with lamotrigine. This indicates that psychosis is a rare adverse event of lamotrigine. Possible risk factors seem to be psychiatric comorbidity and temporal lobe pathology [73]. Another case study of refractory POE found lamotrigine and amisulpride achieved an excellent response [74].

Frontal lobe epilepsy is associated with behavioral changes including fear and agitation. A case study involving two patients presenting with psychosis, observed that treatment with carbamazepine resulted in complete resolution of their psychiatric symptoms [75]. An 11-year-old girl who had been given AEDs for occipital lobe epilepsy was hospitalized with alternative psychosis and dysgraphia. Her epileptic seizures and psychosis disappeared after administration of carbamazepine [76]. Other case studies have supported the therapeutic use of carbamazepine for treating partial epilepsy and psychosis [35].

5.2 Psychosis induced by epilepsy surgery

TLE surgery has become a successful alternative in patients with refractory epilepsy. However, the outcome of epilepsy surgery may be affected by the occurrence of post-surgical psychiatric complications [77]. It is observed that preexisting psychosis usually does not improve after the epilepsy surgery, and there are fears of an exacerbation of psychosis with postsurgical seizure remission [78] or early onset of de novo psychosis with decreased or diminished seizures that might be related to forced normalization. There are case reports regarding the development of psychosis after epilepsy surgery (anterior temporal lobectomy). This adverse event occurred also in patients without a history of previous psychosis [79]. The patients developed a subacute hallucinatory-delusion syndrome, while seizures disappeared [79]. In contrast, late-onset psychosis following temporal lobectomy might be related to synaptic changes due to aberrant reinnervation after temporal lobectomy [78]. Right-sided temporal lobectomy might have a provoking effect on psychosis [79]. A report describing three cases of refractory TLE and hippocampal sclerosis, following anterior temporal lobectomy, presented with acute psychosis. One of them had a history of acute psychosis, and all of them met criteria for Cluster A personality disorder (schizoid/schizotypal) during psychiatric assessment prior to surgery. The three cases had a good seizure outcome, but on follow-up during the first year after surgery, developed acute psychotic episodes compatible with schizoaffective disorder, brief psychotic disorder, and delusional disorder, respectively [77].

Two cases developed mental state changes after right temporal lobectomy and left frontal lesionectomy plus corpus callostomy; a 19-year-old male with mental retardation and medically intractable epilepsy underwent left frontal lesionectomy plus corpus callostomy for seizure control. No intraoperative or immediate postoperative complications were noted [79]. Two weeks after the surgery, he developed aggression, behavioral change, and insomnia despite dramatic improvement of his epilepsy. His psychosis improved after administration of APDs. A 16-year-old female developed de novo acute psychosis characterized by challenging behavior, visual/auditory hallucinations, and delusion one year after right temporal lobectomy. Serial EEGs revealed neither epileptiform abnormalities nor subclinical seizures. There was no intercurrent illness and investigations were normal. Her psychosis began during the tapering off period of carbamazepine as she had been seizure-free for 1 year after the surgery [79]. There was no history or family history of psychosis in either patient prior to surgery. After a few months, their psychosis gradually but significantly improved with APDs [79].

Patients with comorbid psychosis and temporal lobe drug-resistant epilepsy may benefit from epilepsy surgery [28]. Cortico-amygdalohippocampectomy has become an important treatment option for patients with refractory TLE mesial temporal sclerosis (TLE-MTS); it has resulted in a 60%–70% seizure remission rate [28]. Video-EGG monitoring is a safe method to evaluate patients with refractory TLE mesial temporal sclerosis and psychosis [28]. Careful drug selection of AEDs and APDs, dosing, and slow titration can minimize the psychosis after surgery risk, allowing treatment to proceed [80]. The role of the neuropsychiatrist is important in epilepsy surgery with regard to presurgical identification and postoperative support of patients who may be vulnerable to psychosis [78].

6. Clinical assessment and diagnosis

For management of the different presentations of POE, it is important to correctly diagnose the type of epilepsy and cause following a thorough assessment by a neurologist and carrying out appropriate investigations (brain imaging and EEG). Various psychotic symptoms should be identified appropriately and establish their timing in relation to epileptic seizures. Psychotic symptoms in epilepsy that are most frequent are delusions (67%) mainly paranoid and persecutory [81], religious theme or capgrass [82], hallucinations (61%), and thought disturbances (45%) [82]. Studies have found that the diagnosis of hebephrenic schizophrenia had been given mistakenly to patients with CPS [82]. Epileptic patients are deemed to have milder psychotic symptoms than schizophrenic patients [83]. Negative symptoms of schizophrenia are uncommon, although studies have reported negative symptoms in POE. Common negative symptoms reported were alogia (71%), anhedonia (67%), apathy (66%), depressed affect (61%), and affective bluntness (61%) and patients with negative symptoms or mixed (positive and negative symptoms) were the most impaired [9]. POE patients rarely have prodromal symptoms or personality disorganization prior to the onset of POE as normally seen in patients with schizophrenia.

Several studies provide evidence that POE seldom fulfill the Bleulerian concept of schizophrenia, and consequently the term POE/organic psychosis is preferred over "schizophrenia like psychosis" [83]. Organic psychosis/POE are included in the Diagnostic and Statistical Manual of Mental Health Disorders, 5th edition (DSM-V), and improvement in diagnostic criteria is highlighted in Table 1 [82].

A case study using the Wechsler Adult Intelligence Scale, Luria's neuropsychological, test and a quantitative EEG examination on a group of patients with POE concluded that in patients with epilepsy and chronic psychosis, there was decreased performance in verbal abilities thought due to cortical dysfunction of the frontal lobe [83]. Patients with schizophrenia and those with POE had almost identical neuropsychological profiles, with impairments of attention, episodic memory, and executive function [84], compared to controls.

Risk factors associated with POE are chronic epilepsy with a younger age of onset, enduring through puberty, and severity of epilepsy (frequency of seizures, multiple seizure type; a history of status epilepticus/resistance to drug treatment) [5, 7, 18]. Many years (approximately 10–14 years) are said to intervene between the onset of epilepsy and psychosis, although this is variable [18] and could be partially explained by the

Table 1 DSM-V diagnostic criteria of schizophrenia compared with organic psychosis (not substance/medication-induced psychotic disorder)

Schizophrenia 295.90 (F20.9)	Psychotic disorder due to medical condition (e.g., epilepsy) Include the name of the medical condition 293.81 (F06.2) with delusions 293.82 (F06.0) with hallucinations
A. >2 (for at least a month if not successfully treated) **1.** Delusions **2.** Hallucinations **3.** Disorganized speech (e.g., Derailment or incoherence) **4.** Grossly disorganized or catatonic behavior **5.** Negative symptoms **B.** Decline in level of functioning (such as education/work, relationships, personal care). Continuous signs of disturbance persist for at least 6 months, with at least 1 month of symptoms unless successfully treated **C.** Schizoaffective disorder and depression and bipolar disorder with psychotic features have been ruled out **D.** Organic causes of psychosis and substance misuse and medication have been excluded	**A.** Prominent hallucinations or delusions **B.** Evidence from history, examinations, and investigations that disturbance is a direct pathophysiological consequence of the medical condition **C.** The disturbance is not better explained by another mental illness **D.** The disturbance does not occur exclusively during the course of a delirium **E.** The disturbance causes clinical significant distress or impairment in social, occupational, or other important areas of activities of daily living

age of onset of epilepsy tending to be younger compared to mean onset of psychosis, being later around mid-twenties [83]. The frequency of seizures at the time of development of the psychosis is variable; some authors report an improvement, whereas others report a worsening [4]. The psychosocial impact of epilepsy can also act as a trigger for psychosis [29, 85]. There is evidence of overlapping etiological and environmental factors between epilepsy and schizophrenia and recent evidence of a genetic overlap between these disorders [86, 87]. Molecular genetic findings have illustrated that the comorbidity of psychotic symptoms and epilepsy is a product of shared underlying biological mechanisms; specific genomic structural variants have been described that predispose to schizophrenia, autism, epilepsy, and intellectual disability [88]. Of interest are genes encoding ion channels, particularly variation within gene CACNA1C (encoding a subunit of the L-type voltage-dependent calcium channel), which is also associated with schizophrenia as well as recurrent depression and bipolar disorder. Supporting that, individuals might experience both psychosis and epilepsy in part because of underlying genetic vulnerabilities that play a role in the pathogenesis of both epilepsy and psychosis

[88]. TBC1D24 mutations in a family caused expanded dominant and recessive phenotypes that have been seen in POE [89]. It is likely that structural brain abnormalities (e.g.,
similar gene variables associated with both conditions, cortical dysgenesis, or diffuse brain
lesions) underlie both epilepsy and psychosis and that seizures modify the presentation of
psychosis and vice versa, thus producing a clinical picture of both affinity and antagonism
between the two disorders [18].

Table 2 Summary of different groups of psychosis of epilepsy [32]

Psychosis of epilepsy	Feature	Treatment of psychosis
Preictal	EEG important; prodromal symptoms days to hours leading up to a seizure	Psychosis normally resolves without treatment. Aim to control seizures
Ictal	EEG important; often involves a type of nonconvulsive status epilepticus Brief hours–days	If extends beyond days likely to be ictal behavior Psychosis normally resolves without treatment. Aim to control seizures
Postictal	Psychiatric symptoms normally occur within 7 days after a seizure or seizure cluster; after a lucid interval of hours to 1 week Insomnia, aggression, and self-harm are features	Often resolves without treatment, but psychosis can be shortened and normally responds well to antipsychotic treatment, e.g., risperidone, quetiapine, or olanzapine
Interictal (brief/chronic)	Can occur at any time with no relationship to the timing of seizures Common with longstanding complex partial seizures (e.g., temporal lobe epilepsy)	Normally responds well to treatment, e.g., risperidone, quetiapine, or olanzapine. Clozapine has also been effective if other APDs have failed and not exacerbated epilepsy ECT was found to be effective and has emerging anticonvulsive properties
Epileptic treatment	Psychosis may be the expression of adverse effects of AEDs or surgery. But discontinuation of an AED with mood-stabilizing properties can also trigger mania or psychoses Temporal lobectomy is followed by psychosis in a small percent of patients	Medication-induced psychosis by AEDs is more likely in treatment resistant epilepsy Psychosis has been controlled and surgery carried out successfully, responding well to antipsychotic drugs

Family history of psychosis and a family history of epilepsy were significant risk factors for POE [86]. Hence, comprehensive assessment should include exploration of psychosocial factors, including environmental and family factors. In refractory and persistent cases of POE, detailed investigations should include EEG and MRI scan, and blood tests for autoantibodies may be required. Careful evaluation of AEDs and their impact on POE may need consideration. Management of POE depends upon the type of POE and is highlighted in Table 2.

7. Conclusions

Psychosis and epilepsy share similar underlying pathology, with acquired or neurodevelopmental changes making the brain vulnerable, particularly in the mesolimbic structures, which then trigger epileptic seizures. Molecular genetic findings have been found in POE, especially genes encoding ion channels within gene CACNA1C and TBC1D24, which is also associated with schizophrenia as well as recurrent depression and bipolar disorder. The seizures then activate kindling and plastic regenerative changes, affecting DA, glutamate, and GABA pathways, which results in psychosis. This explains why family history and environmental factors play a role and why there is a higher prevalence of psychosis in epileptic patients compared to the general population, with greater prevalence in TLE, hippocampal sclerosis, and frontal lesions, with a chronic history and a high frequency of seizures. It also explains why there is a gap of around 10 years from the onset of epilepsy to developing psychosis. Epilepsy and psychosis have a complex relationship and can be antagonistic of each other ("forced normalization") explaining why the treatment for one (epilepsy or psychosis) can trigger the other. This highlights the importance between collaboration between neurologist and neuropsychiatrist in the management of POE. POE differs from schizophrenia in that it tends to be mainly positive symptoms and premorbid personality is preserved; negative symptoms are very rare and are seen as a poor prognostic factor.

The timing of psychosis in relation to the seizure is important as it effects the management, and for this reason, we have divided the chapter into subsections: preictal psychosis, ictal psychosis, postictal psychosis (of which self-harm and aggression are common features), interictal and AEDs or treatment-induced POE. In preictal and ictal psychosis, seizure control is key in the treatment. In the other sections optimizing seizure control and reviewing the side effects of the AEDs, which may induce psychosis, and treating the psychosis are important. We do this with low doses of APDs (e.g., risperidone, quetiapine, or olanzapine), which have proven to be therapeutic and still maintain epileptic seizure control; even clozapine is used, which is known to be epileptogenic. There is also increasing evidence from case studies to support the use of ECT in the management of POE, although not currently licensed. Also surgery for epilepsy has been successfully carried out in POE with careful management.

References

[1] Clancy MJ, Clarke M, Connor D, Cotter DR, Cannon M. The prevalence of psychosis in epilepsy: a systematic review. Schizophr Bull 2011;37:49.

[2] Sherwin I, Peron-Magnan P, Bancaud J. Prevalence of psychosis in epilepsy as a function of the laterality of the epileptogenic lesion. Arch Neurol 1982;39(10):621–5.

[3] Bredkajer SR, Mortensen PB, Parnas J. Epilepsy and non-organic non-affective psychosis. National epidemiologic study. Br J Psychiatry 1998;172:235–8.

[4] Kandratavicus L, Hallak JE, Leite JP. What are the similarities and differences between schizophrenia and schizophrenia like psychosis of epilepsy? A neuropathological approach to the understanding of schizophrenia spectrum and epilepsy. Epilepsy Behav 2014;38:143–7.

[5] Mendez MF, Grau R, Doss RC, Taylor JL. Schizophrenia in epilepsy: seizure and psychosis variables. Neurology 1993;43(6):1073–7.

[6] van der Feltz-Cornelis CM, Ader HJ, Van Dyck R, Aldenkamp AP, Linszen D, Boenink A. Psychosis in epilepsy patients and other chronic medically ill patients and the role of cerebral pathology in the onset of psychosis: a clinical epidemiological study. Seizure 2008;17(5):446–56.

[7] Irwin LG, Fortune DG. Risk factors for psychosis secondary to temporal lobe epilepsy: a systematic review. J Neuropsychiatry Clin Neurosci 2014;26(1):5–23.

[8] Pal SG, Grillo EB, Salazar GF, Odio SOF. Causas de muerte en pacientes con epilepsia y psicosis asociada. Comparacion con pacientes esquizofrenicos y pacientes no psiquiatricos [Causes of death on patients suffering from epilepsy and associated psychosis. A comparison made with schicophrenic patients and nonpsychiatric patients]. Revista del Hospital Psiquiatrico de la Habana 2005;2(1).

[9] Granieri E, Fazio P. The Lombrosian prejudice in medicine. The case of epilepsy. Epileptic psychosis. Epilepsy and aggressiveness. Neurophysiology 2012;33(1):173–92.

[10] Pearce JMS. Leopold Auenbrugger: camphor-induced epilepsy—remedy for manic psychosis. Eur Neurol 2008;59(1–2):105–7.

[11] Lund, M. Does bromide cause conversion of epilepsy to psychosis? J Hist Neurosci; Apr 1997; vol. 6 (1); p. 61–71

[12] Kawakami Y, Itoh Y. Forced normalization: antagonism between epilepsy and psychosis. Paediatr Neurol 2017;70:16–9.

[13] Kanemoto K, Tsuji T, Kawasaki J. Reexamination of interictal psychoses based on DSM IV psychosis classification and international epilepsy classification. Epilepsia 2001;42(1):98–103.

[13a] Freud S. A seventeenth-century demonological neurosis. Standard Edition of the Complete Psychological Works of Sigmund Freud. 19:London: Hogarth Press; 1923. p. 77–105.

[14] Ovsiew F. A case of epilepsy and psychosis in the seventeenth century. Behav Neurol 1992;5(4):215–7.

[14a] Jackson H. On the anatomical, physiological, and pathological investigations of epilepsies. West Riding Lunatic Asylum Med Rep 1873;3:315–49.

[15] Kasper BS, Taylor DC, Janz D, Kasper EM, Maier M, Williams MR, Crow TJ. Neuropathology of epilepsy and psychosis: the contributions of J.A.N. Corsellis. Brain 2010;133(12):3795–805.

[15a] Hill D, Pond DA, Mitchell W, Falconer MA. Personality changes following temporal lobectomy for epilepsy. J Ment Sci 1957;103(430):18–27.

[15b] Slater E, Beard AW, Glithero E. The schizophrenia-like psychosis of epilepsy. Br J Psychiatry 1963;109:95–150.

[16] Tebartz Van Elst L, et al. Amygdala pathology in psychosis of epilepsy: a magnetic resonance imaging study in patients with temporal lobe epilepsy. Brain 2002;125:140–9.

[17] Adams S, O'Brien TJ, et al. Neuropsychiatry morbidity in focal epilepsy. Br J Psychiatry 2008;192:464–9. https://doi.org/10.1192/bjp.107.046664.

[17a] Mendez MF, Grau R, Doss RC, Taylor JL. Schizophrenia in epilepsy: seizure and psychosis variables. Neurology 1993;43(6):1073–7.

[18] Sachdev P. Schizophrenia-like psychosis and epilepsy: the status of the association. Am J Psychiatry 1998;155:3.

[18a] Crow TJ, Ball J, Bloom SR, Brown R, Bruton CJ, Colter N, Frith CD, Johnstone EC, Owens DG, Roberts GW. Schizophrenia as an anomaly of development of cerebral asymmetry. A postmortem study and a proposal concerning the genetic basis of the disease. Arch Gen Psychiatry 1989;46(12):1145–50.

[19] Gattaz WF, Valente KD, Raposo NRB, Vincentiis S, Talib LL. Increased PLA2 activity in the hippocampus of patients with temporal lobe epilepsy and psychosis. J Psychiatr Res 2011;45 (12):1617–20.

[20] Jibiki I, Maeda T, Kubota T, Yamaguchi N. I-IMP SPECT brain imaging in epileptic psychosis: a study of two cases of temporal lobe epilepsy with schizophrenia-like syndrome. Neuropsychobiology 1993;28(4):207–11.

[21] Bruton CJ, Stevens JR, Frith CD. Epilepsy, psychosis, and schizophrenia: clinical and neuropathologic correlations. Neurology 1994;44(1):34–42.

[21a] Kendrick JF, Gibbs FA. Origin spread and neurosurgical treatment of the psychomotor type seizure discharge. J Neurosurg 1957;14:270–84.

[21b] Heath RG. Common clinical characteristics of epilepsy and schizophrenia. Am J Psychiatry 1962;11:1013–26.

[22] Akiyama T, Tsuchiya M. Study on pathological mechanisms of temporal lobe epilepsy and psychosis through kindling effect. Asian J Psychiatr 2009;2(1):37–9.

[23] Sato M, Hikasa N, Otsuki S. Experimental epilepsy, psychosis, and dopamine receptor sensitivity. Biol Psychiatry 1979;14(3):537–40.

[24] Canuet L, Ishii R, Iwase M, Ikezawa K, Kurimoto R, Takahashi H, Currais A, Azechi M, Aoki Y, Nakahachi T, Soriano S, Takeda M. Psychopathology and working memory-induced activation of the prefrontal cortex in schizophrenia-like psychosis of epilepsy: evidence from magnetoencephalography. Psychiatry Clin Neurosci 2011;65(2):183–90.

[24a] Adachi N, Onuma T, Nishiwaki S, Murauchi S, Akanuma N, Ishida S, Takei N. Inter-ictal and post-ictal psychoses in frontal lobe epilepsy: a retrospective comparison with psychoses in temporal lobe epilepsy. Seizure 2000;9(5):328–35.

[25] Sperling W, Franzek E. Evaluation of 'schizophrenia-like psychosis' in left hemispheric temporal lobe epilepsy. Eur J Psychiatry 1995;9(3):143–50.

[25a] Slater E, Moran PA. The schizophrenia-like psychoses of epilepsy: relation between ages of onset. Br J Psychiatry 1969;115:599–600.

[26] Adachi N, Onuma T, Kato M, Ito M, Akanuma N, Hara T, Oana Y, et al. Analogy between psychosis antedating epilepsy and epilepsy. Epilepsia 2011;52(7):1239–44.

[26a] Schmitz B, Trimble MR, Moriarty J, Costa PC, Ell PJ. Pschiatric profiles and patterns of blood flow in patients with focal epilepsies. J Neurol Neurosurg Psychiatry 1997;62:458–63.

[26b] Trimble M. The Psychoses of Epilepsy. New York, NY: Raven Press; 1991.

[27] Falip, M.; Carreño, M.; Donaire, A; Maestro, I; Pintor, L; Bargalló, N; Boget, T; Raspall, A; Rumià, J; Setoaín, J. Postictal psychosis: a retrospective study in patients with refractory temporal lobe epilepsy. Seizure; Mar 2009; vol. 18 (2); p. 145–149

[27a] Adachi N, Akanuma N, Ito M, Kato M, Hara T, Oana Y, et al. Epilpetic organic and genetic vulnerabilities for timing of the development of interictal psychosis. Br J Psychiatry 2010;196:212–6.

[28] Fenton GW. Epilepsy and psychosis. Ir Med J 1978;71(9):315–24.

[29] Smith PF, Darlington CL. The development of psychosis in epilepsy: a re-examination of the kindling hypothesis. Behav Brain Res 1996;75(1–2):59–66.

[30] Semple D, Smyth R. Oxford handbook of psychiatry. 2nd ed ; 2011.p. 152–4.

[31] David A, Fleminger S, Kopelman M, Lovestone S, Mellers J. Lishman's organic psychiatry—a textbook of neuropsychiatry. 4th ed. Wiley-Blackwell Chapter 6 Epilepsy p. 335.

[32] https://www.epilepsy.com/learn/challenges-epilepsy/moods-and-behavior/mood-and-behavior-101/psychosis.

[33] Bennett J, Dusad A. Non-convulsive status epilepticus in a woman with psychosis and epilepsy treated with clozapine: an EEG and video evidence presentation. J Neuropsychiatry Clin Neurosci 2014;26 (2):10.

[34] Kazis DA, Papaliagkas V, Vlaikidis N, Kiana T, Lialias I. Psychosis or epilepsy? Prolonged events do not always indicate psychosis and should prompt, under certain conditions, further investigation. Epilepsia 2013;54:110–1.

[35] Gandhi P, Ogunyemi B, MacDonald A, Gadit A. Psychosis in temporal lobe epilepsy: atypical presentation. BMJ Case Rep 2012;2012. https://doi.org/10.1136/bcr.11.2011.5169.

[36] Leutmezer F, Podreka I, Asenbaum S, Pietrzyk U, Lucht H, Back C, Benda N, Baumgartner C. Postictal psychosis in temporal lobe epilepsy. Epilepsia 2003;44(4):582–90.

[37] Hilger E, Zimprich F, Jung R, Pataraia E, Baumgartner C, Bonelli S. Postictal psychosis in temporal lobe epilepsy: a case-control study. Eur J Neurol 2013;20(6):955–61.

[38] Alper K, Kuzniecky R, Carlson C, Barr WB, Vorkas CK, Patel JG, Carrelli AL, Starner K, Devinsky O, Flom PL. Postictal psychosis in partial epilepsy: a case-control study. Ann Neurol 2008;63(5):602–10.

[38a] Kanner AM. Postictal psychiatric events during prolonged video-electroencephalographic monitoring studies. Arch Neurol 1996;53:258–63.

[38b] Logsdail SJ, Toone BK. Postictal psychosis: a clinical and phenomenological description. Br J Psychiatry 1988;152:246–52.

[39] Iqbal M, Prasad M, Baxter P. Postictal psychosis: a rare entity in childhood epilepsy. Eur J Paediatr Neurol 2013;17(Suppl 1)S70.

[40] Kanemoto K, Kawasaki J, Mori E. Violence and epilepsy: a close relation between violence and postictal psychosis. Epilepsia 1999;40(1):107–9.

[41] Cleary, RA; Thompson, PJ; Thom, M; Foong, J. Postictal psychosis in temporal lobe epilepsy: risk factors and postsurgical outcome? Epilepsy Res; Sep 2013; vol. 106 (no. 1–2); p. 264–272.

[42] Logsdail SJ, Toone BK. Postictal psychosis: a clinical and phenomenological description. Br J Psychiatry 1988;152:246–52.

[43] Mendez MF, Grau R. The postictal psychosis of epilepsy: investigation in two patients. Int J Psychiatry Med 1991;21(1):85–92.

[44] Pollak TA, Nicholson TR, Mellers JDC, Vincent A, David AS. Epilepsy-related psychosis: a role for autoimmunity? Epilepsy Behav 2014;36:33–8.

[45] Akanuma N, Kanemoto K, Adachi N, Kawasaki J, Ito M, Onuma T. Prolonged postictal psychosis with forced normalization (Landolt) in temporal lobe epilepsy. Epilepsy Behav 2005;6(3):456–9.

[46] Ceri V, Demirpence D, Sen E, Dogangun B. Efficacy of quetiapine in interictal psychosis of epilepsy. Neuropsychiatr Enfance Adolesc 2012;60(5):S184.

[47] Tufan AE, Yilmaz S, Ozel OO, Ugurlu GK, Bilici R, Namli M. Epilepsi ve sinirda entelektuel islevselligi olan bir ergende interiktal psikoz ve tedavisi: Vak'a takdimi Inter-ictal psychosis and its treatment in an adolescent with epilepsy and borderline intellectual functioning: a case report. Yeni Symposium 2011;49(1):51–3.

[48] Baum P, Kopf A, Hermann W, Wagner A. Postictal paranoid-hallucinatory psychosis in cryptogenic epilepsy. Psychiatr Prax 2007;34(5):249–57.

[49] Brown P, Kashiviswanath S, Huynh A, Allha N, Piaggio K, Sahoo S, Gupta A. Lithium therapy in comorbid temporal lobe epilepsy and cycloid psychosis. Oxf Med Case Reports 2016;2016(12).

[50] Besag F, Caplan R, et al. Psychiatric and behavioural disorders in children with epilepsy (ILAE Task Force Report): epilepsy and psychosis in children and teenagers. Epileptic Disord 2016; [Epub ahead of print].

[51] D'Alessio L, Scevola L, Fernandez LM, Oddo S, Konopka H, Seoane E, Kochen S. Two years follow up after epilepsy surgery in patients with a history of presurgical psychosis. Epilepsia 2013;54:179.

[51a] Wolf P. Acute behavioral symptomatology at disappearance of epileptiform EEG abnormality: paradoxical or "forced" normalization. In: Smith D, Treiman D, Trimble M, editors. Neurobehavioral problems in epilepsy: advances in neurology. vol. 55: New York: Raven Press; 1991. p. 127–42.

[52] Adachi N, Matsuura M, Okubo Y, Oana Y, Takei N, Kato M, Hara T, Onuma T. Predictive variables of interictal psychosis in epilepsy. Neurology 2000;55(9):1310–4.

[53] Ramani V, Gumnit RJ. Intensive monitoring of interictal psychosis in epilepsy. Ann Neurol 1982;11(6):613–22.

[54] Flügel D, O'Toole A, Thompson PJ, Koepp MJ, Cercignani M, Symms MR, Foong J. A neuropsychological study of patients with temporal lobe epilepsy and chronic interictal psychosis. Epilepsy Res 2006;71(2–3):117–28.

[55] van der Feltz-Cornelis CM. Treatment of interictal psychiatric disorder in epilepsy. II. Chronic psychosis. Acta Neuropathol 2002;14(1):44–8.

[56] Marsh L, et al. Structural brain abnormalities in patients with schizophrenia, epilepsy, and epilepsy with chronic interictal psychosis. Psychiatry Res 2001;108(10):1–15.

[56a] Reith J, Benkelfat C, Sherwin A, Yasuhara Y, Kuwabara H, Andermann F, Bachneff S, Cumming P, Diksic M, Dyve SE, Etienne P, Evans AC, Lal S, Shevell M, Savard G, Wong DF, Chouinard G, Gjedde A. Elevated dopa decarboxylase activity in living brain of patients with psychosis. Proc Natl Acad Sci USA 1994;91:11651–4.

[57] Cifelli P, Grace A. Psychosis in temporal lobe epilepsy and the modulation of dopamine system activity. In: Biological Psychiatry. vol. 65 (8); 2009.

[58] Gattaz WF, Valente KD, Raposo NR, Vincentiis S, Talib LL. Increased PLA2 activity in the hippocampus of patients with temporal lobe epilepsy and psychosis. J Psychiatr Res 2011;45(12):1617–20.

[58a] Suckling J, Roberts H, Walker M, Highley JR, Fenwick P, Oxbury J, Esiri MM. Temporal lobe epilepsy with and without psychosis: exploration of hippocampal pathology including that in subpopulations of neurons defined by their content of immunoreactive calcium-binding proteins. Acta Neuropathol 2000;99(5):547–54.

[59] Yelmo S, Morera-Fumero AL, González PA, Barrau V. Serum S100B levels in first-episode psychosis and juvenile myoclonic epilepsy. Eur Psychiatry 2012;27:1033. https://doi.org/10.1016/S0924-9338(12)75200-8.

[59a] Monji A, Yanagimoto K, Maekawa T, Sumida Y, Yamazaki K, Kojima K. Plasma folate and homocysteine levels may be related to interictal "schizophrenia-like" psychosis in patients with epilepsy. J Clin Psychopharmacol 2005;25(1):3–5.

[60] Scherer EA, Hallak JEC, Leite JP, Gitai DLG, Brusco J, Moreira JE, Lucio-Eterovic AKB, Andrade VDSS, Carlotti Junior CG. Neurotransmitters related to depression and psychosis in patients with temporal lobe epilepsy. Eur Psychiatry 2011;26:909.

[61] Kanner AM, Rivas-Grajales AM. Psychosis of epilepsy: a multifaceted neuropsychiatric disorder. CNS Spectr 2016;21(3):247–57.

[62] Taylor D, Paton C, Kapur S. The South London & Maudsley NHS Foundation Trust Oxleas NHS Foundation Trust. Prescribing Guidelines in Psychiatry 12th ed. Wiley-Blackwell; Chapter 7 p. 632–635

[63] Oner O, Unal O, Deda G. A case of psychosis with temporal lobe epilepsy: SPECT changes with treatment. Pediatr Neurol 2005;32(3):197–200.

[64] Onuma T, Adachi N, Hisano T, Uesugi S. 10-year follow-up study of epilepsy with psychosis. Jpn J Psychiatry Neurol 1991;45(2):360–1.

[65] Hino K, Tanaka S, Miyajima M, Sakamoto K, Hara K, Watanabe Y, Watanabe M, Takahashi S, Kato M, Onuma T. Status of atypical antipsychotic use for epileptic psychosis in the epilepsy ward of our hospital. Epilepsia 2009;50:249.

[66] Langosch JM, Trimble MR. Epilepsy, psychosis and clozapine. Hum Psychopharmacol 2002;17(2):115–9.

[67] Robertson MM, Trimble MR, Townsend HRA. Phenomenology of depression in epilepsy. Epilepsia 1987;28:364–8.

[68] Reutens DC, Savard G, Andermann F, Dubeau F, Olivier A. Results of surgical treatment in temporal lobe epilepsy with chronic psychosis. Brain 1997;120:1929–36.

[69] Marchetti RL, Fiore LA, Valente KD, Gronich G, Nogueira AB, Tzu WH. Surgical treatment of temporal lobe epilepsy with interictal psychosis: results of six cases. Epilepsy Behav 2003;4(2):146–52.

[70] Chen Z, O'Brien TJ, Kwan P, Lusicic A, Velakoulis D, Adams SJ. Psychosis in epilepsy: role of antiepileptic drugs. Neuroepidemiology 2015;45(4):308–9.

[71] Pasini A, Pitzianti M, Baratta A, Moavero R, Curatolo P. Timing and clinical characteristics of topiramate-induced psychosis in a patient with epilepsy and tuberous sclerosis. Clin Neuropharmacol 2014;37(1):38–9.

[72] Trimble M. Patients with epilepsy and psychosis treated with vigabatrin. J Epilepsy 1998;11(2):61–6.

[73] Brandt C, Fueratsch N, Boehme V, Kramme C, Pieridou M, Villagran A, Woermann F, Pohlmann-Eden B. Development of psychosis in patients with epilepsy treated with lamotrigine: report of six cases and review of the literature. Epilepsy Behav 2007;11(1):133–9.

[74] Needham E, Hamelijnck J. Temporal lobe epilepsy masquerading as psychosis—a case report and literature review. Neurocase 2012;18(5):400–4.

[75] Sinclair DB, Snyder T. Psychosis with frontal lobe epilepsy responds to carbamazepine. J Child Neurol 2008;23(4):431–4.

[76] Hirashima Y, Morimoto M, Nishimura A, Osamura T, Sugimoto T. Alternative psychosis and dysgraphia accompanied by forced normalization in a girl with occipital lobe epilepsy. Epilepsy Behav 2008;12(3):481–5.

[77] Calvet E, Caravotta PG, Scévola L, Teitelbaum J, Seoane E, Kochen S, D'Alessio L. Psychosis after epilepsy surgery: report of three cases. Epilepsy Behav 2011;22(4):804–7.

[78] Matsuura M. Psychosis of epilepsy, with special reference to anterior temporal lobectomy. Epilepsia 1997;38:32–4.

[79] Sanguankiat P, Nabangchang C. The paradox of epilepsy surgery and psychosis: report of two cases. J Neurol Sci 2009;285:S257.

[80] Guarnieri R, Hallak JEC, Walz R, Velasco TR, Alexandre Júnior V, Terra-Bustamante VC, Wichert-Ana L, Sakamoto AC. Pharmacological treatment of psychosis in epilepsy. Rev Bras Psiquiatr 2004;26 (1):57–61 [Sao Paulo, Brazil: 1999].

[81] Benjaminsen S. Temporal lobe epilepsy and schizophreniform psychosis. Ugeskr Laeger 1980;142 (3):168–9.

[82] Arzy S, Schurr R. "God has sent me to you": right temporal epilepsy, left prefrontal psychosis. Epilepsy Behav 2016;60:7–10.

[83] Ito M, Adachi N, Okazaki M, Adachi T, Kato M, Onuma T, Matsubara R, Hara K. Evaluation of psychiatric symptoms in epilepsy psychosis using brief psychiatric rating scale. Epilepsia 2010;51:29.

[84] Mellers JDC, Toone BK, Lishman WA. A neuropsychological comparison of schizophrenia and schizophrenia-like psychosis of epilepsy. Psychol Med 2000;30(2):325–35.

[85] Kandratavicius L, Hallak JEC, Leite JP. Psicose e depressao na epilepsia do lobo temporal psychosis and depression in temporal lobe epilepsy. J Epilepsy Clin Neurophysiol 2007;13(4):163–7.

[86] Clarke MC, Tanskanen A, Huttunen MO, Clancy M, Cotter DR, Cannon M. Evidence for shared susceptibility to epilepsy and psychosis: a population-based family study. Biol Psychiatry 2012;71 (9):836–9.

[87] Shrivastava AK. Psychosis in relation to epilepsy—a clinical model of neuro-psychiatry. Indian J Psychiatry 1996;38(3):120–32.

[88] Xenitidis K, Campbell C. Molecular and the relationship between epilepsy and psychosis. Br J Psychiatry 2010;197:75–7.

[89] Banuelos E, Ramsey K, Belnap N, Krishnan M, Balak C, Szelinger S, Siniard AL, Russell M, Richholt R, De Both M, Piras I, Naymik M, Claasen AM, Rangasamy S, Huentelman MJ, Craig DW, Campeau PM, Narayanan V, Schrauwen I. Case Report: novel mutations in *TBC1D24* are associated with autosomal dominant tonic-clonic and myoclonic epilepsy and recessive Parkinsonism, psychosis, and intellectual disability. F1000Res 2017;6:553.

CHAPTER 18

Epilepsy and psychogenic nonepileptic seizures

Sofia Markoula*, Markus Reuber[†]
*Department of Neurology, University Hospital of Ioannina, Ioannina, Greece
[†]Academic Neurology Unit, University of Sheffield, Royal Hallamshire Hospital, Sheffield, United Kingdom

Contents

1. Introduction

Psychogenic nonepileptic seizures (PNES) are experiential and behavioral responses to internal or external triggers that superficially resemble or can be mistaken for epileptic seizures. They are neither associated with epileptic discharges in the electroencephalogram (EEG) nor other readily identifiable pathophysiological changes [1, 2].

PNES sit uneasily within the current psychiatric classification systems. Most fulfill the diagnostic criteria of a dissociative (conversion) disorder (dissociative convulsions) in the International Classification of Diseases, 10th edition (World Health Organization 1992) or those of a functional neurological symptom (conversion) disorder in the Diagnostic

The Comorbidities of Epilepsy
https://doi.org/10.1016/B978-0-12-814877-8.00018-0

and Statistical Manual of Mental Disorders, 5th edition (DSM-V) (American Psychiatric Association 2013) [3]. However, many patients also meet the criteria for mood and anxiety disorders, posttraumatic stress disorder, and intermittent explosive disorder. Some of these disorders show phenomenological overlap with PNES and may be difficult to distinguish reliably from PNES [4]. The overwhelming majority of PNES are not perceived as or considered to be willfully produced, but a small minority of seizures that are objectively indistinguishable from PNES (experts estimate <5%) [5] are thought to involve intentional processes, for instance, in factitious disorder (i.e., willful fabrication of symptoms to adopt the sick role) or malingering (i.e., willful fabrication of symptoms in the presence of external incentive, not considered a mental disorder) [4, 6].

Together with syncope and epilepsy, PNES are one of the three commonest causes of transient loss of consciousness, accounting for 10%–20% of new presentations in seizure clinics [7]. Unfortunately, PNES continue to represent a serious diagnostic challenge, and most patients eventually receiving the diagnosis are initially told they have epilepsy. In fact, most PNES are only diagnosed correctly several years after their initial manifestation [8]. Diagnostic delay is not limited to complex scenarios in which epilepsy is comorbid with PNES [9].

As a consequence of misdiagnoses, PNES account for approximately 20% of patients referred to specialists with apparently refractory epilepsy and up to 30% of patients with intractable epilepsy referred for consideration of epilepsy surgery [10]. Similarly, 25% of patients referred to a neurological intensive care unit with refractory seizure status turned out to have PNES (pseudostatus) [11].

Diagnostic uncertainty and delay can have serious consequences: Patients with epilepsy and PNES are treated with multiple drugs in higher dosages, and they report more side effects or allergies than patients with epilepsy, with more than 22% of patients found to have drug levels beyond their usual therapeutic range [12]. Patients are at particularly high risk when they present with prolonged PNES. In such scenarios, the inappropriate use of intravenous anticonvulsants, general anesthesia, and intubation can cause iatrogenic injury or even death [13].

The diagnostic difficulties are enhanced by the fact that a proportion of patients have a combination of epilepsy and PNES—either concurrently or sequentially. If one condition follows the other, epilepsy is almost invariably the initial problem. It can, therefore, be considered a risk factor for PNES [14–17]. There is considerable uncertainty about the epidemiology of mixed epileptic and nonepileptic seizure disorders; actively comorbid epilepsy has been described in 6%–60% of patients with PNES [14]. To some extent this broad range is explained by case selection. For instance, the frequency of concurrent epilepsy has been found to be higher in PNES patients with intellectual disabilities (IDs) [18, 19]. Another important factor is the use of different diagnostic criteria for the diagnoses of epilepsy and PNES [20]. Lower frequencies of comorbid epilepsy are found when the criteria include the video-EEG documentation of PNES as well as epileptic seizures [21, 22].

The demographics of patients with PNES in the context of concurrent epilepsy are similar to those of patients with "pure" PNES. Except in particular subpopulations, such as pediatric patients, those with ID, or elderly patients [18, 23, 24], female patients predominate, making up about 75% of the whole patient population [25, 26]. When compared with those with PNES only at group level, patients with PNES and epilepsy may be a little younger at the time of diagnosis [8]. However, overall, the age distribution is similar in both groups; although PNES have been described as initially manifesting in children as young as five or in older patients [1, 27], most PNES disorders start in adolescence or early adulthood [9, 26].

2. Pathogenesis
2.1 Etiological factors

The variability of subjective and objective PNES manifestations and the diversity of commonly associated other psychiatric symptoms suggest the involvement of multiple mechanisms, indicating that PNES disorders are no homogeneous nosological entity [2]. A wide variety of environmental, physical, and psychological stressors may be etiologically relevant [6]. Predisposing/precipitating factors occur before the manifestation of the disorder and perpetuating/triggering after symptom onset. Different factors typically interact with each other, and particular stressors may only become pathogenic in the presence of other contributing factors [28].

Epilepsy can act as a predisposing, precipitating, perpetuating, or trigger factor: Epileptic seizures may contribute directly to the development of PNES [29]. For instance, it has been demonstrated that focal seizures without impaired consciousness may trigger PNES [30]. Epilepsy may also be one of several manifestations of an underlying brain disorder, with other manifestations putting patients at increased risk of developing PNES [31]. What is more, epilepsy is highly associated with stress and psychiatric disorders, such as anxiety and depression, potentially facilitating PNES [29, 32]. In some patients with epilepsy, mood disorders (or psychotic symptoms) linked to the development of PNES may be related to the use of antiepileptic drugs (AEDs) with negative psychotropic effects [32, 33]. Epilepsy can also cause stigmatization and adversely affect social inclusion [34]. Furthermore, it can reduce patients' self-esteem [35]. Having said all this, there is only limited knowledge about the special characteristics of the etiology of PNES in those with comorbid epilepsy. Trauma/sexual abuse is likely to be a less important etiological factor in this subgroup of PNES patients [23]. Like in those without previous epileptic seizures, PNES are more likely to develop in women than men with epilepsy [16]. A later onset of epileptic seizures [36] and right hemispheric brain lesion [37, 38] have been proposed as additional risk factors for the development of PNES in patients with epilepsy, although these findings were not confirmed in a study by Reuber et al. [14], which suggested that, apart from female gender, mental retardation and lower

IQ are the main factors associated with an increased risk of PNES in those with epilepsy. Low IQ could predispose patients to the development of PNES because of more limited problem-solving and communication skills or greater difficulties with verbalizing emotional distress [19]. However, even in the subgroup of the PNES patient population with additional epilepsy factors also found in patients with "pure" PNES, disorders are likely to be relevant.

Stressful or traumatic life events have been identified in the majority of PNES patients, and there is some evidence to suggest that a history of predisposing traumatic experiences is more common in patients with PNES than in patients with other functional neurological symptoms [28]. Trauma, particularly sexual abuse, has been proposed by many authors as a major factor in the pathogenesis of PNES, and high rates of posttraumatic stress disorder (PTSD) have been reported among PNES patients [39, 40]. Other factors that may be relevant include severe environmental stress, problems in the family or close social environment, bereavement, bullying, and separation anxiety [28]. Stressful or traumatic experiences have also been reported as precipitants of PNES disorders [41]. In fact, Bowman et al. identified a precipitating event in all but 9% of patients in their series [42]. Factors that have been described as precipitating PNES include rape [39], injury [43], "symbolic" traumatic experience in adulthood after childhood abuse [39], head injury [44], intracranial surgery [44, 45], death of or separation from family members or friends [46], job loss [42], road traffic and other accidents [42], relationship difficulties [42], and legal action [47].

In children with PNES, studies have demonstrated that challenging family settings, difficulties in school (including bullying, specific learning difficulties, or unrealistic expectations), and interpersonal conflicts such as bullying predispose to or precipitate PNES [23, 48]. Seizure or illness models (reflected by a positive family history of epilepsy or psychiatric illness) are also a frequently reported [23]. In children, a previous history of epilepsy appears to be a more important risk factor for the development of PNES than in adults [23].

PNES disorders with onset in older age are equally common in men and women and less likely to be related to reported emotional trauma or sexual abuse [27]. Physical illnesses or health anxieties seem to be particularly important factors in this patient group, who are often experiencing other physical health problems (including epilepsy) [24] leading to health-related traumatic experiences [27, 48].

PNES can be associated with physical brain disorders and ID, and such conditions are a risk factor for the development of PNES [18, 19, 31]. Patients with ID and PNES form a subgroup with a particular clinical and etiological profile. Studies reveal that the proportion of patients with PNES and comorbid ID is similar to that of patients with PNES and additional epilepsy [49]. In those with PNES and ID, there is a trend toward a male preponderance and a relative paucity of antecedent sexual abuse [18]. Immediate situational or emotional triggers preceding individual PNES may be identified more commonly in those who develop PNES in the context of ID [18], and such patients may be particularly likely to present with recurrent PNES status [18].

Once PNES have become established, perpetuating factors often pose a major hindrance to patients' recovery or improvement. Many patients with PNES are frequent users of health care services, and their frequent health care contacts can exacerbate the problem [50]. Such contacts may lead to traumatic experiences with health care professionals or simply disrupt effective treatment by causing confusion through the involvement of many different health professionals [50]. Recurrent PNES have been reported as being triggered by medical encounters in scanners and during consultations. Excessive or inappropriate use of AEDs and AED toxicity has been shown to exacerbate PNES disorders [51]. The social/financial illness gain with financial or social benefits related to PNES may play a perpetuating role. A number of studies have demonstrated that outcomes are poorer in patients receiving health benefits, although this observation may simply reflect the fact that these patients are more unwell [52].

2.2 Mental and personality disorders

There is a complex relationship between PNES and comorbid mental and personality disorders, regardless of whether PNES are co-occurring with epilepsy or not. PNES can also cause other mental health symptoms directly (including panic, flashbacks, more prolonged dissociative states, functional motor symptoms) or, conversely, PNES may be precipitated or triggered directly by mental health symptoms such as panic or flashbacks. PNES can be facilitated by arousal or rumination associated with mental disorders. However, they may also coexist with mental disorders in the same patient without such a direct connection. The same is true for features of personality disorders such as emotional dysregulation or compulsivity.

Studies have found high rates of different psychiatric and personality disorders in patients with PNES [43], with almost all patients with PNES having at least one current and recognizable additional psychiatric illness categorized in DSM-IV [2, 53]. Depression is associated with this condition particularly closely in adolescents and more than half of patients with PNES have significant depressive symptoms, as measured by the Beck Depression Inventory [54]. Similarly, more than half the patients with PNES meet criteria for an anxiety disorder, including PTSD [55]. In general, patients with PNES score higher on emotional dysregulation tests than healthy and epileptic controls and have, more often, dissocial behavior and inhibitedness [56]. Personality traits considered pathological are frequently found in PNES patients—in some studies in as many as 75%–90% of patients [56]. There is evidence that certain premorbid personality traits and coping styles are associated with PNES, for example, a relationship has been found between PNES and cluster B disorders (borderline personality disorder and histrionic personality disorders), cluster C disorders (dependent personality disorder), and alexithymia [57].

A few studies have compared the psychiatric profile of patients with pure PNES and those with mixed epileptic and nonepileptic seizure disorders, revealing differences and similarities [14, 29, 53]. Kuyk et al. reported higher rates of somatoform and anxiety disorders in pure PNES patients with dissociative symptoms (dissociative amnesia, fugue, depersonalization disorder), somatoform symptoms, generalized anxiety, panic attacks, PTSD symptoms (flashbacks), paroxysmal anger, and motor agitation. Compared to those with only PNES, they found higher rates of personality disorders in patients with epilepsy and PNES, who were more often characterized by cluster C traits, resembling the pattern of personality pathology found in epilepsy-only patients [29]. However, compared to the findings in patients with epilepsy alone, personality pathology was more marked in those with PNES and epilepsy [29]. In accordance with the previous study, Devinsky et al. identified more than twice as many DSM-III Axis II personality disorders in a mixed PNES and epilepsy group compared with a pure PNES group [16]. Having said that, these findings were not replicated by Galimberti et al. who found that patients with PNES alone and those affected by PNES and epilepsy shared the same psychological profile, which differed from that of patients with epilepsy alone [53]. In their study, most of the patients with PNES or PNES and epilepsy were diagnosed with a somatoform disorder, with conversion disorders being the most frequent, followed by anxiety disorders [53], while in those with epilepsy, mood disorders were the most frequent diagnosis. At personality pathology level, patients affected by PNES (with or without additional epilepsy) were more likely to be diagnosed with cluster B personality disorders than those with epilepsy alone [53].

2.3 The integrative cognitive model of PNES

The previously discussed factors may confer an increased risk of developing PNES, but none are necessary or sufficient to explain the occurrence of PNES. What is more, they are not specific to PNES but could also be relevant in many other mental health disorders. The integrative model by Brown and Reuber incorporates previous theories and acknowledges that PNES are a particularly dramatic manifestations of a disorder that is also characterized by abnormal functioning between seizures [58]. According to this model, the preconscious activation of a rogue mental representation, the seizure scaffold, by internal or external triggers is common to all PNES (with the exception of those that result from patients' willed action). These rogue representations consist of cognitive-emotional-behavioral action programs that combine elements of inherent schemata (such as how to respond to fear) with the results of learning and experience across multiple contexts. Activation of the scaffold may be associated with abnormal arousal, emotion, or cognitive processing, accounting for the wide range of different PNES manifestations [58]. Comorbid or previous epilepsy fits into this model as a potential contributor to the seizure scaffold but also as a trigger for a threat response, a stressor leading to chronically

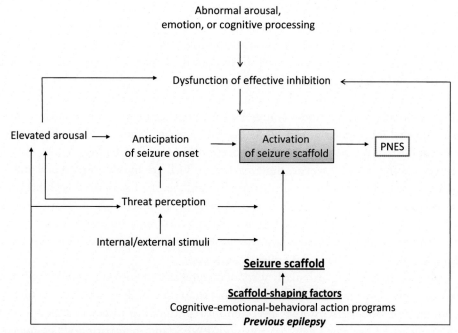

Fig. 1 The integrative cognitive model of PNES.

increased physiological arousal and a factor interfering with effective inhibition (for instance by giving rise to rumination about possible seizures) (Fig. 1).

3. Diagnostic evaluation

3.1 Clinical features

The diagnosis of PNES is still largely made on clinical grounds. It is important not to think of the diagnosis as a single event that takes place before treatment is started but as an ongoing process. This is particularly true in those with PNES and comorbid epilepsy in whom the relative frequency of epileptic and nonepileptic seizures may fluctuate. As PNES almost invariably develop after the onset of epilepsy [26], the initial diagnosis of PNES in such patients will often be prompted by the emergence of a new seizure type. Alternatively, diagnosticians may be alerted to the development of PNES by an unexpected change in seizure frequency or severity. Sometimes the diagnosis of additional PNES may be suggested by unusual seizure occurrence patterns, for instance, a complete absence of seizures during the summer holidays.

Although there are certain features that should alert clinicians to the possibility of PNES, it is important to stress that no single semiological feature is pathognomonic for this seizure disorder. Typical features of PNES, such as pelvic thrusting or asymmetric limb movements, can also be observed in epileptic seizures, and certain clinical features considered characteristic of epilepsy often occur in PNES [59]. Such features include autonomic manifestations (e.g., tachycardia, flushing, and sweating [60]), incontinence, and injury including tongue biting [1], provocation by specific triggers such as flashing lights [61], and nocturnal attacks [62].

Evidence of flailing or thrashing alone cannot be used to distinguish between PNES and epileptic seizures since these complex movements can also occur as ictal manifestations in frontal lobe epilepsy (FLE) [63]. Side-to-side head movements or body turning can occur during PNES, but they can also occur during focal epileptic seizures, especially FLE seizures [63, 64]. However, most seizures in FLE are highly stereotyped and brief (5–45 s), have a tendency to occur nocturnally, and are often associated with prominent axial body movements that begin abruptly [64]. In focal seizures of temporal origin, seizures may also be "bland," only associated with impairment of awareness and behavioral arrest [64]. Consequently, the absence of motor features does not allow a certain distinction of PNES and epileptic seizures.

Clinicians have to be particularly wary of features that are only reported by witnesses. Unfortunately, some aspects of the history that should be of diagnostic use according to the findings of video-EEG studies are often misreported. For instance, although PNES very rarely arise from true sleep, patients with PNES (and their partners/caregivers) are similarly likely to report seizures from sleep as those with epilepsy (when sleep-associated PNES are captured on video-EEG they typically arise from "pseudosleep," a state in which the patient seems to be asleep but is in fact awake or shortly after the patient has woken from sleep) [62]. Although video-EEG studies demonstrate that persistent eye-closure during a seizure is a strong indicator of PNES [65], this ictal sign is so often misreported by witnesses [66] that it cannot be used as a strong diagnostic indicator when it has not been captured on video. Ictal injuries are more common in those with epilepsy but reports of injuries (or incontinence) do not differentiate well [1]. However, despite the fact that single seizure features in the patient's history are of limited diagnostic value, seizure manifestation profiles can help distinguish between epileptic and nonepileptic seizures [9]. The diagnostic value of such profiles is increased when they are combined with similar profiles of witness observations.

A number of conversation analytic studies have demonstrated that clinicians should not only listen out for particular symptoms but also note how patients describe these symptoms. Patients with epilepsy have been shown to focus on their subjective seizure symptoms and to work hard to explain their nature whereas patients with PNES tend to focus on the situations in which the seizures have occurred or the consequences of their seizures. When prompted, patients with PNES resist the doctor's efforts to focus on one particularly memorable seizure (like the first, last, or worst) and do not provide more detail about what exactly any symptoms they have volunteered feel like [67].

Unfortunately, even careful history-taking from patients and witnesses is likely to leave clinicians and patients uncertain about the distinction of epileptic and nonepileptic seizures in some cases. The diagnosis of PNES can be made with greater certainty if clinicians are able to examine patients during a seizure or see a recording of a typical event (for instance on video) [65]. Examination findings suggesting a PNES rather than an epileptic seizure include the observation of responsiveness to environmental stimuli (including the presence of others, speech, or eyelid tickle—the use of painful stimuli is discouraged!), persistently closed eyes, resistance to eye-opening, and a normal pupillary light response. Cyanosis is likely to be absent. In a PNES involving flaccidity of the limbs, a hand held over the patient's head may drop to their side rather than onto their face. A review of semiological observations that may be useful in the differentiation of PNES and epileptic seizures suggested that the most reliable signs evident on video recordings of seizures are long duration, occurrence from apparent sleep with EEG-verified wakefulness, fluctuating course, asynchronous movements, pelvic thrusting, side-to-side head or body movement, closed eyes during the episode, ictal crying, memory recall, and absence of postictal confusion [63].

However, other observations may be very helpful as well. For instance, shaking movements in PNES typically have the characteristics of tremor (alternating agonist/antagonist activity) and not of clonic activity (rapid contractions of agonists followed by relaxation). The frequency of these movements tends not to change during the course of a PNES (only the amplitude varies) while it diminishes gradually in tonic-clonic epileptic seizures [68]. PNES often stop more suddenly than epileptic seizures.

Seizures involving complex movements such as writhing, flailing, and whole-body thrashing are likely to be PNES, especially if this activity persists for longer than 3 min [69]. In fact, writhing and thrashing movements have been shown to occur in 45% of patients with PNES but only in 17% of patients with focal epileptic seizures [65]. Asynchronous body movements, side-to-side head or body movement, rhythmic pelvic movements and fluctuating course with discontinuous motor patterns are often observed in PNES [69]. Opisthotonic posturing has been shown to be present in up to 28% of patients with PNES and is rarely observed in epileptic seizures [63].

Swooning attacks in which patients collapse in a limp, still, and unresponsive state are unlikely to be epileptic seizures, especially if prolonged [3].

Moaning or weeping during a seizure is much more common in PNES than epileptic seizures [60]. If ictal speech is observed, it tends to have more emotional content during PNES than epileptic seizures, in which speech has a monotone quality, is often "empty," and typically comprises repeated meaningless phrases or sounds [64]. Speech during PNES is often intelligible (patients with PNES often respond to questions during episodes) or stuttering [4].

Recent studies have suggested that visible (or subjective) semiological PNES elements are not combined randomly, but there may be several distinct PNES types in patients with PNES alone. One study based on clustering features identified five different PNES types, including dystonic attacks with primitive gestural activity, pauci-kinetic attacks with preserved responsiveness, episodes of pseudosyncope, hyperkinetic prolonged attacks with hyperventilation and auras, and axial dystonic prolonged attacks [70]. Other authors have described somewhat different categories and subdivided PNES into a moderate number of alternative discrete semiological groups [71, 72]. Little is known about why PNES look different in different patient subpopulations, although there is evidence that at least some of the semiological variability is explained by previous experiences, as patients with sexual abuse have been shown to be more likely to present with convulsive PNES, nocturnal attacks, ictal injuries, incontinence, seizures prodromes, flashbacks, and emotional triggers [73]. Possible differences in the semiology of PNES between those with purely nonepileptic seizures disorders and those with additional epilepsy remain unexplored. In the framework of the integrative cognitive model, the experience of epileptic seizures (or its recall during the process of history-taking) could affect the PNES scaffold and lead to modeling of PNES on at least some aspects of epileptic seizures. Studies on PNES patients with comorbid epilepsy have suggested that PNES semiology is similar to that of epileptic seizures in about one third of cases [14, 16]. This can make it very difficult to distinguish between the semiology of PNES and epileptic seizures in these patients. Such difficulties have been highlighted in a recent report, presenting patients with epileptic seizures and PNES captured with intracerebral EEG recordings in which the two seizure types showed a striking resemblance [74].

3.2 Video-EEG findings

Ultimately, the diagnosis of PNES is based on the integration of data from a range of different sources, including information obtained from the patient, seizure witnesses, and investigations. Although home video recordings can be useful [65], they often miss the seizure onset or other important seizure elements, and the additional information provided by simultaneously recorded EEG can be crucial. Even if ictal EEG changes are obscured by muscle artifacts, this test can help by showing EEG activity just before the onset of visible seizure manifestations (e.g., epileptic discharges in focal seizures or EEG manifestations of sleep at seizure onset), and demonstrate the lack of postictal EEG changes immediately after the cessation of convulsive seizure activity.

What is more, the concomitant ECG recording, which is routinely included in video-EEG recordings, may demonstrate a more rapid heart rate (HR) increase in an epileptic seizure than would be expected in PNES [75–77]. The peak ictal HR during motor epileptic seizure is also greater than the peak ictal HR during motor PNES [77], with generalized tonic-clonic seizures having the highest peak heart rate [77]. An ictal HR elevation of 30% or greater above the preictal baseline has been shown to have a positive predictive value for an epileptic seizure of 97% [75]. However, it has also been noted that ictal HR does not differentiate between frontal seizures and PNES, although a preictal HR increase in PNES and a rapid postictal HR reduction in frontal seizures distinguished PNES from frontal seizures [76].

While video-EEG recordings are the best test available for the differentiation of epileptic and nonepileptic seizures, they can still give rise to interpretation errors. For instance, too much weight may be placed on the absence of epileptiform EEG changes when a seizure has not involved loss of awareness. If such seizures were caused by epilepsy, 70%–90% would not have a definite EEG correlate in scalp recordings [78].

The misdiagnosis of FLE as PNES has also been reported as a common error, although in most cases this should only pose a major challenge if diagnosticians are unaware of the typical ictal features of FLE and if they do not realize that up to one third of frontal lobe seizures are unassociated with epileptiform activity in scalp EEG recordings [16]. Nevertheless, the fact that some frontal lobe epileptic automatisms seem "bizarre" (for instance, the production of moaning or humming sounds, automatisms of mimicry, fear, laughter, or crying) may lead to the misdiagnosis of nonconvulsive frontal lobe seizures as PNES [36]. However, seizures in FLE are more likely than PNES to start in childhood, are predominantly or exclusively sleep-related in many patients, often involve asymmetric posturing with partial awareness, are typically very short, often highly stereotyped, and have a tendency to occur in clusters [16].

There may be a greater risk of misdiagnosing parietal lobe seizures as PNES. The diversity of parietal lobe semiology, including polysensory auras and heterogeneous motor manifestations, such as dystonia and hyperkinetic behavior, may even cause experienced epileptologists to make diagnostic errors in the absence of the documentation of ictal EEG discharges.

Despite these diagnostic challenges, noninvasive video-EEG recordings with scalp electrodes should allow clinicians to differentiate clearly between epileptic seizures and PNES in most cases, especially when patients' subjective seizure experiences are taken into account and when ictal testing and examination of recall for the ictal testing has taken place. Ideally, the ictal examination should include testing of responsivity to verbal and tactile stimuli (such as eyelash tickle), the encouragement to remember a small number of words, and postictal testing of recall of the ictal examination procedure (patients are more responsive during PNES than epileptic seizures with apparent loss of awareness and show greater recall of the testing procedure) [79]. Testing for avoidance, such as resistance to eye-opening or a controlled fall of the hand when it is dropped over the patient's face, may demonstrate muscle tone and volitional movement in apparently atonic or dialeptic attacks [1, 80, 81].

Although it has been argued that only intracranial EEG recordings can reliably differentiate between PNES and epileptic seizures in some cases, invasive EEG recordings cannot be recommended for the overwhelming majority of cases and should be reserved for exceptional diagnostic dilemmas and for when surgery would be a treatment option if epilepsy was proven [74, 82]. Wyler et al. presented six patients whose scalp EEG recordings were unchanged from baseline during seizures, considered as PNES, but who had deep frontal or temporal electrographic seizures during intracranial EEG [82], while Ostrowsky-Coste et al. presented two cases with remarkably similar epileptic seizures and PNES [74].

Especially when patients have comorbid epilepsy and PNES, it is of great importance to ensure that the recorded episodes were typical of the patients' habitual attacks. In order to do this, it is best practice to document detailed descriptions of all seizure types of interest before the video-EEG recording and to show recordings to witnesses of habitual attacks after they have been recorded to confirm that the seizures captured were the reason for the investigation. This may involve asking the patient and showing the recording to patients and relatives/friends or carers as well [82], since caregivers may be better able to distinguish between seizure types than patients [83].

3.3 Suggestion and provocation techniques

The majority of patients with PNES will experience an event within the first few hours of video- EEG recording [84]. However, in those with suspected comorbid epilepsy and PNES, it is of great help for the patient's further treatment if all habitually occurring seizure types have been recorded and the relative frequency of epileptic and nonepileptic seizures quantified, so the recording should not be discontinued after the first seizure has been captured. This also means that seizure suggestion/provocation techniques have less of a role in patients with mixed seizure disorders involving PNES and epileptic seizures, although such techniques are used in many centers to shorten video-EEG monitoring and to increase the "yield" of this procedure, and these procedures have been endorsed in principle by the PNES Task Force of the International League Against Epilepsy when habitual PNES have not been captured during routine video-EEG recording [80]. Suggestion/provocation techniques include measures that direct the patient's attention to their seizures or increase physiological arousal. Simply taking a detailed history of seizure manifestations is likely to have a suggestive effect, perhaps enhanced if the recording physiologist takes notes and reviews aloud to clarify details [85]. Such simple measures allow practitioners to capture PNES in one to two thirds of patients [86]. Somewhat more suggestive force may be exerted, for instance, by stating how often routine activation techniques (such as photic stimulation or hyperventilation) elicit a typical attack. Relatively brief outpatient EEGs lasting 1–2 h, which include hyperventilation, photic stimulation, and suggestion, have been shown to capture typical PNES in up to 66% patients suspected to have this disorder [87].

In addition to EEG activation procedures and verbal suggestion, practitioners have used a range of placebo interventions to provoke seizures when PNES are suspected, with the injection of IV saline being the method used most commonly. Studies suggest that the diagnostic yield of such more invasive procedures may be higher, but the use of these methods is subject to ethical debate. Furthermore, more forceful suggestion techniques are likely to be associated with a greater risk of patients having atypical attacks leading to diagnostic errors [88].

3.4 PNES biomarkers

Many biomarkers have been assessed as candidates in the differentiation of epileptic seizures from PNES [89]. However, all of these tests are of limited utility in the diagnosis or management of PNES, especially in the context of comorbid epilepsy. Prolactin (PRL) is the best studied postictal blood tests with diagnostic potential. Propagation of epileptic discharges from mesial temporal structures to the hypothalamus during an epileptic seizure may result in postictal serum PRL level elevations from 10–20 min to about 2 h after a seizure [89]. Although PRL levels are more likely to be elevated after epileptic than nonepileptic seizures, especially when the seizure was convulsive, false positive and negative results occur, and the diagnosis of a PNES should never be based entirely on this test. One study found elevated postictal PRL in up to 20% of the PNES cohort [90], while a second group, recruiting patients with complex focal seizures with or without generalization, found no statistically significant difference in postictal PRL between epileptic seizures and PNES subjects [91].

4. PNES and epilepsy surgery

PNES may be recognized as comorbidity in patients with epilepsy who are considered candidates for epilepsy surgery; PNES may exist as an unrecognized comorbidity of epilepsy before epilepsy surgery but only be diagnosed after surgical intervention, or they may newly manifest after epilepsy surgery.

The association of epilepsy and PNES poses particular challenges when surgery is considered as a treatment for medication-resistant epilepsy. For a start, an additional diagnosis of PNES calls into question how resistant epileptic seizures really are to AED treatment and how many of the patient's seizures are actually due to their PNES disorder rather than their epilepsy. Further difficulties may arise because of the common comorbidities of PNES, including anxiety, depression, PTSD, other somatoform, dissociative, and personality disorders, all of which are relative contraindications to epilepsy surgery if they are sufficiently severe to interfere with a patient's ability to cope with the presurgical evaluation process, the procedure itself, and a successful recovery from it [92]. Nevertheless retrospective epilepsy surgery case series from centers where patients with PNES were not excluded from surgical intervention have reported that 1.3%–3.2% of the patients operated to stop epilepsy were known preoperatively to have coexisting PNES [92, 93], and there is evidence from such centers that epilepsy surgery can be associated with good outcomes, potentially including the improvement or cessation of PNES [92].

To date, there are no clear guidelines detailing how decisions about epilepsy surgery in patients with refractory epilepsy and PNES should be made and how these patients are best managed. Indeed, in view of the heterogeneity of both epileptic and nonepileptic seizure disorders, it would be difficult to come up with universal rules taking account of the different contributions of epileptic and nonepileptic seizures to a particular patient's disabilities, the relative clinical importance of psychological, medical, and surgical treatments, and the optimal sequence of different interventions [93]. One retrospective study of patients with mixed seizure disorders who underwent epilepsy surgery suggested that surgical and psychiatric outcomes may be poor if there is evidence of chronic and multiple somatoform symptoms and in patients exhibiting behaviors suggesting factitious disorder [92]. Frequent PNES and a history of nonepileptic seizure status were also identified as predictors for poor surgery outcome [92]. However, epilepsy surgery may be considered in this patient group after careful epileptological, psychiatric, and psychological assessment. In some cases it may be important to treat PNES and psychiatric comorbidity before considering surgery. In others initial surgical treatment may be more appropriate. Epilepsy surgery should be offered to patients predominately disabled by epileptic rather than nonepileptic seizures. However, patients should be informed preoperatively about the diagnoses of epileptic and nonepileptic seizures and that surgery is an intervention for their epilepsy and not for PNES [92].

The de novo development of PNES has been described after brain surgery unrelated to seizures [45], but the phenomenon is more likely to occur after epilepsy surgery, reportedly complicating 1.8%–8.8% of excisional surgical treatment procedures for epilepsy [38, 94–99]. Postoperative PNES have not been well studied. They may well be underdiagnosed and confound the assessment of postsurgical seizure outcomes and clinical management. The highest frequency has been reported by Glosser (8.8%), but it is possible that some of the patients who were found to have PNES postoperatively actually also had mixed seizure disorders preoperatively, although the diagnosis of PNES was only confirmed after epilepsy surgery [38].

A review combining data from all cases reported in the literature found that female gender is the most prominent risk factor for postepilepsy surgery PNES followed by the presence of a preoperative psychiatric disorder. Postoperative PNES may be more common in patients who suffer physical complications of their surgery [94]. In a study by Markoula et al. [94], female patients with a preoperative psychiatric disorder had an 8.5% chance of developing PNES. Furthermore, the study indicated that patients who have experienced postoperative complications may be at greater risk. The study also showed that postoperative PNES development was not associated with epileptic seizure outcome [94], although it has been postulated that, in some patients who develop PNES after becoming free of epileptic seizures, the "burden of normality" could be etiologically relevant [100].

Postoperative PNES may emerge within the first year following epilepsy surgery [38, 93] but have also been reported as starting 10 years later [94]. It has been reported that postoperative PNES tend to resemble "motor" seizures [94] and that they usually do not resemble the patient's habitual epileptic seizures [95].

In view of the likely underdiagnosis of PNES in patients in whom seizures continue or reemerge after epilepsy surgery, postoperative seizures should be carefully evaluated. The development of "atypical seizures" with motor manifestations, especially in female patients with presurgical psychiatric disorders should be interpreted as "red flags" for possible postoperative PNES.

5. Management

5.1 Communicating the diagnosis

The communication of the diagnosis of PNES is often challenging, especially when PNES coexist with epileptic seizures. Unfortunately, much of what we know about this can only be extrapolated from studies exclusively (or predominately) based on the explanation of the diagnosis of PNES to patients with no other types of seizures. A number of communication strategies have been published [101–104], however, only one of these has been subjected to a prospective study confirming that patients found the approach acceptable and that the strategy was effective at communicating the possibility of a "psychological" etiology of PNES, but patients with coexisting epilepsy were excluded from this study [102].

Patients with PNES tend to not perceive themselves as needing psychiatric care or psychological treatment, to have a more external locus of control, and to be resistant to psychosocial explanations of their disorder [52]. Because of PNES patients' resistance to receiving a psychiatric label, the benefits of a team approach and the availability of positive diagnostic tests (such as video EEG) is of great value, especially if results are not merely presented as having "ruled out" epilepsy but as having demonstrated ictal phenomena typical of PNES. Establishing the diagnosis of PNES as securely as possible is the first step toward managing the disorder.

No research has established whether it is effective to involve the patients' family members in the discussion of the diagnosis. However, having family members present during the presentation may facilitate understanding and allow the neurologist to challenge unhelpful or incorrect ideas about PNES potentially held by family members. Family members or carers of patients with PNES have been shown to be slightly more accepting of the idea that PNES may be linked to challenging emotions, and they may be able to help patients understand links that they do not readily perceive themselves [105].

While there are no studies exploring outcomes of patients with epilepsy and PNES who have had the diagnosis of PNES explained to them, studies of patients with exclusively nonepileptic seizures suggest that about one third of patients will report that their seizures have stopped 3–6 months after diagnosis with no further intervention [106], and that most patients who became PNES-free stopped having seizures immediately after the explanation of the condition [107]. In those with PNES only, the continued prescription of AEDs is associated with poorer outcome than the discontinuation of AEDs [108]. However, in patients with concurrent PNES and epilepsy it may not be possible to stop AEDs because of the additional epilepsy.

Apart from the explanation of the diagnosis in patients with epilepsy and PNES, health care professionals will need to invest time and effort to educate patients (and caregivers) about the differences between their PNES and epileptic seizures, for instance, by showing patients and caregivers video recordings of typical seizures. It is also essential that the diagnosis is communicated clearly to other doctors involved in the patient's care.

Although in patients with pure PNES disorders the communication of the diagnosis typically has an immediate (lasting) effect on healthcare utilization with reductions in health care expenditure and emergency service use [25], in those with additional epilepsy it may not be possible to advice caregivers not to involve emergency medical services. Having said that, caregivers would ideally learn to distinguish between epileptic emergencies, requiring medication and perhaps a call to emergency services, and nonepileptic seizure emergencies, which should be managed by minimizing patients' injury risk followed by offering verbal reassurance and avoiding ambulance call outs or other intervention likely to exacerbate anxiety. It is advisable to check whether the process of education has been successful by encouraging families to video attacks they observe at home, so that the diagnosis (and the families' abilities to distinguish between PNES and epilepsy) can be checked. Some patients may need to be investigated with video EEG repeatedly.

5.2 Treatment

A comprehensive psychiatric assessment should be carried out early in the diagnostic workup to examine psychiatric symptomatology (comorbid mental health disorders are expected in the majority of patients), developmental history, character traits, and psychosocial environment [52]. However, psychiatrists are not part of the routine care team in many specialist epilepsy centers [109]. Mental health professionals unfamiliar with epilepsy or PNES may struggle to recognize relevant but "subthreshold" psychopathology and to engage patients who are not at all convinced that they will benefit from seeing a psychiatrist.

Unfortunately, there is only very limited information about the optimal treatment of patients with PNES and even less evidence for the treatment of those with PNES and epilepsy who were typically excluded from PNES treatment studies. Nevertheless, psychoeducational or psychotherapeutic interventions are likely to be most effective [110, 111]. In view of the heterogeneity of relevant etiological factors, it is likely that an individualized approach is most appropriate, although this may consist of a sequence of scripted/standardized interventions. The planning of such an intervention is likely to require a psychological or psychotherapeutic assessment aiming to develop a diagnostic and treatment formulation for each individual patient [5]. If patients can learn clearly to distinguish between their PNES and epileptic seizures, psychological treatment for PNES can be delivered along similar lines as treatment for PNES in the absence of epilepsy [52]. If PNES and epileptic seizure cannot be differentiated, psychological treatment may still be possible, but it may have to focus on less specific aims, such as improvement of stress/stressor recognition, optimization of stress management techniques, mindfulness, or enhanced tolerance of unpleasant emotions [112].

There is no agreement as to the type of psychotherapy that is likely to achieve the best results in patients with PNES, and it is likely that different approaches are most suitable for different groups of patients [113]. A number of treatments (e.g., cognitive behavioral, psychodynamic therapy, family therapy) have been used in patients with PNES. Two CBT approaches have been evaluated in open-label studies and multicenter pilot randomized controlled trials (RCTs), showing reduction in seizure frequency and improvement of comorbid depression, anxiety, and psychosocial functioning [55, 114, 115]. One recent study of patients with the combination of temporal lobe epilepsy and mesial temporal sclerosis and PNES suggested a positive impact of CBT-based group psychological intervention on levels of alexithymia, anxiety/depression symptoms, and quality of life (primary outcomes), as well as seizure frequency (secondary outcome) [109].

Clearly treatments such as psychoeducation or psychotherapy also need to take account of the intellectual capacity of patients. In those with ID approaches aiming to reduce environmental stressors or purely behavioral measures may be more effective than traditional psychotherapeutic interventions.

While psychological treatments are currently the treatment of first choice for those with PNES, there may be a role for pharmacological treatment, especially in those with additional epilepsy. There is some evidence of (potential) effectiveness of antidepressant drugs in patients with PNES [114]; a small RCT evaluating the effect of sertraline showed a 45% reduction in PNES frequency from baseline to final visit [114]. Psychopharmacologic intervention may also be considered a treatment for PNES-associated other somatoform symptoms or the common psychiatric comorbidities of this seizure disorder [41]. In patients with psychogenic movement disorder who received citalopram, paroxetine, or venlafaxine, the primary conversion symptoms, depression, or anxiety responded to treatment with antidepressants [116]. Of course, when using antidepressants in patients with epilepsy, clinicians should avoid high doses, rapid titration, and antidepressants with particularly well-documented proconvulsant effects at therapeutic doses (clomipramine, bupropion, amoxapine, and maprotiline). They should also consider potential pharmacodynamic and pharmacokinetic interactions of antidepressants with AEDs [32].

Perhaps more importantly, alterations of patients' AED treatment may be helpful in those with PNES and additional epilepsy. In view of evidence that AED toxicity is common in those with PNES and that AEDs can exacerbate PNES, AED treatment should be reduced in terms of dose and drug number as much as possible [49]. Furthermore, clinicians should aim to avoid or consider withdrawing AEDs with negative psychotropic effects (i.e., topiramate, levetiracetam, zonisamide, and perampanel) [33]. The use of sedative drugs or agents with marked negative effects on cognition should also be minimized (this includes GABAergic AEDs, such as barbiturates and benzodiazepines, and opiate pain killers) [33]. In contrast to the previously listed AEDs, others may have potentially useful psychotropic effects [32]. These include AEDs with mood-stabilizing properties, such as valproic acid, carbamazepine, oxcarbazepine, and lamotrigine, and anxiolytic effect, such as valproate, lamotrigine, pregabalin, clobazam, and clonazepam [33].

5.3 Outcome

Our understanding of the prognosis of patients with PNES remains incomplete. Some patients become PNES-free when the diagnosis has been explained to them and remain so, others develop chronic disorders in which PNES are the key cause of disability. There is still much to learn about the prognostication of where on this spectrum individual patients will end up. In general, studies tend to show a discrepancy between relatively encouraging short-term outcomes and a poorer prognosis in the longer term.

One outcome study of patients with PNES only showed that half of the patients were free of attacks 3 months after PNES diagnosis, while, at 6 months, some patients had relapsed and 44.4% reported no further attacks [107]. In a longer-term study in which PNES patients were reevaluated 4–6 years after diagnosis, 7 of 22 patients were in remission and 3 patients had occasional seizures.

Outcomes other than seizure frequency may be important in patients with PNES, such as the use of emergency medical services [25] and dependence on social benefits [117]. McKenzie et al. reported that 49.7% of 260 PNES patients had used emergency medical services at baseline and 15.5% had used them at 12 months postdiagnosis [25]. A retrospective cohort study of 164 PNES patients captured a mean period of 11.9 years after manifestation and 4.1 years after diagnosis of PNES, 71.2% of patients continued to have seizures and 56.1% were dependent on social benefits [117]. It is possible that the discrepant findings between short- and long-term outcome studies are, at least in part, due to differences in outcome measures or patient selection [41].

Unfortunately, most PNES outcome studies have excluded patients with confirmed or suspected comorbid epilepsy [83]. There is a suggestion that outcomes may be better in less complex patients who receive the diagnosis of PNES quickly [107]. On the other hand, large retrospective outcome studies have not demonstrated a clear difference in prognosis between those thought to have PNES only and those with mixed seizure disorders who are likely to have had more complex disorders [117].

Several studies have demonstrated that outcome is better in children with PNES than in adults [118]. Younger age has also been found to be associated with better prognosis in adult patient populations [117], possibly because of intervention (even if only in the form or making and explaining the diagnosis) at an earlier stage of life [118]. This emphasizes the importance of avoiding diagnostic delays and mistreatment of PNES as epilepsy. The importance of early intervention is also demonstrated by studies showing better prognosis in patients with recent-onset PNES [107].

6. Conclusion

The overwhelming majority of patients with PNES only have PNES and no additional epilepsy. However, epilepsy is a risk factor for the development of PNES. When PNES occur in the context of epilepsy, patients and clinicians face a number of challenges. The initial diagnosis of both disorders in the same patient often causes difficulties (and may be significantly delayed), since there are many superficial similarities between the manifestations of PNES and epileptic seizures. Even after the initial diagnosis, there is an ongoing need to differentiate between the two seizure types as the effects of different interventions are evaluated and treatment modifications considered. Video EEG can help with this task by providing materials that can be used to teach patients and caregivers to distinguish epileptic seizures from PNES, but additional diagnostic methods such as careful and repeated history-taking during follow-up and home video recordings will have to be employed. The treatment of PNES in the context of comorbid epilepsy is easier and can be more specific when patients, caregivers, and clinicians are able to distinguish between these two types of seizures. However, less specific interventions, such as reducing AED toxicity or negative psychotropic effects of AEDs or psychotherapeutic interventions aiming to increase mindfulness or tolerance of challenging emotions or physical sensations, may help patients even when PNES and epileptic seizures cannot be differentiated. More research focusing on etiology, treatment, and outcome in this patient group is badly needed, although the heterogeneity of both epilepsy and PNES will pose a significant methodological challenge to researchers.

References

[1] Reuber M, Elger CE. Psychogenic nonepileptic seizures: review and update. Epilepsy Behav 2003; 4(3):205–16.

[2] D'Alessio L, Giagante B, Oddo S, Silva WW, Solis P, Consalvo D, Kochen S. Psychiatric disorders in patients with psychogenic non-epileptic seizures, with and without comorbid epilepsy. Seizure 2006;15(5):333–9.

[3] Oto M, Reuber M. Psychogenic non-epileptic seizures: aetiology, diagnosis and management. Adv Psychiatr Treat 2014;20:13–22.

[4] Bodde NM, Brooks JL, Baker GA, Boon PA, Hendriksen JG, Aldenkamp AP. Psychogenic non-epileptic seizures-diagnostic issues: a critical review. Clin Neurol Neurosurg 2009;111(1):1–9.

[5] Doss RC, LaFrance WC. Psychogenic non-epileptic seizures. Epileptic Disord 2016;18(4):337–43.

[6] Brown RJ, Reuber M. Psychological and psychiatric aspects of psychogenic non-epileptic seizures (PNES): a systematic review. Clin Psychol Rev 2016;45:157–82.

[7] Malmgren KR, Appleton R. Differential diagnosis of epilepsy. In: Shorvon S, editor. Oxford textbook of epilepsy and epileptic seizures. Oxford: Oxford University Press; 2012. p. 81–94.

[8] Mari F, Di Bonaventura C, Vanacore N, Fattouch J, Vaudano AE, Egeo G, Berardelli A, Manfredi M, Prencipe M, Giallonardo AT. Video-EEG study of psychogenic nonepileptic seizures: differential characteristics in patients with and without epilepsy. Epilepsia 2006;47(Suppl. 5):64–7.

[9] Reuber M, Fernandez G, Bauer J, Helmstaedter C, Elger CE. Diagnostic delay in psychogenic nonepileptic seizures. Neurology 2002;58(3):493–5.

[10] Angus-Leppan H. Diagnosing epilepsy in neurology clinics: a prospective study. Seizure 2008; 17(5):431–6.

[11] Walker MC, Howard RS, Smith SJ, Miller DH, Shorvon SD, Hirsch NP. Diagnosis and treatment of status epilepticus on a neurological intensive care unit. QJM 1996;89(12):913–20.

[12] Hantke NC, Doherty MJ, Haltiner AM. Medication use profiles in patients with psychogenic nonepileptic seizures. Epilepsy Behav 2007;10(2):333–5.

[13] Reuber M, Baker GA, Gill R, Smith DF, Chadwick DW. Failure to recognize psychogenic nonepileptic seizures may cause death. Neurology 2004;62(5):834–5.

[14] Reuber M, Qurishi A, Bauer J, Helmstaedter C, Fernandez G, Widman G, Elger CE. Are there physical risk factors for psychogenic non-epileptic seizures in patients with epilepsy? Seizure 2003;12(8):561–7.

[15] Cuthill FM, Espie CA. Sensitivity and specificity of procedures for the differential diagnosis of epileptic and non-epileptic seizures: a systematic review. Seizure 2005;14(5):293–303.

[16] Devinsky O, Sanchez-Villasenor F, Vazquez B, Kothari M, Alper K, Luciano D. Clinical profile of patients with epileptic and nonepileptic seizures. Neurology 1996;46(6):1530–3.

[17] Krumholz A. Nonepileptic seizures: diagnosis and management. Neurology 1999;53(5 Suppl. 2): S76–83.

[18] Duncan R, Oto M. Psychogenic nonepileptic seizures in patients with learning disability: comparison with patients with no learning disability. Epilepsy Behav 2008;12(1):183–6.

[19] Silver LB. Conversion disorder with pseudoseizures in adolescence: a stress reaction to unrecognized and untreated learning disabilities. J Am Acad Child Psychiatry 1982;21(5):508–12.

[20] Reuber M, Fernandez G, Bauer J, Singh DD, Elger CE. Interictal EEG abnormalities in patients with psychogenic nonepileptic seizures. Epilepsia 2002;43(9):1013–20.

[21] Lesser RP, Lueders H, Dinner DS. Evidence for epilepsy is rare in patients with psychogenic seizures. Neurology 1983;33(4):502–4.

[22] Martin R, Burneo JG, Prasad A, Powell T, Faught E, Knowlton R, Mendez M, Kuzniecky R. Frequency of epilepsy in patients with psychogenic seizures monitored by video-EEG. Neurology 2003;61(12):1791–2.

[23] Vincentiis S, Valente KD, Thome-Souza S, Kuczinsky E, Fiore LA, Negrao N. Risk factors for psychogenic nonepileptic seizures in children and adolescents with epilepsy. Epilepsy Behav 2006; 8(1):294–8.

[24] Kellinghaus C, Loddenkemper T, Dinner DS, Lachhwani D, Luders HO. Non-epileptic seizures of the elderly. J Neurol 2004;251(6):704–9.

[25] McKenzie P, Oto M, Russell A, Pelosi A, Duncan R. Early outcomes and predictors in 260 patients with psychogenic nonepileptic attacks. Neurology 2010;74(1):64–9.

[26] Baroni G, Piccinini V, Martins WA, de Paola L, Paglioli E, Margis R, Palmini A. Variables associated with co-existing epileptic and psychogenic nonepileptic seizures: a systematic review. Seizure 2016;37:35–40.

[27] Duncan R, Oto M, Martin E, Pelosi A. Late onset psychogenic nonepileptic attacks. Neurology 2006;66(11):1644–7.

[28] Reuber M, Howlett S, Khan A, Grunewald RA. Non-epileptic seizures and other functional neurological symptoms: predisposing, precipitating, and perpetuating factors. Psychosomatics 2007;48(3):230–8.

[29] Kuyk J, Swinkels WA, Spinhoven P. Psychopathologies in patients with nonepileptic seizures with and without comorbid epilepsy: how different are they? Epilepsy Behav 2003;4(1):13–8.

[30] Devinsky O, Gordon E. Epileptic seizures progressing into nonepileptic conversion seizures. Neurology 1998;51(5):1293–6.

[31] Lelliott PT, Fenwick P. Cerebral pathology in pseudoseizures. Acta Neurol Scand 1991;83(2):129–32.

[32] Kanner AM. The treatment of depressive disorders in epilepsy: what all neurologists should know. Epilepsia 2013;54(Suppl. 1):3–12.

[33] Piedad J, Rickards H, Besag FM, Cavanna AE. Beneficial and adverse psychotropic effects of antiepileptic drugs in patients with epilepsy: a summary of prevalence, underlying mechanisms and data limitations. CNS Drugs 2012;26(4):319–35.

[34] Baker D, Eccles FJR, Caswell HL. Correlates of stigma in adults with epilepsy: a systematic review of quantitative studies. Epilepsy Behav 2018;83:67–80.

[35] Kwong KL, Lam D, Tsui S, Ngan M, Tsang B, Lai TS, Lam SM. Self-esteem in adolescents with epilepsy: psychosocial and seizure-related correlates. Epilepsy Behav 2016;63:118–22.

[36] Henry TR, Drury I. Non-epileptic seizures in temporal lobectomy candidates with medically refractory seizures. Neurology 1997;48(5):1374–82.

[37] Devinsky O, Mesad S, Alper K. Nondominant hemisphere lesions and conversion nonepileptic seizures. J Neuropsychiatr Clin Neurosci 2001;13(3):367–73.

[38] Glosser G, Roberts D, Glosser DS. Nonepileptic seizures after resective epilepsy surgery. Epilepsia 1999;40(12):1750–4.

[39] Bowman ES. Etiology and clinical course of pseudoseizures. Relationship to trauma, depression, and dissociation. Psychosomatics 1993;34(4):333–42.

[40] Harden CL. Pseudoseizures and dissociative disorders: a common mechanism involving traumatic experiences. Seizure 1997;6(2):151–5.

[41] Reuber M. Psychogenic nonepileptic seizures: answers and questions. Epilepsy Behav 2008; 12(4):622–35.

[42] Bowman ES, Markand ON. The contribution of life events to pseudoseizure occurrence in adults. Bull Menn Clin 1999;63(1):70–88.

[43] Bowman ES, Markand ON. Psychodynamics and psychiatric diagnoses of pseudoseizure subjects. Am J Psychiatry 1996;153(1):57–63.

[44] Pakalnis A, Paolicchi J. Psychogenic seizures after head injury in children. J Child Neurol 2000; 15(2):78–80.

[45] Reuber M, Kral T, Kurthen M, Elger CE. New-onset psychogenic seizures after intracranial neurosurgery. Acta Neurochir 2002;144(9):901–7 [discussion 7].

[46] Gardner DL, Goldberg RL. Psychogenic seizures and loss. Int J Psychiatry Med 1982;12(2):121–8.

[47] Guberman A. Psychogenic pseudoseizures in non-epileptic patients. Can J Psychiatr 1982;27(5):401–4.

[48] Duncan R, Oto M. Predictors of antecedent factors in psychogenic nonepileptic attacks: multivariate analysis. Neurology 2008;71(13):1000–5.

[49] Krumholz A, Niedermeyer E. Psychogenic seizures: a clinical study with follow-up data. Neurology 1983;33(4):498–502.

[50] Lacey C, Cook M, Salzberg M. The neurologist, psychogenic nonepileptic seizures, and borderline personality disorder. Epilepsy Behav 2007;11(4):492–8.

[51] Niedermeyer E, Blumer D, Holscher E, Walker BA. Classical hysterical seizures facilitated by anticonvulsant toxicity. Psychiatr Clin 1970;3(2):71–84.

[52] LaFrance Jr. WC, Reuber M, Goldstein LH. Management of psychogenic nonepileptic seizures. Epilepsia 2013;54(Suppl. 1):53–67.

[53] Galimberti CA, Ratti MT, Murelli R, Marchioni E, Manni R, Tartara A. Patients with psychogenic nonepileptic seizures, alone or epilepsy-associated, share a psychological profile distinct from that of epilepsy patients. J Neurol 2003;250(3):338–46.

[54] Ettinger AB, Devinsky O, Weisbrot DM, Ramakrishna RK, Goyal A. A comprehensive profile of clinical, psychiatric, and psychosocial characteristics of patients with psychogenic nonepileptic seizures. Epilepsia 1999;40(9):1292–8.

[55] LaFrance Jr. WC, Miller IW, Ryan CE, Blum AS, Solomon DA, Kelley JE, Keitner GI. Cognitive behavioral therapy for psychogenic nonepileptic seizures. Epilepsy Behav 2009;14(4):591–6.

[56] Reuber M, Pukrop R, Bauer J, Derfuss R, Elger CE. Multidimensional assessment of personality in patients with psychogenic non-epileptic seizures. J Neurol Neurosurg Psychiatry 2004;75(5):743–8.

[57] Bewley J, Murphy PN, Mallows J, Baker GA. Does alexithymia differentiate between patients with nonepileptic seizures, patients with epilepsy, and nonpatient controls? Epilepsy Behav 2005; 7(3):430–7.

[58] Brown RJ, Reuber M. Towards an integrative theory of psychogenic non-epileptic seizures (PNES). Clin Psychol Rev 2016;47:55–70.

[59] Reuber M, Jamnadas-Khoda J, Broadhurst M, Grunewald R, Howell S, Koepp M, Sisodiya S, Walker M. Psychogenic nonepileptic seizure manifestations reported by patients and witnesses. Epilepsia 2011;52(11):2028–35.

[60] Goldstein LH, Mellers JD. Ictal symptoms of anxiety, avoidance behaviour, and dissociation in patients with dissociative seizures. J Neurol Neurosurg Psychiatry 2006;77(5):616–21.

[61] Meierkord H, Will B, Fish D, Shorvon S. The clinical features and prognosis of pseudoseizures diagnosed using video-EEG telemetry. Neurology 1991;41(10):1643–6.

[62] Duncan R, Oto M, Russell AJ, Conway P. Pseudosleep events in patients with psychogenic non-epileptic seizures: prevalence and associations. J Neurol Neurosurg Psychiatry 2004;75(7):1009–12.

[63] Avbersek A, Sisodiya S. Does the primary literature provide support for clinical signs used to distinguish psychogenic nonepileptic seizures from epileptic seizures? J Neurol Neurosurg Psychiatry 2010; 81(7):719–25.

[64] Saygi S, Katz A, Marks DA, Spencer SS. Frontal lobe partial seizures and psychogenic seizures: comparison of clinical and ictal characteristics. Neurology 1992;42(7):1274–7.

[65] Chen DK, Graber KD, Anderson CT, Fisher RS. Sensitivity and specificity of video alone versus electroencephalography alone for the diagnosis of partial seizures. Epilepsy Behav 2008;13(1):115–8.

[66] Syed TU, Arozullah AM, Suciu GP, Toub J, Kim H, Dougherty ML, Wehner T, Stojic A, Syed I, Alexopoulos AV. Do observer and self-reports of ictal eye closure predict psychogenic nonepileptic seizures? Epilepsia 2008;49(5):898–904.

[67] Schwabe M, Reuber M, Schondienst M, Gulich E. Listening to people with seizures: how can linguistic analysis help in the differential diagnosis of seizure disorders? Commun Med 2008;5(1):59–72.

[68] Vinton A, Carino J, Vogrin S, Macgregor L, Kilpatrick C, Matkovic Z, Kilpatrick C, Matkovic Z, O'Brien TJ. "Convulsive" nonepileptic seizures have a characteristic pattern of rhythmic artifact distinguishing them from convulsive epileptic seizures. Epilepsia 2004;45(11):1344–50.

[69] Devinsky O, Gazzola D, LaFrance WC. Differentiating between nonepileptic and epileptic seizures. Nat Rev Neurol 2011;7(4):210–20.

[70] Hubsch C, Baumann C, Hingray C, Gospodaru N, Vignal JP, Vespignani H, Maillard L. Clinical classification of psychogenic non-epileptic seizures based on video-EEG analysis and automatic clustering. J Neurol Neurosurg Psychiatry 2011;82(9):955–60.

[71] Szabo L, Siegler Z, Zubek L, Liptai Z, Korhegyi I, Bansagi B, Fogarasi A. A detailed semiologic analysis of childhood psychogenic nonepileptic seizures. Epilepsia 2012;53(3):565–70.

[72] Seneviratne U, Reutens D, D'Souza W. Stereotypy of psychogenic nonepileptic seizures: insights from video-EEG monitoring. Epilepsia 2010;51(7):1159–68.

[73] Selkirk M, Duncan R, Oto M, Pelosi A. Clinical differences between patients with nonepileptic seizures who report antecedent sexual abuse and those who do not. Epilepsia 2008;49(8):1446–50.

[74] Ostrowsky-Coste K, Montavont A, Keo-Kosal P, Guenot M, Chatillon CE, Ryvlin P. Similar semiology of epileptic and psychogenic nonepileptic seizures recorded during stereo-EEG. Seizure 2013;22 (10):897–900.

[75] Opherk C, Hirsch LJ. Ictal heart rate differentiates epileptic from non-epileptic seizures. Neurology 2002;58(4):636–8.

[76] Reinsberger C, Perez DL, Murphy MM, Dworetzky BA. Pre- and postictal, not ictal, heart rate distinguishes complex partial and psychogenic nonepileptic seizures. Epilepsy Behav 2012;23(1):68–70.

[77] Tatum WO, Acton EK, Langston ME, Yelvington K, Bowman C, Shih JJ, Shih JJ, Cheshire WP. Multimodality peak Ictal vital signs during video-EEG monitoring. Seizure 2016;40:15–20.

[78] Verma A, Radtke R. EEG of partial seizures. J Clin Neurophysiol 2006;23(4):333–9.

[79] Reuber M, Kurthen M. Consciousness in non-epileptic attack disorder. Behav Neurol 2011; 24(1):95–106.

[80] LaFrance Jr. WC, Baker GA, Duncan R, Goldstein LH, Reuber M. Minimum requirements for the diagnosis of psychogenic nonepileptic seizures: a staged approach: a report from the International League Against Epilepsy Nonepileptic Seizures Task Force. Epilepsia 2013;54(11):2005–18.

[81] Lesser RP. Psychogenic seizures. Neurology 1996;46(6):1499–507.

[82] Wyler AHB, Blumer D, Richey ET. Pseudopseudoepileptic seizures. In: Rowan AJ, Gates JR, editors. Nonepileptic seizures. Boston: Butterworth-Heinemann; 1993. p. 73–84.

[83] Gordon PC, Valiengo Lda C, Proenca IC, Kurcgant D, Jorge CL, Castro LH, Marchetti RL. Comorbid epilepsy and psychogenic non-epileptic seizures: how well do patients and caregivers distinguish between the two. Seizure 2014;23(7):537–41.

[84] Ettinger AB, Devinsky O, Weisbrot DM, Goyal A, Shashikumar S. Headaches and other pain symptoms among patients with psychogenic non-epileptic seizures. Seizure 1999;8(7):424–6.

[85] Whitehead KKN, Wardrope A, Kandler R, Reuber M. Proposal for best practice in the use of video-EEG when psychogenic non-epileptic seizures are a possible diagnosis. Clin Neurophysiol Pract 2017;2:130–9.

[86] McGonigal A, Russell AJ, Mallik AK, Oto M, Duncan R. Use of short term video EEG in the diagnosis of attack disorders. J Neurol Neurosurg Psychiatry 2004;75(5):771–2.

[87] Benbadis SR. Provocative techniques should be used for the diagnosis of psychogenic nonepileptic seizures. Epilepsy Behav 2009;15(2):106–9 [discussion 15-8].

[88] Walczak TS, Williams DT, Berten W. Utility and reliability of placebo infusion in the evaluation of patients with seizures. Neurology 1994;44(3 Pt 1):394–9.

[89] Sundararajan T, Tesar GE, Jimenez XF. Biomarkers in the diagnosis and study of psychogenic nonepileptic seizures: a systematic review. Seizure 2016;35:11–22.

[90] Alving J. Serum prolactin levels are elevated also after pseudo-epileptic seizures. Seizure 1998; 7(2):85–9.

[91] Shukla G, Bhatia M, Vivekanandhan S, Gupta N, Tripathi M, Srivastava A, Pandey RM, Jain S. Serum prolactin levels for differentiation of nonepileptic versus true seizures: limited utility. Epilepsy Behav 2004;5(4):517–21.

[92] Reuber M, Kurthen M, Fernandez G, Schramm J, Elger CE. Epilepsy surgery in patients with additional psychogenic seizures. Arch Neurol 2002;59(1):82–6.

[93] Gonzalez Otarula KA, Tan YL, Dubeau F, Correa JA, Chang E, Hall JA, Knowlton RC, Kobayashi E. Psychogenic nonepileptic seizures in patients with surgically treated temporal lobe epilepsy: presurgical and de novo postsurgical occurrence. Epilepsy Behav 2017;75:252–5.

[94] Markoula S, de Tisi J, Foong J, Duncan JS. De novo psychogenic nonepileptic attacks after adult epilepsy surgery: an underestimated entity. Epilepsia 2013;54(12):e159–62.

[95] Parra J, Iriarte J, Kanner AM, Bergen DC. De novo psychogenic nonepileptic seizures after epilepsy surgery. Epilepsia 1998;39(5):474–7.

[96] Krahn LE, Rummans TA, Sharbrough FW, Jowsey SG, Cascino GD. Pseudoseizures after epilepsy surgery. Psychosomatics 1995;36(5):487–93.

[97] Montenegro MA, Guerreiro MM, Scotoni AE, Stella F, Leone AA, Honorato DC, Damasceno BP, Guerreiro CA, Cendes F. De novo psychogenic seizures after epilepsy surgery: case report. Arq Neuropsiquiatr 2000;58(2B):535–7.

[98] Ferguson SM, Rayport M. The adjustment to living without epilepsy. J Nerv Ment Dis 1965;140:26–37.

[99] Ney GC, Barr WB, Napolitano C, Decker R, Schaul N. New-onset psychogenic seizures after surgery for epilepsy. Arch Neurol 1998;55(5):726–30.

[100] Wilson S, Bladin P, Saling M. The "burden of normality": concepts of adjustment after surgery for seizures. J Neurol Neurosurg Psychiatry 2001;70(5):649–56.

[101] Duncan R. Psychogenic nonepileptic seizures: diagnosis and initial management. Expert Rev Neurother 2010;10(12):1803–9.

[102] Hall-Patch L, Brown R, House A, Howlett S, Kemp S, Lawton G, Mayor R, Smith P, Reuber Ml. Acceptability and effectiveness of a strategy for the communication of the diagnosis of psychogenic nonepileptic seizures. Epilepsia 2010;51(1):70–8.

[103] Mellers JD. The approach to patients with "non-epileptic seizures" Postgrad Med J 2005; 81(958):498–504.

[104] Shen W, Bowman ES, Markand ON. Presenting the diagnosis of pseudoseizure. Neurology 1990; 40(5):756–9.

[105] Whitehead K, Stone J, Norman P, Sharpe M, Reuber M. Differences in relatives' and patients' illness perceptions in functional neurological symptom disorders compared with neurological diseases. Epilepsy Behav 2015;42:159–64.

[106] Arain AM, Hamadani AM, Islam S, Abou-Khalil BW. Predictors of early seizure remission after diagnosis of psychogenic nonepileptic seizures. Epilepsy Behav 2007;11(3):409–12.

[107] Duncan R, Razvi S, Mulhern S. Newly presenting psychogenic nonepileptic seizures: incidence, population characteristics, and early outcome from a prospective audit of a first seizure clinic. Epilepsy Behav 2011;20(2):308–11.

[108] Oto M, Espie CA, Duncan R. An exploratory randomized controlled trial of immediate versus delayed withdrawal of antiepileptic drugs in patients with psychogenic nonepileptic attacks (PNEAs). Epilepsia 2010;51(10):1994–9.

[109] de Barros ACS, Furlan AER, Marques LHN, de Araujo Filho GM. Effects of a psychotherapeutic group intervention in patients with refractory mesial temporal lobe epilepsy and comorbid psychogenic nonepileptic seizures: a nonrandomized controlled study. Seizure 2018;58:22–8.

[110] Kuyk J, Siffels MC, Bakvis P, Swinkels WA. Psychological treatment of patients with psychogenic non-epileptic seizures: an outcome study. Seizure 2008;17(7):595–603.

[111] LaFrance Jr. WC, Rusch MD, Machan JT. What is "treatment as usual" for nonepileptic seizures? Epilepsy Behav 2008;12(3):388–94.

[112] Dewhurst E, Novakova B, Reuber M. A prospective service evaluation of acceptance and commitment therapy for patients with refractory epilepsy. Epilepsy Behav 2015;46:234–41.

[113] Reuber M, House AO, Pukrop R, Bauer J, Elger CE. Somatization, dissociation and general psycho-pathology in patients with psychogenic non-epileptic seizures. Epilepsy Res 2003;57(2-3):159–67.

[114] LaFrance Jr. WC, Baird GL, Barry JJ, Blum AS, Frank Webb A, Keitner GI, Machan JT, Miller I, Szaflarski JP. Multicenter pilot treatment trial for psychogenic nonepileptic seizures: a randomized clinical trial. JAMA Psychiat 2014;71(9):997–1005.

[115] Goldstein LH, Chalder T, Chigwedere C, Khondoker MR, Moriarty J, Toone BK, Mellers JD. Cognitive-behavioral therapy for psychogenic nonepileptic seizures: a pilot RCT. Neurology 2010;74(24):1986–94.

[116] Voon V, Lang AE. Antidepressant treatment outcomes of psychogenic movement disorder. J Clin Psychiatry 2005;66(12):1529–34.

[117] Reuber M, Pukrop R, Bauer J, Helmstaedter C, Tessendorf N, Elger CE. Outcome in psychogenic nonepileptic seizures: 1 to 10-year follow-up in 164 patients. Ann Neurol 2003;53(3):305–11.

[118] Wyllie E, Friedman D, Luders H, Morris H, Rothner D, Turnbull J. Outcome of psychogenic seizures in children and adolescents compared with adults. Neurology 1991;41(5):742–4.

CHAPTER 19

Nursing issues in managing comorbidities of epilepsy

Shelly Brett

Department of Neurology, Kingston Hospital NHS Foundation Trust, London, United Kingdom

Contents

Abbreviations

AED	antiepileptic drug
CBZ	carbamazepine
ESN	epilepsy specialist nurse
ID	intellectual disability
MCM	major congenital malformation
MHRA	Medication and Healthcare products Regulatory Authority
NICE	National Institute of Clinical Excellence
PHT	phenytoin
QOL	quality of life
SVP	sodium valproate
SVP	sodium valproate
WWE	women with epilepsy

The Comorbidities of Epilepsy
https://doi.org/10.1016/B978-0-12-814877-8.00019-2

1. Introduction

Epilepsy is a very common neurological condition affecting approximately 65 million people worldwide, with up to 75% live in developing countries with little or no access to diagnostic facilities or medical treatment demonstrating a huge treatment gap. In developed countries, the incidence of epilepsy is around 50 per 100,000, but in developing countries it may increase to 190 per 100,000 [1].

Doctors should be confident that with sophisticated diagnostic tools (MRI, EEG), if they are available, diagnosis of epilepsy is secure, and following commencement of treatment and a period of monitoring the person's response to the treatment, the outcome should be reasonably predictable based on studies that demonstrate response rates [2]. However, the management of epilepsy is not straightforward, and many people with the condition do not respond to treatment or they develop comorbidities that can have a severely negative impact on their quality of life (QOL). Furthermore, the original diagnosis may not be secure, and differential diagnosis should be considered in patients that are not responding to treatment. As yet epilepsy is not curable and individual response to the diagnosis and treatment is unpredictable and multifactorial. Many comorbidities are age related, predictable, and manageable, and a key role of the ESN is to understand the individual's response to the condition and recognize underlying comorbidities that may not be obvious initially.

2. Epilepsy specialist nurses: Background information

In the United Kingdom the first epilepsy specialist nurses (ESNs) were located in Doncaster in 1988. However, it was some time before they gained recognition for their role and funding became more widely available to develop new posts across the United Kingdom. This remains haphazard, and many locations and health care trusts in the United Kingdom still do not employ ESNs. It is clear that more research is required to provide evidence for the value of the role [3]. Internationally there is even more discrepancy with some countries not recognizing the role at all. The global economic crises has forced governments around the world to reassess their health care expenditure, and specialist nurses are being more widely recognized as playing a vital and cost-effective part in the management of people with epilepsy. Ridsdale et al. looked at the effectiveness of specific epilepsy services and concluded that although nurse-led clinics did not show any evidence of reduction of seizure frequency or severity in comparison with usual care (general practitioner and neurologist), there was evidence of reduced rates of depression and improvement in patient satisfaction [4]. In the United Kingdom the majority of ESNs practice in secondary care in nurse-led hospital outpatient clinics under the clinical supervision of a neurologist, with or without specialist interest in epilepsy. There are a number ESNs employed in primary care who practice autonomously referring back to secondary care when appropriate. Pediatric specialist nurses require very specific skills to manage the complex needs of children with epilepsy, but this chapter will focus on care of adults. There are no specific qualifications for the role, but once established in post, ESNs have the responsibility to develop their knowledge and skills to provide the expertise that comes with experience. Many ESNs are also qualified nurse prescribers and therefore can manage the drug titrations that are so crucial to effective treatment. A key role for the ESN is to provide information and educate individuals and their families and carers to help them live with epilepsy, particularly for those people with poorly controlled epilepsy. The delivery of health care is multidisciplinary. The patient with epilepsy is exposed to a variety of health care professionals during their pathway, including the paramedic who manages the first fit, MRI radiographers, EEG neurophysiologists, and the consultant who delivers the diagnosis and starts treatment. The ESN is often the last person they meet on this journey, but ESNs are usually able to provide continuity of care that supports the person with epilepsy. They should also be able to access other team members and health care professionals when appropriate. The National Institute of Clinical Effectiveness (NICE) recommends the following:

> Epilepsy specialist nurses (ESNs) should be an integral part of the network of care of children, young people and adults with epilepsy. The key roles of the ESNs are to support both epilepsy specialists and generalists, to ensure access to community and multi-agency services and to provide information, training and support to the child, young person or adult, families, carers and, in the case of children, others involved in the child's education, welfare and well-being.
> Ref. [5].

Traditionally the role of the nurse has been a caring one and this continues, providing a holistic approach. The role of individual ESNs will depend very much on their experience and the setting in which care is delivered. One of the criticisms of the role is that there is no recognized training for the job and no clear framework or guidelines to support the role. Roach defines competence as "the state of having the knowledge, judgement, skills, energy, experience and motivation required to respond adequately to the demands of one's professional responsibilities." A framework has been developed in the United Kingdom together with the Royal College of Nursing to identify the key areas of care delivered by ESNs as novice, competent, or advanced nurse practitioners [6]. Neurologists need to understand that the primary role of the ESN is to support the patient who lives with the condition and their families and carers who look after them.

3. The nursing assessment for comorbidities

Every clinical appointment should be an opportunity for the ESN to complete an assessment of the patient. The majority of patient interaction occurs within a hospital outpatient clinic but may be in the community. The length of the appointment will vary from

15 min to 1 h. If possible, clinic templates should reflect the requirements of the patients with complex patients being allocated more time. The review should always be structured with a clear methodology of questioning and documenting [7]. Primarily the appointment will be a review of the person's epilepsy but should also include a comprehensive overview of the person's general health focusing on the high risk areas of potential comorbidity. The assessment should include the person's past medical history, family history, and social situation. Over time the ESN will establish a caseload of patients with epilepsy and one of the key factors of the role is the continuity of care and the development of a collaborative therapeutic relationship with the majority of patients. The cohort will comprise of a variety of people with specific needs in terms of management, particularly comorbidities. Shakespeare describes the seven stages of man in his play *As You Like It* (see Appendix), and epilepsy presents through each phase reliably. From infantile, childhood, and juvenile generalized epilepsies to later onset focal or symptomatic epilepsy there are special considerations and care required to avoid preventable comorbidities. Epilepsy is a spectrum disorder and is indiscriminate, affecting all ages and races, which makes management both challenging and interesting with each phase bringing specific recognizable risks to the individual [8].

4. Somatic comorbidities

The English Oxford University dictionary defines comorbidity as "the simultaneous presence of two chronic conditions in a patient." Strictly applied the term "comorbidity" is a condition that preexists the diagnosis of epilepsy or arises during the course of the disease but does not occur as a consequence of the epilepsy [9]. However, as discussed in this book, the relationship is more complex than that. Every system has the potential to develop a condition that may pose comorbidity problems if occurring with the person with epilepsy. Comorbidities fall into two broad recognizable areas; the inevitable, which are mainly genetic, and the preventable, which are mainly acquired. They may be chronic, acute, or episodic. Some patients may have epilepsy with other conditions that have been explored in more depth in previous chapters. Registered nurses have the background training to be familiar with other health conditions and recognize the risk factors for new onset and possibly preventable comorbidities in people with epilepsy (Table 1).

All comorbidities may have severe consequences for the person's health if not recognized and treated promptly. Renal and hepatic disease need special consideration; due to the complexity of the pharmacokinetics and pharmacodynamics of the antiepileptic drugs (AEDs), the medications prescribed for renal and kidney failure may pose potential problems, and prescribers need to be vigilant to reduce the risk of harm to the patient. Neurological comorbidities, such as stroke, brain tumors, and arteriovenous malformations, may be the underlying cause of a patient's epilepsy and may be considered part of the condition (i.e., focal epilepsy). Seizures may be the first presenting sign of an underlying

Table 1 Risk factors for potential somatic comorbidities of epilepsy

System	Potential comorbidity	Risk factors
Neurological	Vascular disease, stroke	Age, weight, smoking
	Headache, migraine	Age, sex, stress
	Dementia	Age, genetic
	Brain tumor	Not predictable
	Intellectual disability	Syndromic, brain injury
Cardiovascular	Hypertension	Age, weight, smoking
	Heart disease	Genetic, age
Gastrointestinal	Celiac disease/IBS	Genetic
	GI bleeding	Medication, stress
	Obesity/anorexia	Psychological
Respiratory	Asthma	Genetic, environmental
	Carcinoma of the lung	Smoking, environmental
	TB	
Muscular-skeletal	Rheumatoid arthritis	Genetic, environmental
	Osteoarthritis	Age, obesity
	Osteopenia/osteoporosis	Medication, age, genetic
	Fibromyalgia	Unknown
Skin	Allergy	Sodium channel blockers
	Neurocutaneous (tuberous sclerosis)	Genetic
	Psoriasis	Genetic, environmental
Endocrine	Diabetes	Genetic, obesity
	Thyroid dysfunction	Genetic
Reproductive system	Sexual dysfunction	Psychosocial, medication
	Pregnancy complications	Tonic-clonic seizures

neurological disorder. Any endocrinological disorder that disrupts biochemistry may have an effect on seizure frequency; for example, people with epilepsy and diabetes may see a correlation between their blood glucose levels and their seizure control. Thyroid dysfunction is a common cause of fatigue that may be attributed incorrectly to an AED. All autoimmune diseases such as rheumatoid arthritis or psoriasis may require treatment with biological therapies that can interact with AEDs. Treating women with epilepsy requires special considerations due to the impact of hormones on the seizures and medication interactions. People with epilepsy who have an established somatic comorbidity need their health care practitioners to have an effective communication route between each other, particularly regarding medication changes in case there are interactions. In the United Kingdom it is the role of the general practitioner in primary care to coordinate this, but this is not necessarily the case internationally. There is a strong argument for the patients being responsible for their own electronic record in the developed world, as so many people possess smartphones, and this is an area for future research and development to ensure quality and safety of the data [10].

5. Psychiatric comorbidities

Epidemiological studies confirm that the major determinants of QOL, which are employment, social interactions, family relationships, and experiential activities, are at considerable risk in people with epilepsy and these risks are multifaceted. People with epilepsy who experience psychosocial problems are often more disabled by these than by the epilepsy [11]. Furthermore, poor mental health can have a negative effect on seizure control. We are aware that psychiatric comorbidities in people with epilepsy may be twofold to threefold higher than in the general population with up to 50% of people with epilepsy experiencing reduced mental health in a lifetime history, with depression being the most common [12]. There is evidence that certain cognitive and psychiatric conditions may precede the onset of epilepsy and that there may be shared mechanisms that contribute to the emergence of epilepsy and a psychiatric condition in the patient [13]. Risk appears to be higher in focal epilepsies over those with a generalized epilepsy syndrome [14]. Ictal and postictal psychosis is not a comorbidity per se, but people who experience this often feel the consequences and experience postictal anxiety, particularly if they have insight into the episode. Depression can not only affect the QOL but also increase the risk of suicide.

Psychotic illnesses such as schizophrenia and also personality disorders can be challenging to the epilepsy health care practitioner and will usually also involve a psychiatrist with a special interest. Many of the medications used in psychiatry have a powerful interaction with the AEDs reducing the seizure threshold in many cases.

It is often the ESN who the patient first starts to talk about their feelings. Probably the most important question to ask someone with epilepsy is, "How are you feeling?" This is a good indicator of the QOL for that individual. More formal screening tools can be implemented if depression is suspected. The most commonly used by ESNs in the United Kingdom is the Neurological Disorders Depression Inventory for Epilepsy, which can be easily utilized in a busy clinic [15].

Scores over 15 are considered positive for depression and question four (e.g., "I'd be better off dead") is a valid suicidality screening instrument in Ref. [16]. This can open discussion about their wellbeing and QOL. Although the role of the ESN is primarily the management of the person's epilepsy, many ESNs will provide a forum for the person to discuss the problems they have as a consequence of their epilepsy. Being a good listener is crucial to the role; sometimes all the person needs is a sympathetic ear to listen to how they are feeling and help them seek the professional help they may require.

Stress and anxiety are also extremely common. Both developed and developing worlds have very different environmental factors that can trigger anxiety, which can be extremely disabling. Anxiety can manifest with somatic symptoms, and people may experience breathlessness, palpitations, nausea, abdominal churning, dry mouth, dizziness, and sweating [17]. People cite stress and anxiety as clear triggers for seizures, and frequency of seizures often increases in stressful periods of peoples' lives. Although stress is subjective, recommending stress reduction methods and referring to therapists is a reasonable adjunct to standard treatments methods for people with epilepsy and anxiety [18].

The impact of living with epilepsy can have far-reaching consequences; people with epilepsy may not achieve their full educational potential due to ongoing seizures, missing class, and side effects of medication. Gaining employment may be difficult for people with epilepsy as there remains a stigma about the condition. This can have an effect on housing and independent living. The person should be encouraged to develop skills and seek further education or voluntary work experience to provide structure and meaning to their life and help build confidence. Many people with epilepsy are able to form healthy personal relationships and social networks, but for those who are depressed, anxious, sad, and lonely, this may seem like an impossible achievement due to their own negative perception of their self-worth resulting in lack of confidence and low-esteem. The ESN is often best placed to recognize potential psychiatric comorbidity and refer to the appropriate health care professional as early as possible as early interventions are more likely to have a positive effect on the outcome.

6. Nonepileptic attacks

It is worth briefly discussing nonepileptic attacks. This complex condition is well known to neurologists, neuropsychiatrists, and ESNs and has been explored in Chapter 18. The ESN will develop a relationship with the person diagnosed with epilepsy, particularly those with poorly controlled epilepsy as they will attend clinic more frequently. With experience, the ESN can often suspect if the patient is having nonepileptic attacks. Nonepileptic attacks usually present as treatment resistant. If a patient is not responding to treatment and there are other indications that there is no organic cause (negative EEG/MRI) and the seizure descriptions are inconsistent, then nonepileptic attacks may be suspected. If this is the case, prompt referral to a neuropsychiatrist with experience in nonepileptic attacks is the most effective treatment for this condition. The ESN should support the person and help them accept this diagnosis as there is usually a denial period before acceptance, and sensitive management may help improve the outcome.

7. Cognitive dysfunction

Cognitive dysfunction is a common comorbidity for people with epilepsy and is multifactorial. Earlier age of seizure onset may be associated with poorer cognitive dysfunction, and early life seizures may be associated with a lower IQ, developmental delay, and poor academic performance [13]. In people without intellectual disability (ID) poor memory is one of the most common presenting complaints epilepsy clinicians hear from their patients. Memory deficits can be categorized into four main areas, listed in Table 2.

Table 2 Memory deficits in epilepsy
Identifying memory deficits in epilepsy

- Underlying pathology that leads to impaired encoding and storage of memory, including posttraumatic, postsurgical, and epilepsy syndromes
- Ongoing seizures and status epilepticus may interfere with the process of memory consolidation.
- AED side effects
- The consequence of psychological and social comorbidities that cause memory impairments

Early recognition and evaluation of deficits may improve outcomes as identifying the cause will always remain the most important factor in the management of cognitive dysfunction. Simple assessment tools, such as the mini mental state examination, are available to clinicians and are quick and easy to perform. These are assessments that an ESN would be able to undertake in a nurse-led clinic. Referral for psychometry to formally assess the person with suspected reduced cognition will identify the severity of the problem and possibly the underlying cause; unfortunately there are not enough psychologists with appropriate skills for this service to be widely available. Poor seizure control will remain a major contributory factor and more likely result in an impaired memory [19].

If the poor cognition is drug related, reduction or withdrawal should be considered. In some cases this is a difficult decision as the drug may be controlling seizures. Careful counseling for the person will involve reviewing the risks versus the benefits, with many people accepting some reduced cognition as the price to pay for seizure freedom. Alternatively some people will accept seizures (mainly simple focal) if they are treatment resistant and the cognitive side effects affect their QOL. Treatment options for poor cognition remains limited.

8. Intellectual and developmental disabilities

An ID may be defined as a person with an IQ of less than 70 and is caused by a range of different pathological processes and syndromes. The incidence of epilepsy in people with IDs is much higher than in the general population, occurring in about 6% of people with mild ID (IQ 50–70), 24% of people with severe ID (IQ <50), and 50% of people with profound ID (IQ <20) [20]. Many people with intellectual difficulties have complex comorbidities and are surviving into adulthood and old age. People with epilepsy and severe and profound intellectual difficulties may have syndromic diagnoses with associated comorbidities. These are usually identified in childhood, but some problems may arise as the person ages. If the person is nonverbal, it is the responsibility of family members, carers, and allied health care professionals to be diligent to ensure that health care checks are undertaken regularly. Measuring weight can identify fluctuations that could indicate underlying health care conditions, such as cancer or obesity. Blood screenings for cholesterol, diabetes, and bone health should be performed at regular intervals for early detection of any problems. People with ID should not be excluded from general health checks, such as dental examinations, vision checks, and mammograms for females. If they live in a residential care facility, staff are not necessarily registered nurses; however, they should be trained not only in the management of the person's epilepsy, such as first aid and seizure observation and recording, but also in the maintenance of regular health screening to monitor for potential comorbidities. People with ID will often display a change of behavior or demonstrate nonverbal clues of distress, and care staff need to be vigilant about their observation and seeking professional help if there are concerns.

9. Drug interactions and side effects

Epilepsy is a long-term condition and most people with epilepsy require treatment for life, and many will develop one or more of the comorbidities requiring treatment with drugs. Formal drug interaction studies have now become a requirement of clinical trials [21]. Anticipating and predicting metabolic drug interactions is a key skill required by the ESN to avoid prescribing errors that may reduce the seizure threshold or result in adverse side effects due to increased serum levels of an AED. In the electronic age of prescribing, warnings of potential interactions should be given to prescribers to prevent potential interactions and should contain prompts to monitor for liver disease where appropriate. Electronic systems are being implemented globally at an increasing rate and a systematic review by Anneworth et al. concluded that they can reduce adverse drug errors by 25%; however, the study did not identify which of these were potential interaction errors, and they proposed further research [22]. Patients should be informed of potential interactions, particularly those that may occur with over-the-counter medication, such as St John's wort, an herbal remedy for depression that is a powerful enzyme inducer and may reduce the seizure threshold.

Side effects of medications may occur in people with epilepsy without taking concurrent medications for other conditions, but the likelihood will increase if the person is taking other medications. All antiepileptic medications have the potential to produce side effects, and this is unpredictable apart from the increased risk of carbamazepine (CBZ) prescribed to people of the Han Chinese population who have a genetic susceptibility to Stevens-Johnsons syndrome and should be screened prior to prescribing [23].

Side effects are defined as common (1:10) and rare (1:1000) [24] and may occur as soon as the person starts taking the medication. It is the responsibility of the prescriber to make sure that the patient clearly understands the potential side effects, particularly the most serious ones, such as rash. In the United Kingdom all medication prescribed has a patient information leaflet that describes all the potential side effects. Although this is best practice many patients do not understand the data and can be discouraged from taking the medication when they see the list of side effects, so this needs clear explanation. Many of the drugs have adverse effects on mood and can be a common cause of depression, anxiety, and, in rare cases, psychosis and suicide (see Table 3).

In people with ID who are nonverbal it is often a behavior change that will demonstrate that they are experiencing side effects. As discussed before, cognitive impairment is a common side effect of many drugs and may be dose related or associated with long-term use. Careful consideration of the person's existing comorbidities must be considered when prescribing AEDs. All practitioners should be aware of the risk of poor bone health and screen for Vitaminosis D if appropriate. Vitamin D is cheap and well tolerated, and it should be considered as a supplement for all people taking enzyme-inducing AEDs [25].

It is also worth considering the positive side effects of AEDs, as the adverse effects most often receive the attention. Sodium valproate (SVP), CBZ, and lamotrigine are all mood stabilizers and so may improve QOL with an improved sense of wellbeing. People who have the comorbidity of a high BMI or who suffer from migraine may benefit from topiramate or zonisamide. Prescribing gabapentin to people with associated neuropathic pain may be beneficial [26].

10. The XX factor: Pregnancy and childbirth

Women with epilepsy (WWE) of childbearing age account for approximately 25% of patients with epilepsy. Although not a comorbidity as such, WWE present with specific issues. Contraception, preconceptual care, and management in pregnancy, labor, and the postnatal period can present challenging problems and increased risks to mother and baby. Providing contraception advice to WWE can be challenging as there are many issues to be considered, particularly the interaction of some AEDs and oral contraceptives, and the ESN must be able to research the latest evidence as new contraceptive methods are being developed.

In the early 1990s, emerging evidence demonstrated that WWE taking AEDs were at an increased risk over the background population of having a baby with a major congenital malformation (MCM) from 2%–3% to 4%–7% and specific concerns had been raised around SVP [27]. At around the same time studies showed that the mean IQ was significantly lower in children born to mothers taking certain AEDs (CBZ and phenytoin) resulting in special educational needs [28]. With the increase in AEDs in the 1990s, awareness of potential problems increased. This resulted in the development of international pregnancy registries with the aim of providing outcome data

Table 3 An overview of side effects of commonly used antiepileptic drugs

Drug	Common	Rare/idiosyncratic	Long term
Carbamazepine	Dizziness Sedation Diplopia Cognitive problems	Rash Stevens-Johnson syndrome Aplastic anemia Sexual dysfunction	Osteoporosis Hepatatoxicicity Hyponatremia Bone loss
Clobazam	Fatigue Drowsiness	Rash	Dependence
Clonazepam	Fatigue Drowsiness	Rash	Dependence Thrombocytopenia
Ethosuxemide	Nausea	Lupus, psychotic episodes	Aplastic anemia
Gabapentin	Fatigue Weight gain Nausea	Ataxia Oedema	Poorly controlled seizures
Lacosamide	Dizziness	Prolonged PR interval Rash	
Lamotrigine	Skin rash Drowsiness Insomnia	Stevens-Johnson syndrome Lupus	Aplastic anemia
Leviteracetam	Depression Irritability	Psychosis Suicidal ideation	
Phenobarbital	Fatigue Irritability (in (children)	Rash Stevens-Johnson Syndrome Hyperkinesia Sexual dysfunction	Osteomalacia Hepatatoxiciity
Phenytoin	Nystagmus Nausea Ataxia	Stevens-Johnson syndrome Lupus Bradycardia	Gingival hyperplasia Facial coarseness Blood dyscrasias Hepatatoxicicity Bone loss
Sodium valproate	Weight gain Hair loss Cognitive dysfunction	Pancreatitis, Hepatatoxicicity	Tremor (dose related) Polycystic ovaries Thrombocytopenia Bone loss
Topiramate	Weight loss Cognitive problems Mood disorder Reduction in verbal IQ	Extreme dysphasia Renal calculi Metabolic acidosis	Osteomalacia Hepatatoxicicity
Vigabatrin	Visual field disturbance	Ataxia	Tremor
Zonisamide	Dizziness	Renal calculi Myeloma Hyperhidrosis/ hyperthermia	Aplastic anemia

on large numbers of pregnancies in WWE. All of the registries have confirmed that valproate is associated with the greatest risk with 6%–14% pregnancies resulting in a child with a MCM [29]. There is a clear dose response with doses over 800 mg within in a twenty-four hour period posing the higher risk. There was no relevance to the formula; it was the daily dose rather than the peak effect that was significant [30]. Furthermore, studies showed that taking folic acid 5 mg significantly reduced the risk of MCMs, particularly of neural tube defects and could also possibly be neuro protective preserving the IQ. Although results are inconsistent and further research is required, routine prescribing of folates is recommended, particularly in the peri-conceptual period and first trimester [31]. All practitioners looking after WWE who are pregnant should have access to recruiting into the registers and women should be encouraged. Many ESNs help WWE join the studies so robust data can be maintained. With this evidence in mind, care of young women who are potentially going to become pregnant should be considered early on when the girl is diagnosed. In the United Kingdom the Medication and Healthcare products Regulatory Authority has put out an alert to all practitioners who prescribe SVP. The medication is dispensed with warnings on the label alerting to the risks in pregnancy and robust media campaigns have increased awareness of the problem. All women of childbearing age should be on a documented pregnancy prevention program. Not only will this protect the woman, it will also protect the prescriber from litigation [32]. A key role of the ESN is to provide preconceptual counseling so that evidence-based medication changes can be completed before pregnancy as once the person is pregnant it is too late.

Pregnancy with epilepsy carries a risk to the mother and the fetus. There are specific predictable issues that may arise, and these need to be managed effectively to reduce the risk to mother and baby. Reducing seizure frequency during pregnancy, particularly tonic-clonic seizures, is the goal but may not be achievable. There is evidence that due to pharmacokinetic alterations, including increased volume of distribution, elevated renal clearance, serum levels of some medications can reduce [33]. Labor and birth can present problems, but the actual risk of seizures in labor is low. Although there are detectable levels in breast milk as the baby has been exposed to medication in utero breastfeeding is not contraindicated and should be recommended [34]. Organizations that provide health care to women should produce guidelines for the management of pregnancy in women with comorbidities such as epilepsy. In the United Kingdom the National Health Service uses the NICE guideline, which is available free online as a resource for clinicians [35].

11. Mortality

Epilepsy is associated with a risk of mortality three times that of the general population. Analysis of mortality in epilepsy is complicated due to methodology difficulties.

Death certificates may not be reliable sources of data, and the cause of death may not represent the association with epilepsy [36]. Broadly there are four main categories that represent the increased risk: accidents, directly related to epilepsy, not directly epilepsy related, and sudden unexpected death in epilepsy (SUDEP) (see Table 4).

Many of these deaths are preventable and health care professionals have a duty of candor to discuss the risks and talk openly with the patients and their families and carers to reduce the risk. Educating and counseling people with epilepsy will be discussed later in the chapter; however, the ESN plays an important part in this activity. Discussions about death may be difficult, but clinicians must not censor information due to their own discomfort [8]. Accidents and injuries as a result of seizures remain common, particularly for those with poorly controlled tonic-clonic or atonic seizures, and it is imperative that safety guidelines are discussed with this group of patients. Information about potential accidental risks should be given to people as soon as they are diagnosed and ideally after the first seizure to reduce the risk. The risk of death may be much higher in high-risk patient groups, particularly those with comorbidities. People with a psychiatric morbidity have a dramatically increased risk of dying of suicide and accidental overdose with opiates [37]. SUDEP may not be preventable as there is not always a clear cause of death found postmortem, and there may or may not be evidence of a seizure. Usually the events are unwitnessed in an otherwise well person, the majority occur at night, and the person is found dead in bed. Tragically the incidence is much higher in young people with poorly controlled tonic-clonic seizures. Young men living alone have the highest risk, and this may be due to other factors, such as poor adherence to medication (often polytherapy) and alcohol or substance abuse. Nashef et al. investigated risk factors for SUDEP and concluded that larger studies in ECG changes and QT intervals, the association with syncope, and associated arrhythmias in people with epilepsy should all be considered, and all people with epilepsy should be screened with an ECG [38].

12. Practical advice and crisis management

The ESN role should extend beyond the clinic room and the hospital appointment. People with epilepsy live with an unpredictable condition; there are times of crisis between appointments, and they need a point of contact for help and support. A key role of the ESN is to be available to the individual with epilepsy particularly at times of crisis. We live in the digital age; telephone clinics and even FaceTime or Skype appointments are becoming more feasible as technology permits, particularly for people who cannot drive or live in remote or rural areas where transport to hospital appointments may be difficult. A systematic review of health care delivery via telemedicine methods concluded that this method can improve outcomes for patients and health care providers [10].

Epilepsy care plans play a very important role for specific issues, particularly individual care plans for vulnerable people and people with specific needs, such as the administration of emergency benzodiazepine for prolonged seizures. Developing care plans is a key role for the ESN.

Table 4 Prevention strategies to prevent accidents and death in epilepsy

Risk	Cause	Prevention strategies
Accidents	Drowning	Advise to shower and not bathe alone
	Swimming	Never swim alone, use flotation equipment
	Falling from heights	Advise not to climb ladders or rocks
	Burns	Safety information for kitchen
	Machinery	Not to use power tools
	Driving	Follow driving regulations
	Head Injury	Wear protective headgear
	Falls	Avoid waterfronts, road sides, and train platforms
	Extreme sports	No scuba-diving, no rip-cord parachuting, paragliding, or solo white water rafting
Directly epilepsy related	Status epilepticus	Maximize treatment of tonic–clonic seizures
		Emergency treatment plan in situ (Benzos) so early treatment can be implemented
	Cardio-vascular	Regular monitoring and treatment
	Medical complications	
	Drug reactions	Advise patient to be diligent in reporting adverse side effects as soon as possible
Nondirectly epilepsy related	Suicide	Observe for depression, refer to psychiatrist early when detected
	Comorbidities	Vigilant observation of potential comorbidities
SUDEP	Unknown	Control tonic–clonic seizures, ensure adherence, cohabitation

Table 5 A sample entry of a seizure diary

Date	Time	Length of seizure	What happened (description)	Notes (how you were feeling, triggers)

Seizure diaries remain the mainstay of managing poorly controlled epilepsy. As well as monitoring seizure activity, the diary entry should include a section to identify feelings or potential triggers (see Table 5). Reviewing the diary at appointments may help identify psychosocial comorbidities. These may be obtained from epilepsy charities or pharmaceutical companies or printed out to give to the person.

The millennial generation has grown up with technology and will use smartphones, and epilepsy charities provide free apps to monitor seizures and provide medication alarms. Future technology will embrace safety devices such as wristbands that will monitor a seizure and send alarms to family members or carers.

13. Education and training

The diagnosis of epilepsy, although given to an individual, affects the entire family and other relationships, partners, and friends. Studies show that people with epilepsy want to learn more about their condition as they usually only have the minimal knowledge of epilepsy that the general public has, and this is usually limited and often inaccurate. Linsdale et al. asked patients if a nurse intervention can help people with newly diagnosed epilepsy, and patients reported that learning about epilepsy was easier when more time was provided by the epilepsy nurse [39]. Educating people with epilepsy and their carers and families is key so that they become partners in the management of their own health care. Each appointment is an opportunity to further the education, which should be delivered with literacy and cultural sensitivity. Visual aids can be used as most clinical areas have access to a computer and the internet. People should be advised to be cautious about gathering unregulated information from the internet and guided to appropriate websites. People with epilepsy who have a better understanding and knowledge of their condition will have an improved QOL, and this also may reduce hospital admissions. In the United Kingdom the epilepsy charities provide patient information books and pamphlets that cover many different aspects of living with epilepsy [40]. Online self-management programs are being developed so people with epilepsy can obtain a better understanding of their condition. In the United Kingdom there are many regional support groups that are facilitated with the support of epilepsy charities, such as Epilepsy Action. These are an opportunity for people with epilepsy to meet other people with epilepsy in nonclinical surroundings for informal discussions. ESNs should be familiar with options in their local area and advise people how to access what may be available to them. In the United Kingdom families and residential care facilities may be trained in the administration of emergency benzodiazepines to prevent status epilepticus in individuals who are high risk. Training families and carers in the safe administration and the writing of clear guidelines often falls upon the ESN (Table 6).

As well as teaching patients, once established in post and having gained expertise in the management of people with epilepsy, the ESN should be available to educate and train others who may be less experienced or need to learn more about epilepsy. Emergency departments, schools, residential facilities, undergraduate nurses, and allied health care professionals all have learning needs if they provide care in the community for people with epilepsy, and ESNs should have the skills to educate by developing and participating in education programs [41].

14. Health care economics

The delivery of a cost-effective health care service is crucial in the context of today's world of global financial inequality. In the United Kingdom we have the National Health Service and all care is delivered free at point of contact so patients have an advantage in as much as they do not have to worry about cost of care or whether or not they have insurance. This model may place a burden on the government and tax-payer but ensures equal health care for all. Epilepsy is an expensive condition requiring a lifetime of treatment with medication, ongoing tests, and interventions. The key questions relating to epilepsy are: "How much does it cost?" and "Could we do it more cost effectively?" As well as the direct costs of providing hospital appointments, investigations, medication, and emergency and paramedic services, there are the indirect costs, which include unemployment, reduced productivity, and the cost of comorbidities [42].

It is difficult to produce accurate figures for the percentage of people attending emergency departments with seizures as the quality of coding for data analysis is poor and many episodes that may be a result of a seizure, such as head injury, burns, or fractures, would not be recorded as neurological. Paramedics do not attach diagnostic codes to their data. However, we know that people with seizures are frequent attendees at emergency rooms. This may be due to injury, but often it is due to the paramedics not being clinically confident to manage resolving seizures, with preference to take the person to hospital to "be checked out" [43]. Whether or not having access to an ESN can reduce emergency room visits was looked at by Ridsdale et al., and they found that it did not reduce admissions [44].

Table 6 Areas of self-management education for epilepsy, knowledge, and skills

Epilepsy specific	Example of knowledge and skills
Seizures	• Knowledge: specific seizure types and first aid response • Recognition and treatment plans for seizure emergencies • Skills: recording seizures; keeping a seizure diary • Identifying triggers
Medication and treatment	• Knowledge: medication name, dosage, possible medication interactions, and side effects • Consequences of missed doses, alcohol, drug interactions • Skills: keeping track of medication intake, tracking medication dose changes and titrations, managing prescription refills, responding promptly to adverse side effects and allergic reactions
Safety	• Knowledge: risks for injury related to seizures and treatment • Strategies for reducing injury, risks for mortality (including SUDEP) • Skills: assessing risks in environment • Modifying lifestyle to reduce risks yet maintain QOL
Comorbid conditions	• Knowledge: symptoms of common comorbidities • Skills: recognizing symptoms and knowing when to seek advice • Managing treatment of comorbidities

Long term	Example of knowledge and skills
Maintaining a healthy lifestyle • Physical activity • Adequate sleep • Pleasurable activity • Physical health • Emotional health	• Knowledge: how seizures and everyday life interact • The importance of a healthy lifestyle and behavior • Consequences of unhealthy lifestyle • Skills: assessing the impact of seizures on daily life and making modifications • Developing strategies for maintaining a healthy lifestyle • Learn to cope with stressful situations • Seeking help and support when needed
Active partnership with health care team	• Knowledge: need for active partnership with health care providers • Effective communication strategies • Skills: communicating effectively, problem solving, decision making, goal setting, and care planning
Independent living	• Skills: environmental support, resources, implement social services if required, assessing and evaluating resources, handling emergencies, and ensuring action plans in place

15. Conclusion

For the readers who do not have access to an ESN on their team, it is worth considering a business plan to develop a post, and there is an example with guidelines available online [45]. It is widely recognized that clinical nurse specialists across all specialities are valuable, particularly for long-term conditions with potential comorbidity. However, with budget restraints and financial cutbacks internationally, the argument for creating new posts may be a difficult one. Quantitative studies have demonstrated cost-effectiveness, and qualitative studies and patient surveys have confirmed the value that the nurse plays in the management. The responsibility is twofold: nurses should be more proactive in developing career pathways so that they are able to develop roles, and physicians need to support with clinical supervision. Organizations that deliver health care for long-term conditions should all be looking at successful models of care delivery, and the ESN role is an excellent example.

In India where there is a huge treatment gap due to a shortage of neurologists, particularly in rural areas, a pilot study of an epilepsy nurse-led clinic concluded that it is feasible for nurses to run epilepsy follow-up clinics and that patients are likely to be satisfied with this [46].

We have seen the impact that living with comorbidities can have on the individual with epilepsy; both physical and mental health can be affected, which will have a profound impact on QOL and wellbeing. Further research is required to identify risk factors for comorbidities of epilepsy. Epilepsy is a spectrum disorder with no clear disease pathway progression and management may be complex and prolonged. At present epilepsy in adults is usually a lifelong condition requiring ongoing treatment with AEDs, and the consequences are multifactorial and far-reaching. The individual with epilepsy will interact with a variety of different health care professionals from diagnosis through long-term management. However, it is recognized that an ESN can provide a valuable role as part of a multidisciplinary team providing care to people with epilepsy. The ESN should be able to develop a positive therapeutic relationship with the patient and their family, understanding the baseline of the patient's health status so changes and potential comorbidities can be identified early and managed so other investigations and treatments can be initiated as promptly as possible to improve outcomes and prevent further deterioration.

Studies have shown that clinical specialist nurses in all areas of health care delivery can provide a cost-effective way of providing health care to people living with long-term conditions. Registered nurses should be encouraged to develop their clinical skills and access postgraduate education and mentorship programs to become advanced practitioners. In the United Kingdom the Epilepsy Specialist Nurse Association (ESNA) is a recognized professional body of nurses that provides ongoing education and research to ensure that the role maintains viability.

Furthermore, we understand that there is a global treatment gap in the delivery of care to people with epilepsy, particularly in rural areas of the developing world due to a shortage of doctors. Promoting the role of the ESN could be the best way to bridge this gap, helping to improve the health care of people with epilepsy worldwide.

Appendix

Shakespeare's Seven Ages of Man

All the world's a stage,
And all the men and women merely players,
They have their exits and entrances,
And one man in his time plays many parts,
His acts being seven ages. At first the infant,
Mewling and puking in the nurse's arms.
Then, the whining schoolboy with his satchel
And shining morning face, creeping like snail
Unwillingly to school. And then the lover,
Sighing like furnace, with a woeful ballad
Made to his mistress' eyebrow. Then a soldier,
Full of strange oaths, and bearded like the pard,
Jealous in honour, sudden, and quick in quarrel,
Seeking the bubble reputation
Even in the cannon's mouth. And then the justice
In fair round belly, with good capon lin'd,
With eyes severe, and beard of formal cut,
Full of wise saws, and modern instances,
And so he plays his part. The sixth age shifts
Into the lean and slipper'd pantaloon,
With spectacles on nose, and pouch on side,
His youthful hose well sav'd, a world too wide,
For his shrunk shank, and his big manly voice,
Turning again towards childish treble, pipes
And whistles in his sound. Last scene of all,
That ends this strange eventful history,
Is second childishness and mere oblivion,
Sans teeth, sans eyes, sans taste, sans everything.

William Shakespeare; AS You Like It Act II. Scene VII

References

[1] Neligan A, Sander SL. The incidence and prevelance of epilepsy. In: ILAE, from bedside to benchside. Oxford Press; 2009. p. 15–9 [Chapter 1].

[2] Brodie MJ, S B. Patterns of treatment response in newly diagnosed epilepsy. Neurology 2012; 78(20):1548–54.

[3] Goodwin M, Higgins S. The role of the clinical nurse specialist in epilepsy. A national survey. Seizure 2004;13:87–94.

[4] Ridsdale L, McCrone P, Morgan M. Can an epilepsy nurse specialist-led self management intervention reduce attendance at emergency departments and promote well-being for people with severe epilepsy? A non-randomised trial with a nested qualiativ ephase. London: NIHR; 2013.

[5] NICE. Epilepsies: diagnosis and management [CG137. 1.8.3 Management]. National Institute of Ciinical Excellence; 2017.

[6] Leavy Y, Goodwin M, Higgins S, Myson V. The adult epilepsy specialist nurse competancy framework. London: Royal College of Nursing; 2013.

[7] Bickley S, Szilasyi P. Bates guide to physical examination and history taking. Philadelphia: Lippincott, Williams and Wilkins; 2017.

[8] England MJ, Liverman CT, Schultz AM, Strawbridge L, editors. Epilepsy across the spectrum. Promoting health and understanding. Washington, DC: Institute of Medicine; 2012 [Public health report].

[9] Ording AG, Sorenson HT. Concepts of comorbidities, multiple morbidities, complications and their clinical epidemiologic analogs. Clin Epidemiol 2013;(5):199–2013. https://doi.org/10.2147/CLEP.S34305.

[10] Krishna S, Boren S, Bales EA. Healthcare via cell phones: a systematic review. Telemed J E Health 2009;15(3):231–40.

[11] Sherman E. Maximizing quality of life for people living with epilepsy. Can J Neurol Sci 2009;36 (Suppl. 2):S17–24.

[12] Josephson C, Jette N. Psychiatric comorbidities in epilepsy. Int Rev Psychiatry 2017; 29(5):409–24.

[13] Lin J, Mula M, Hermann B. Uncovering the neurobehavioral comorbidities of epilepsy over the life-span. Lancet 2012;380:1180–92.

[14] Edeh J, Toone B. Relationship between interictal psychopathology and the type of epilepsy. Results of a survey in gerneral practice. Br J Psychiatry 1987;151:95–101.

[15] Friedman D, Kung D, Lowattana KJ. Identyfying dperession in epilepsu in a busy clinical setting is enhanced with systematic screening. Seizure 2009;03:001.

[16] Mula M, McGonigal A, Micoulud-Franchi J-A, May TW, Labudda K, Brandt C. Validation of rapid suicidality screening in epilepsy using the NDDIE. Epilepsia 2016;57(6):949–55.

[17] Moriarty J. Introduction to epilepsy: Chapter 112. Anxiety disorders and epilepsy. Cambridge University Press; 2012.

[18] McKee H, Privitera M. Stress as a seizure precipitant: identification, associated factors and treatment options. Seizure 2016; https://doi.org/10.1016/j.seizure.2016.12.009.

[19] Elwes R, Johnson A, Reynolds EH. The course of untreated epilepsy. BMJ 1988;297:948–50.

[20] Lhatoo SD, SAnder JW. The epidimiology of epielpsy and learning difficulty. Epilepsia 2007; https://doi.org/10.1046/j.1528-1527.2001.00501.

[21] Patsalos PN. Antiepileptic drug interactions. A clinical guide. 2nd ed. Chalfont: Springer; 2013.

[22] Ammerworth E, Schnell-Indest P, Machan C, Siebert U. The effect of electronic prescribing of med-ication errors and adverse drug events: a systematic review. J Am Med Inform Assoc 2008;15:585–600.

[23] Locharerernkul C, Loplumlert J, Limotai C, Korkij W, Desudchit T. Carbamazepine and phenytoin induced Stevens-Johnson syndrom is associated with HLA-B* 1502 allele in Thai population. Epilepsia 2008;49(12):2087–91.

[24] The Royal Pharmaceutical Society. Adverse reactions to drugs. In: The British National Formulary. 2018.

[25] Cock H. Bone health in eplepsy. London: International League Against Epilepsy; 2009 [From Bench-side to Bedside].

[26] Walia K, Khan E, Ko DH, Raza S, Khan Y. Side effects of antiepileptics a review. Pain Pract 2004; 4(3):194–203.

[27] Devinsky O, Feldmann E, Hainline B. Epilepsy and pregnancy. In: Neurological complications in pregnancy. Raven Press; 1994 [Chapter 5].

[28] Scitnik D, NulmanI, Rover J, Gladstone D, et al. Neurodevelopment of children exposed in utero to phenytoin and carbamazepine monotheraly. JAMA 1994;271:767–70.

[29] Campbell E, Kennedy F, Russell A, Smithson W, Parsons L, Morrison PJ, Liggan B, Irwin B, Delanty N, Hunt SJ, Craig J, Morrow J. Malformation risks of antiepileptic drugs monotherapies in pregnancy:updated results from the UK Pregnancy register. J Neurol Neurosurg Psychiatry 2014;85:1029–34.

[30] Tomson E, BAttino D, Bonnizzoni E, Craig J, Lindhout D, et al. Dose dependent risk of malformation with anti epileptic drugs:an analysis of the data from the EURAP pregnancy register. Lancet Neurol 2011;10:609–12.

[31] Morrow J, Hunt SJ, Russell AJ, et al. Folic acid use and major congenital malformations in offspring of women with epilespy:a prospevtive study from th eUK epilepsy and pregnancy register. J Neurol Neurosurg Psychiatry 2009;80:506–11.

[32] MHRA. Valproate and developmental disorders:new alert for review and further consideration or risk minimisation measures. London: Drug Safety Update; 2018 [Issued 24th April].

[33] Venescu P. Leviteracetam, topirimate and oxcarbazepine clearance changes during pregnancy. Neurology 2018;90(15 Suppl).

[34] Page B. Antiepileptic drug pharmokintetics during pregnancy and lactation. Neurology 2003; 61(6 Suppl. 2):S35–42.

[35] NICE. Epilepsies: diagnosis and management [CG137. 1.15.3 Pregnancy]. London: National Institute of Clinical Excellence; 2017.

[36] Nashef L. Mortality in epilepsy. In: Valantino A, Alarcon G, editors. Introduction to epilepsy. Cambridge: Cambridge University Press; 2012. p. 340–3 [Chapter 62].

[37] Gorton C, Webb R, Carr M. Risk of unnatural mortality in people with epilepsy. JAMA Neurol 2018; https://doi.org/10.1001/jamaneurol.2018.0333.

[38] Nashef L, Hindocha MA. Risk factors in sudden death in epilepsy (SUDEP): the quest for mechanisms. Epilpepsia 2007;48(5):859–71.

[39] Ridsdale L, Kwan I, Morgan M. How can a nurse intervention help people with newly diagnosed epilepsy? Seizure 2003;12:69–73.

[40] Altrup U, Elgar CE, Reuber M. Epilepsy explained. A book for people who want to know more about epilepsy. Lienen: Medicine Explained Publishing; 2005.

[41] Hayes C. Clincal skills; a practical guide for managing adults with epilepsy. Br J Nurs 2004;13(7):380–7.

[42] Heaney D, Begley CE. Health economic evaluation of epilepsy treatment:a review of the literature. Epilepsia 2002;43(Suppl. 4):10–7.

[43] Burrell L, Noble A, Ridsdale L. Decision making by ambulance clinicians in London when managing patients with epilepsy; a qualiative study. Emerg Med J 2012;30:236–40 [Published online: 20.3.12].

[44] Ridsdale L, McCrone P, Morgan M, Goldstein L, Seed P, Noble A. Can an epilepsy nurse specialist-led self management intervention reduce attendance at emergency departments and promote well-being for people with severe epilepsy? A non-randomised trial with a nested qualiativ ephase. In: Health services delivery and research. London: NIHR; 2013.

[45] Long Term Conditions Delivery Support. Guide to writing a business case for an epilepsy nurse specialist, https://www.epilepsy.org.uk.

[46] Paul P, Agrawal M, Bhatia R, Vishnubhatoa, Singh M. Nurse-led epilepsy follow up clinic in India: is it feasible and acceptable to patients? A pilot study. Seizure 2014;23(1):74–6.

Index

Note: Page numbers followed by *f* indicate figures and *t* indicate tables.

Printed in the United States
By Bookmasters